The Case Manager's Training Manual

David W. Plocher, MD
Vice President
Cap Gemini Ernst & Young
Minneapolis, Minnesota

Patricia L. Metzger, RN, BSN, MHA
Chief of Care Management
Memorial Hermann Healthcare System
Houston, Texas

AN ASPEN PUBLICATION®
Aspen Publishers, Inc.
Gaithersburg, Maryland
2001

Library of Congress Cataloging-in-Publication Data

Plocher, David W.
The case manager's training manual/David W. Plocher, Patricia L. Metzger.
p. cm.
Includes bibliographical references and index.
ISBN 0-8342-1930-1
1. Hospitals—Case management services—Handbooks, manuals, etc. 2. Managed care plans (Medical care)—Handbooks, manuals, etc. I. Metzger, Patricia L. II. Title.
RA975.5.C36 P56 2001
362.1'068—dc21
2001022633

Orders: (800) 638-8437
Customer Service: (800) 234-1660

Editorial Services: Denise Hawkins Coursey
Library of Congress Catalog Card Number: 2001022633
ISBN: 0-8342-1930-1

Printed in the United States of America

1 2 3 4 5

To my wife, Michelle; our children, Jessica, David, and Joseph;
and my parents, Edward and Paula

David W. Plocher

To my husband, Dale, and our daughter, Adrianne,
with my undying gratitude for their love, support, and
encouragement in all I do

Patricia L. Metzger

Contents

Contributors

Sara Atwell
Manager
Cap Gemini Ernst & Young
Detroit, Michigan

G. David Baker, MSW
Regional Director
Home Care Services
St. John Health System
Detroit, Michigan

Carol L. Belmont, RN, BS, MEd
Vice President
Cap Gemini Ernst & Young
Cleveland, Ohio

Kathryn W. Bradshaw, RN, BSN
Manager
Cap Gemini Ernst & Young
Richmond, Virginia

Nancy L. Brennan, RN, BSN, MBA
Manager
Cap Gemini Ernst & Young
Dallas, Texas

Sharon E. Brodeur, RN, BS, MPA
Manager
Consulting Services
Cap Gemini Ernst & Young
Washington, DC

Anne C. Dye, MHSA
Manager
Health Care Consulting
Cap Gemini Ernst & Young
Tampa, Florida

Darlene D. Dymond, BSN, MEd, JD
Director
Case Management/Performance Improvement
Memorial Hermann Hospital System
Memorial Hermann The Woodlands Hospital
Houston, Texas

Nancy H. Fullerton, MBA
Senior Consultant
Health Care Consulting
Cap Gemini Ernst & Young
Chicago, Illinois

Barbara Gray, BSN, MBA
Director for Managed Care Services
Ernst & Young LLP
Washington, DC

Geri Hempel, RN, BA
Senior Manager
Cap Gemini Ernst & Young
Tampa, Florida

Magdalen M. Hunssinger, RNC
Midwest Alliance for Nursing Informatics
Healthcare Information and Management Systems Society
Chicago, Illinois

Mary Ellen Kripp, BSN, MS
Manager
Cap Gemini Ernst & Young
Chicago, Illinois

June M. Laing, BA, BMedS
Registered Health Information Administrator
American Health Information Management Association
Atlanta, Georgia

Hilary M. Lawn, MBA, MHA
Consultant
Cap Gemini Ernst & Young
Atlanta, Georgia

Leslie A. McGregor, RN, BSN, MEd
Manager
Cap Gemini Ernst & Young
Washington, DC

Kathleen L. Meredith, RN, MBA, MSN
Senior Manager
Cap Gemini Ernst & Young
Philadelphia, Pennsylvania

Patricia L. Metzger, RN, BSN, MHA
Chief of Care Management
Memorial Hermann Healthcare System
Houston, Texas

Dale H. Metzger II, RN, RNC, BA
Case Manager
Memorial Hermann Healthcare System
Continuing Care Corporation
Houston, Texas

Carole Neff, MS-MIS, MBA
Manager
Health and Managed Care Practice
Cap Gemini Ernst & Young
Pittsburgh, Pennsylvania

Lana S. Peters, BSN, MBA, MHA
Manager
Cap Gemini Ernst & Young
St. Louis, Missouri

David W. Plocher, MD
Vice President
Cap Gemini Ernst & Young
Minneapolis, Minnesota

Peggy H. Rodebush, RN, BS, MSN
Vice President
Health Care Consulting
Cap Gemini Ernst & Young
Tampa, Florida

Timothy J. Rowell, MS
Principal
Cap Gemini Ernst & Young
Cleveland, Ohio

Cindy J. Urbancic, RN, BSN, MBA
Senior Manager
Cap Gemini Ernst & Young
Cleveland, Ohio

Laura L. Waltrip, RN, BSN
Manager
Consulting Services
Cap Gemini Ernst & Young
Tampa, Florida

Judith M. Wilczewski, RN, BSN, MBA
Senior Consultant
Cap Gemini Ernst & Young
Detroit, Michigan

Wendy L. Wilson, MD, MSE
Senior Manager
Cap Gemini Ernst & Young
Cleveland, Ohio

James D. Witt, RN, MBA, CHE
Senior Manager
Health Care Consulting
Cap Gemini Ernst & Young
Chicago, Illinois

Preface

Case managers are enjoying increased market demand. This is occurring in the provider world more than the payer environment due to several developments, and, hence, the provider orientation for this book.

- Payers are minimizing their medical management activities and staffing, in general, due to the health maintenance organization backlash. This applies especially to the precertification functions within utilization management, which appear to have a negative or breakeven ROI.
- Payers are starting to move their utilization review employees into hospitals, partly for better information access; residual roles for the payer-based case manager have centered around negotiations, such as extra contractual benefits, per diem rates at facilities, or durable medical equipment.
- Payers have shifted varying amounts of risk to providers, thereby motivating providers to attend to a larger continuum of care; where payers keep most of the risk, hospitals are still rewarded for reducing length of stay on case rate contracts and for reducing cost per day on their per diem or business.
- Providers have learned that, even as a fee-for-service medical center, a broader investment in case management can improve profit margin per admission (anecdotally, the chronic patient readmitted after improved ambulatory care is less morbid) and reduce denial rates, and, that a full hospital, succeeding at length of stay control, can increase revenue through larger admission volume.
- There is a race among payers, providers, and various carve-out vendors for an analysis of populations for risk and subsequent outreach activities, culminating in disease management programs. To date, the finishing order shows payers in first place, carve-out vendors in second, and providers a distant third. Payers are recently more willing to outsource this function to carve-out vendors.

Case management is not primary prevention, although this book will address member risk assessment and the role of the community-based case manager. Neither is case management disease management, although this book will address the interaction between case managers and disease managers.

The intent for this volume is to produce a step-by-step "how-to" training manual that bridges from the classroom to practical assistance in daily case management workflow. We hope this meets your needs, as you alone will judge whether we have achieved this goal.

David W. Plocher, MD

Acknowledgment: The authors thank Paulette Land for her major contribution to manuscript preparation.

Part I

The Fundamentals

Chapter 1

Organizational Structure of Case Management Programs

Patricia L. Metzger and Carol L. Belmont

TAKE THIS TO WORK

1. The old adage of "form follows function" is one that should be invoked in the selection, development, and implementation of any model for case management. Key stakeholders should be asked to define program performance expectations and articulate the indicators against which they will measure program success or failure.
2. Organizational structure and reporting lines must be consolidated in order to avoid competition among departments.
3. Close communication with financial leadership is necessary to determine how far to expand across the continuum of care.
4. Role definitions will occupy most of the initial design efforts.
   - scope of responsibilities
   - activity in emergency department admitting
   - assignment to service line or physician
   - interaction with social work
   - prioritization by patient risk
   - caseload options
   - minimization of interaction with payers
5. Where goals are poorly defined, we have seen staff stressed beyond reasonable expectation with constant reprioritization of work and a minimal sense of purpose.

There is no single right answer on how best to assign case managers (i.e., service line, unit based, or physician). Each organization will need to look introspectively to determine the best choice, based on culture, organizational structure, unit configuration, technology, and patient populations served.

The debate concerning the optimal structure for case management has been a long-standing one. There are schools of thought that view case management as strictly a nursing function, one that is overseen and managed by nurses. Other schools of thought envision case management as a distinct department whose purpose is to coordinate and expedite care for patients during an acute hospital stay. Others see case management as strictly a function of third-party payers, where resources are managed to deal with catastrophic or complex cases. The purpose of this chapter is to discuss, from the vantage point of a hospital/health system, the process for selecting a structure that will most effectively address patient need while managing the increasingly high cost of care.

FORM AND FUNCTION

It is important to understand the current environment and unique characteristics of the individual provider or health system before any attempt is made to drive toward a best practice in case management. We often see an organization try to make determinations about reporting structure, departmental structure, and role definition long before it has clearly articulated what it expects a case management program to do for the organization. Decisions regarding structure and reporting are often based on the individuals who currently hold positions in the organization, or who are well known to leadership, rather than on the goals, objectives, and expected results for case management. This kind of decision making has led to rework, unachieved outcomes, and the challenges associated with trying to re-implement programs that, from the medical staff vantage point, have proven to be less than successful.

Migration to a more continuum-based, integrated provider system is new for many organizations. Unfortunately, several integrated delivery networks have combined utilization management (UM)/discharge planning, case management, and social work under one reporting structure without comprehensive integration. As a result, roles and responsibilities of the persons performing these functions frequently have not been clearly defined, nor have utilization review (UR), case management, and discharge planning functions been incorporated into one role. This creates confusion and a lack of coordination among the multidisciplinary team. Under this system, there are multiple persons involved in reviewing the patient's chart and in interacting with the family and the physician.

Often, relationships between case managers and physicians are fragmented and are characterized by inconsistent collaboration. Staff may not be organized in a way that enables them to build relationships with physicians or allows them to expedite care with attention to utilization effectiveness and quality. Many organizations have spent a great deal of time on compliance documentation (clerical tasks) as opposed to collaborating with physicians to expedite care and provide for the efficient use of clinical resources.

The availability of case management services is suboptimal to meet today's level of clinical demand. Departmental operations are based on an eight-hour day, Monday through Friday. Case management triage has not been universally employed in many emergency departments (EDs) or other access entry points (e.g., patient admissions and observation units). Case manager roles have been widely varied, and the qualifications for case manager selection have been equally varied. For case management to work, case manager roles and responsibilities must be defined based on organizational needs and expectations. A lack of clarity concerning roles and responsibilities will continue to result in a duplication of effort and rework.

Enterprisewide infrastructure and capabilities typically do not exist to provide continuum-based case management. Most of these functions are at the local (departmental or unit) level, but are not serving the needs of the entire system and its component parts. Multiple handoffs are required to move patients efficiently through the continuum (i.e., home health coordinator, skilled nursing facility (SNF) placement coordinator, rehabilitation nurse evaluators, hospice). Tools and processes to support standardization and efficient workflow processes are underdeveloped. A lack of physician leadership and involvement often limits the effectiveness of current case management models. Physicians frequently do not fully understand the role and functions of the case manager. Physicians do not perceive the current model to be physician driven and physician focused.

The old adage of "form follows function" is one that should be invoked in the selection, development, and implementation of any model for case management. Key stakeholders should be asked to define program performance expectations and to articulate the indicators against which they will measure program success or failure. The key stakeholder group needs to include representatives from across the organization and, in particular, the physicians, who are critical to program success or failure. In designing a high-performance case management approach to care, an organization ultimately moves toward managing a total population's health and provides cost-effective care. The design needs to focus on care across the continuum and lay the foundation for the organization to accept financial risk and improve denial and clinical resource management.

KEY CONSIDERATIONS

Some of the key questions that need to be answered prior to making a determination about the case management structure best suited for an organization include the following:

- What does the organization hope to achieve through the implementation of a case management program? In our experience, organizations have undertaken the implementation of a case management program without clearly defining realistic goals for the program and articulating these goals to key stakeholders and staff.
  1. Is the organization moving to a case management model because it is the trend?
  2. Have key stakeholders clearly agreed to implement the redesigned case management model suited to meet the needs of the organization?
  3. Is the goal to manage payer expectations or to provide care facilitation for patients?
  4. Is the organization prepared to make an investment in resources, if required, to match the model with the needs of the organization?
  5. Have the goals for the case management program been clearly articulated?

  Where goals are poorly defined, we have seen staff stressed beyond reasonable expectation with constant reprioritization of work and a minimal sense of purpose. Insufficient time is allowed to demonstrate success, and the associated staff frustrations of never having a sense of accomplishment result in high turnover and little measurable success. For others, case management was entered into with a sense of purpose and planning for the future. Regardless of the reason, it is essential that each organization clearly articulate and document the organizational expectations of a case management program in order to set realistic, achievable, measurable targets for success.
- Are there preexisting, defined organizational needs that must be addressed through the program?
  1. Is a financial imperative driving the movement to case management?
  2. If this is being driven by a financial imperative, is there a specific time frame within which results must be achieved?
  3. Is case management being viewed by the organization as a way to mitigate financial risk and resolve a fiscal crisis?
  4. Does the organization recognize the interdependency of departments in taking out costs in order to realize the benefits of case management?
- Is the model for case management intended to be a fully integrated model, or are there organizational boundaries within which the design of the program must flow?
  1. Are there current staff roles that are prohibited from consideration as part of a new case management model redesign?
     –social work
     –transplant/trauma coordinators
     –home health coordinators
  2. Are there union considerations or employment agreements that may be prohibitive or restrictive in the development of a new model, necessitating in-depth discussion with those constituencies?
     –union leaders
     –physicians
- Is the model intended to span the continuum of care?

1. Will program implementation encompass the full continuum at the outset, or will the program be implemented in phases?
2. Are there any special timing considerations surrounding implementation?

- Is the organization prepared to make the investment in resources required to make the program successful?
  1. Is this initiative intended to be budget neutral?
  2. Are there capital restrictions that could impact program design?

After initial evaluation of these preliminary questions, a go/no go decision needs to be made. If the organization is sufficiently confident that, based on the answers to the questions outlined above, they are still willing and prepared to proceed, the work begins.

ROLES AND RESPONSIBILITIES

Here are some key elements to consider when addressing the roles and responsibilities of case managers.

- Will all patients be case managed?
- Will the case manager role be a fully integrated role, including UM, discharge planning, and care facilitation?
- Will case managers be responsible to provide direct, hands-on care for patients in addition to case managing them?
- Will case managers be expected to coordinate quality management activities in addition to managing a caseload?
- How will case managers be assigned (i.e., service line, physician, unit, other)?
- Will case managers manage patients along the full continuum, including in the ambulatory setting, ED, and so on?
- What are the expectations of physicians in the new model?

Will All Patients Be Case Managed?

There are different schools of thought regarding the answer to this question. Some organizations feel the need to manage only the high-cost, high-risk, complex patients and then create a separate UM function to manage the routine cases throughout the organization. This is certainly one effective way of addressing payer and provider considerations related to the effective use of resources. The challenge in this scenario is the potential it presents for rework, the possibility of duplication of effort, and the greater risk that patient needs may be overlooked.

Other organizations assign case managers to oversee patients by payer. Although this may seem pertinent, it is important to identify the clinical issues driving the decision to manage by payer in order to avoid the risk of being accused of managing patients based strictly on payer class. The financial penalties associated with even the suggestion of this type of practice can be severe.

A third approach, for purposes of simplicity, is to say that all patients will be case managed, but to varying degrees. The expectation, in this scenario, is for all patients to be evaluated by a case manager in order to

- determine clinical necessity for admission and continued stay
- evaluate potential discharge planning needs
- identify any other issues that might impact the plan of care, discharge, or reimbursement
- prioritize the level of any additional intervention based on patient need and/or payer requirement

Once the case manager has completed the initial evaluation and identified the patient need, the case manager is expected to prioritize work based on patient need. Even when no patient intervention is required, it is still the responsibility of the case manager to make certain that payer needs receive the required level of emphasis and that payer expectations are met.

This third scenario minimizes the potential risk of not identifying key patient needs early in the acute care stay. It also sets the stage for discussions and negotiations with payers, should the need arise.

Although there is no "one size fits all" answer to the question of which patients will be case managed, each case manager should answer the above questions honestly in order to determine the best approach for the organization.

Will the Case Manager Role Be a Fully Integrated Role?

There has been wide variability among organizations surrounding this question. The variability often arises out of territorialism associated with certain functions that have traditionally become the responsibility of a specific group of individuals. If we look historically at who has had primary responsibility for discharge planning in an organization, we will see that it has traditionally been the social worker. When we look at training and preparation, we find that social workers have been educationally prepared to address

- the psychosocial and emotional needs of the patients they serve
- high-social-risk case finding and screening
- information and referral needs of patient populations
- preadmission planning
- financial counseling
- health education
- postdischarge follow-up
- outpatient continuity of care
- patient and family advocacy[1]

By default, in addressing these needs, which are so closely connected to the discharge planning process, members of the multidisciplinary team have typically delegated primary and almost sole responsibility for discharge planning to social workers. Organizations that rethink these functions as being the primary responsibility of social workers will inevitably experience some organizational distress. As in any circumstance, when individuals are taken out of their comfort zone and faced with role changes, individual reactions are varied but emotionally charged under the best of circumstances.

In developing a model of case management, each organization must clearly define the working relationships between nurses at the bedside and the case manager. As discussed earlier, nursing has historically viewed "case management" as a nursing function. Nurses play a pivotal role in the care facilitation process, having been trained to look comprehensively at patient need. Although nurses at the bedside are integral to the overall care facilitation process, because of competing agendas and limited resources, nurses at the bedside often cannot focus sufficient time to provide direct care and simultaneously respond to provider and payer needs. Transitions have occurred that have moved nurses from the bedside into case manager roles in order to meet organizational needs. In their roles as case managers, these nurses work to facilitate care, expedite care, serve as the vehicle for communication among the various disciplines, and serve as the liaison between the patient and the payer.

The UM role for the case manager has evolved over time. Most organizations have had a UR function in place to deal specifically with payer demands. The UR function, prior to the advent of diagnosis-related groups (DRGs), was one focused on justifying the length of stay (LOS). With the advent of DRGs, it became less imperative to justify LOS and more critical to justify the need for inpatient admission. Payer demands are not the only utilization issue that case managers should be focusing on. As organizations try to position themselves better for contracting, they must be able to demonstrate that they can manage resource utilization effectively. When we speak of effective resource utilization, we refer to managing the level of care, use of diagnostics, use of pharmaceuticals, use of supplies, and LOS. Case managers must be sufficiently well versed in all of these aspects of resource utilization in order to communicate effectively with the team regarding the development of a comprehensive plan of care designed to meet patient need.

To be effective, a fully integrated case manager role is imperative. The patient, the physician, and the organization benefit from a point person who has a clear understanding of the global picture—from both a care perspective and a reimbursement perspective. The person ideally suited for this type of position is one who is (1) clinically excellent, (2) assertive and self-confident, and (3) known for excellent communication skills. We will discuss these characteristics in greater depth later, but it is important to acknowledge the characteristics needed to function effectively in the very challenging role of a case manager.

Although the case manager should be responsible for discharge planning, the case manager should not be the individual solely responsible for discharge planning. It is essential to recognize that discharge planning is a collaborative effort with the entire team, and the case manager's role in the process is to coordinate activities and facilitate the discharge planning arrangements.

Will Case Managers Be Responsible To Provide Care?

This is a frequently debated issue and has become more so with the identified nursing shortage throughout the country. Case managers, if they continue their reporting relationship with nursing services, can be and frequently are pulled into the ranks of staffing for daily care. The pressures of trying to respond to immediate staffing needs can, at times, negate the critical responsibilities that the case managers have for ensuring that clinical necessity criteria are being met and those considerations pertinent to reimbursement are reviewed on a daily basis. We have also found that case managers will assume responsibility for patient teaching. They do so for a variety of reasons, not the least of which is to expedite patient discharge, recognizing that nursing staff are under pressure to meet the daily demands of caring for patients whose LOS is shorter and whose care is increasingly more complex. Removing the case managers from staff nurse duties and direct patient education is not intended to minimize the importance of the work that needs to get completed on a daily basis at the bedside. However, it is critical to recognize that when case managers do not have sufficient time to focus on their primary roles of UM, discharge planning, and facilitation of care, the end result will impact both clinical and financial outcomes. It is essential to recognize that the roles of professional nurse at the bedside and case manager are complementary, and that the organization cannot be successful without the distinct roles of both.

Will Case Managers Be Expected To Coordinate Quality Management Activities?

In addition to integrating the activities of UM, discharge planning, and care facilitation, many organizations have included aspects of quality management and performance improvement in the case manager's role. Organizations considering this type of integration should thoroughly evaluate the workload associated with these activities. It would seem important to involve case managers in the collection and management of data for performance improvement activities. Case managers routinely review records and are well positioned to communicate performance improvement opportunities and sentinel events in a timely way. To the extent that the organization expects case managers to support medical staff and hospital performance improvement committee activities, consideration must be given to determining required staffing levels.

For case management programs that are in their early start-up phase, it is best to consider separating case management from performance improvement activities and to provide dedicated staff to deal with quality and performance improvement. This will allow case managers sufficient time to concentrate on their primary areas of responsibility and will minimize the possibility that quality and performance improvement activity might not be receiving sufficient attention to create a positive impact for the organization. Case managers are frequently responsible for the variance tracking for clinical pathways, analyzing these data, and reporting the results.

How Will Case Managers Be Assigned?

This is another question with no single right answer. Each organization will need to look introspectively to determine the best choice for assigning case managers, based on culture, organizational structure, unit configuration, technology, and patient populations served.

Service Line Case Management

Service line case management can be effective when patients and resources are in close proximity and the case manager is readily available to physicians and staff alike. Under this configuration, the reduced variability in patients allows the case manager to concentrate on leading practices within the service line and to more effectively track and trend results by population. In a true service line structure, where each service line operates as its own cost center, there are challenges associated with having case managers report up through the service line structure. Case managers in service line structures have reported that they are more likely to be pulled into direct caregiver roles, which decreases the amount of time they devote to managing care and resource utilization. We have seen direct financial impact to the organization when this occurs. We have seen service line-oriented organizations fail to provide case managers with sufficient information and support regarding rules, regulations, payer expectations, and corporate compliance. Additionally, we have seen decentralized case management in the service line structure suffer from the absence of sufficiently well-trained staff to provide coverage when the designated case manager is off duty. This absence of information and support has led to increased variability of practice and subsequent variability of clinical and financial performance in the service lines.

If the organization is moving to a service line structure, it is best to consider some type of centralized case management support system to ensure that fragmentation of comprehensive services does not occur. This centralized support can take on a variety of configurations. For example, the organization can elect to have a resource center designated to serve all case managers and communicate changes in rules, regulations, and procedures to the case managers at large. The disadvantage of simply providing a resource center for information is that there is still no single point of accountability to ensure compliance. Another alternative is to centralize case management and provide it as a support or contract service to each service line. This increases the likelihood of compliance with rules and regulations; it provides a source of skilled, well-trained coverage to the service line, in the absence of the designated case manager; and it increases the likelihood of the case manager being more in tune with changes that directly impact issues of clinical necessity and reimbursement.

Service line case management can also present challenges around issues of patient movement. As patients transition quickly from one unit to another, and from one level of care to another, each organization is faced with some key considerations concerning the following:

- continuity of care by allowing the case manager to follow the patient during the entire course of treatment
- availability of the case manager to the care team when the case manager is expected to travel from unit to unit and manage patients
- ability of the case manager to interact with physicians when the case manager is expected to travel from unit to unit and manage patients

Case Management by Diagnosis

In larger organizations, the clustering of patients with similar diagnoses is more likely to occur. Patient volumes generally support the placement of patients with like diagnoses in close proximity. In smaller facilities, it becomes more challenging to approach things from a service line perspective because patient volumes generally do not support a dedicated case manager. The organization must carefully weigh and acknowledge the challenges associated with the above-mentioned considerations in making the decision to provide service line case management.

Case Management by Physician

Other organizations initially elect to assign case managers to specific physicians or physician groups. Although these organizations may see some initial positive impact, the impact generally has not been sustainable. Case managers who are assigned to specific physicians experience a particular set of challenges that are often difficult to overcome. Under this arrangement, physician-based case managers tend to lose objectivity about their roles and responsibilities. As they develop strong working relationships with the physicians to whom they are assigned, they are often reluctant to challenge practice and raise issues regarding clinical necessity and clinical decision making. We have also seen case managers assume responsibilities that, except in cases of the advanced practice nurse, may well exceed the scope of nursing practice. Both sets of circumstances are difficult to overcome and, unless carefully monitored, can quickly erode any potential gains that the organization hopes to realize from effective case management.

Unit-Based Case Management

Unit-based case management does afford the organization some advantages. Case managers who are unit based are generally easily accessible and readily available to the physicians and care team. The physicians and team for any given unit are quickly able to identify the case manager with whom they can interact on clinical and financial fronts. Strong working relationships develop, with the team often anticipating the needs of each member in facilitating the care process.

Technology may play a key role in determining how best to assign case managers. The availability of work reports, census reports, and priority lists may be limited by the systems used. The ease of access to information for case managers is essential to allow them to complete daily tasks. Absence of an organized approach to providing this information can introduce a substantial level of complexity into daily work and increase the potential for error.

Will Case Managers Manage Patients along the Full Continuum?

Any model of case management currently presumes a strong emphasis on inpatient care. In fact, the true strength of any model is its ability to flex and respond to care in the ambulatory setting. The challenge for an organization is to determine whether a single case manager can effectively manage patient populations in both the inpatient and the outpatient setting. Suffice it to say that some organizations have developed and implemented models in which a single case manager is responsible for segments of both inpatient and outpatient populations. Although this may seem optimal from a continuity standpoint, from a workload management perspective, it is challenging at best. To effectively concentrate on patients in the ambulatory setting, the case manager must have sufficient time to work with patients, families, and community resources to implement a plan of care that allows the patient to function optimally in the ambulatory arena and minimizes the potential for frequent readmission.

The clinical and payer requirements and compliance standards associated with an inpatient stay can compete significantly for the case manager's time if he or she is trying to manage the gap between acute inpatient and the ambulatory setting. Generally, although a handoff or transition to another case manager is not ideal, the reality is that, with competing initiatives in the inpatient and ambulatory settings, no single case manager can effectively balance the work in both settings.

The case manager in the inpatient setting typically carries a caseload of 25–30 adult patients and 20–25 pediatric patients. Acute inpatient case managers must ensure coordinated handoffs in order to efficiently and effectively transfer patient care from the acute setting to alternative levels of care along the continuum.

What Are the Expectations of Physicians in the New Model?

The successful development and management of a case management program is highly dependent on a "partnership" between the health system and its affiliated physicians. Physicians remain the primary providers of patient care services and, as such, do the following:

- Manage the overall health of their patients.
- Act as critical elements in providing patients with information related to wellness programs.
- Determine diagnoses, care settings, treatment plans, and follow-up.

Physicians drive the utilization of clinical resources within the organization. Therefore, it is essential that the physicians provide leadership and direction to the development and implementation of a leading practice case management model.

Although case management requires a multidisciplinary team composed of physicians, other clinical practitioners, administrative personnel, and external (e.g., payer) representatives, physicians actually lead the team and direct a number of critical processes in case management.

- Physicians must collaborate with the patient care team regarding the overall plan of care.
- Physicians retain the technical knowledge needed to develop various tools used in case management (e.g., pathways and guidelines).
- Physicians are a primary user of case management systems.
- Physicians document care, and so generate a considerable amount of data that should be retained within the case management program. Ongoing management and improvement of the case management program depends, in part, on information access and information management.
- Physicians act as advisors within the case management system to resolve clinical practice issues and serve as clinical resources for case managers.
- Physicians are primary, proactive intermediaries with payers. In this role, physicians provide clinical information that is critical to resolving care and benefit issues.
- Physicians have clinical leadership and administrative roles within the health system. In these roles, physicians help define the direction and priorities of the health system.

CASE MANAGEMENT MODELS

Once an organization has successfully addressed each of the considerations outlined so far, the likelihood of success in selecting a structural model for case management is high.

The next few pages will summarize several structures that can work effectively, depending on the needs of the organization.

Unit-Based Case Management

Figure 1–1 represents a fully integrated, unit-based model that can span the full continuum of care. It reflects case management evaluation and assessment of all patients to best determine patient need. It is designed around the use of case managers, social workers, and support staff. The concept is based on an understanding that approximately 20 percent to 30 percent of the patients managed will require intense case management, but the case manager will review his or her entire caseload to make certain that resources are being correctly used and that patient needs are being met. This model incorporates the use of a resource center. The resource center provides support to case management functions for all case managers. Typical functions include clerical support, postacute service arrangements, benefit and eligibility verification, concurrent and retrospective denial management, and data entry, analysis, reporting, and tracking.

Although this model presumes a strong emphasis on inpatient care, it is easily transferable to the ambulatory setting. In essence, the ambulatory processes become interwoven with the acute care model and the resource center functions to both expedite and facilitate care.

Continuum Case Management Model

Figure 1–2 illustrates a model similar to Figure 1–1, but that incorporates the use of an outcomes specialist in the ambulatory setting.

- The *outcomes specialist* assumes responsibility for the oversight of select patient populations in the ambulatory environ-

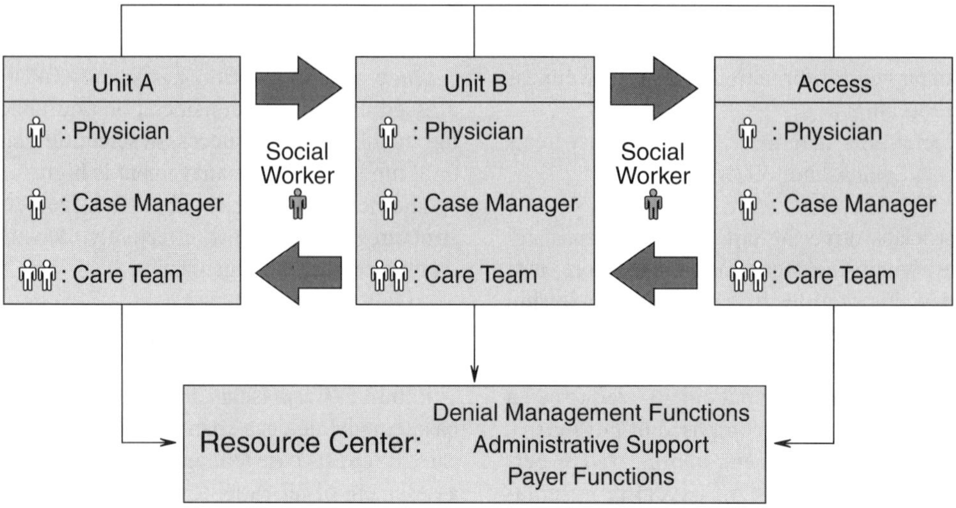

Figure 1–1 Unit-Based Case Management with Resource Center Support

ment. This role serves as the conduit to ensure that continuity of care is maintained and that compliance with medication and plans of care are followed by patient and family. This role manages the collection and analysis of data (e.g., access/service, satisfaction/health status, utilization/cost, and morbidity/mortality) relevant to the patient population. The outcomes specialist participates in the development of ambulatory clinical pathways that address wellness and prevention.

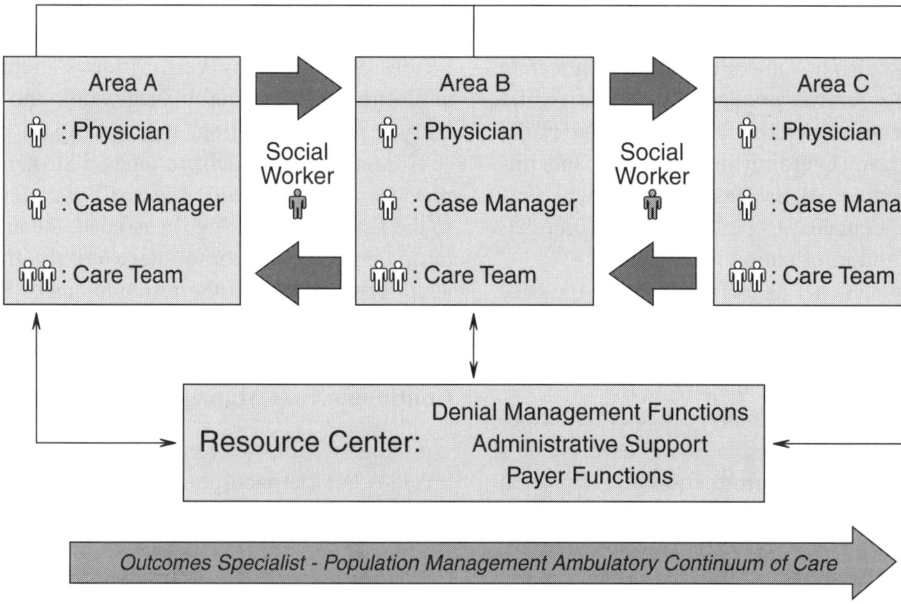

Figure 1–2 Continuum Case Management Model

- The *case manager* carries a consistent caseload consisting of both low-risk and high-risk patients and is expected to prioritize work based on patient need. The case manager is responsible for the coordination of UM, discharge planning, and care facilitation. The case manager also screens all admissions for clinical necessity, concurrently monitors resource utilization, and completes continued stay reviews. This role provides coordination of care in a collaborative effort with physicians, nursing, and the multidisciplinary team to manage the patient's plan of care across the continuum.
  - The *ED case manager* is responsible for screening all potential patient admissions to determine that they meet admission or observation criteria and linking them to the applicable inpatient case manager. The ED case manager also facilitates services for those patients in the ED requiring postdischarge follow-up or transfers/referrals to nonacute services.
  - The *admitting department case manager* is responsible for screening all inpatient admissions to ensure that they meet clinical and financial admission criteria. In the absence of the ED case manager, the admitting case manager will also provide screening services for the ED. This case manager also assists with communication and collaboration between the payer and the physician to obtain authorizations for admission and other alternate care delivery services.
- The *social worker* typically provides intervention/assistance to patients throughout multiple levels of care, focusing on crisis intervention and psychosocial counseling. In cases of suspected abuse/neglect, the social worker initiates referrals to protective services as required by law. The social worker also serves as a consultant for processing issues such as guardianship, power of attorney, health care surrogate, advance directives, and financial/health program coverage.
- *Resource center* staff serve as support for the case management program by improving the efficiency of case managers. The staff assume responsibility for time-consuming, nonclinical functions associated with facilitating care and discharge (e.g., communication to payers, arrangement of simple nonacute services, administrative/secretarial functions). The presence of a resource center allows the case managers and social workers to focus on the care facilitation, patient/family issues, and concurrent UM components of these roles.

Clinical Care Coordination Model

Figure 1–3 represents a comprehensive model that spans the full continuum of care and places an emphasis on optimizing the use of resources across all levels of care. It addresses the points of access and discharge and captures the need to put support mechanisms in place to allow case managers to optimize the time they have available for patients, families, physicians, and the care team.

In this model, the outcomes manager, case manager, and social worker function as a team and are assigned by service line or by a specific patient population. This team partners with the physician and the multidisciplinary team members to coordinate care of these patients. Patients are case managed through multiple levels of care (i.e., ED, medical–surgical, rehabilitation/SNF, and the outpatient setting).

- The *outcomes case manager* typically carries a caseload consisting of patients whose care is "high-risk, high-cost, and complex." These patients have serious physiological disease processes, often chronic in nature; profound psychosocial needs; multiple physician consultants; a variety of interdisciplinary care providers; and, often, changes in their functional abilities (e.g., ability to perform activities of daily living). Extended LOS and frequent planned or unplanned readmissions are also prevalent in these high-risk patients. They have tedious

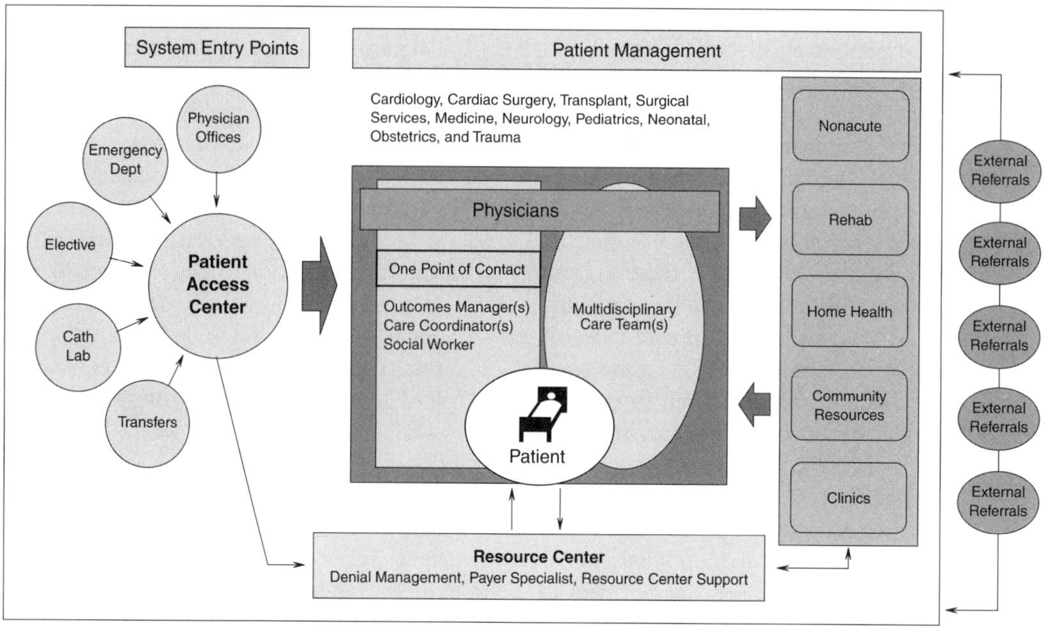

Figure 1–3 Clinical Care Coordination Model

discharge requirements (e.g., financial assistance with medications, compliance issues, and transportation) that require coordination and overall facilitation of care across the continuum. The outcomes case manager performs continued stay reviews and clinical resource utilization on the 20 percent of the patient population they manage. The outcomes case manager is also responsible for programmatic development for the service line, is in partnership with key physicians, and links the patient to disease management/external or community care management, as needed.

- The *case manager* typically carries a caseload consisting of patients whose care is "lower risk"—those patients who typically follow clinical pathways/protocols, whose acute care episode/illness is somewhat predictable or routine, and who have the benefits and resources to manage nonacute care requirements. Patients managed by case managers typically require less intensive services but have discharge planning needs. The case manager ensures handoffs to efficiently transfer patient care from the acute to nonacute sites. This role also screens all admissions for clinical necessity, concurrently monitors resource utilization, and performs continued stay reviews. The case manager works with physicians, nursing, and the multidisciplinary team to manage the patient's plan of care across the continuum.
  - The *ED case manager* is responsible for screening all patients to ensure that they meet admission or observation criteria and linking their status to the applicable inpatient outcomes manager/case manager. The ED case manager also facilitates patient care for those patients in the ED requiring postdischarge follow-up or transfers/referrals to nonacute services.
  - The *admitting department case manager* is responsible for screening all nonelective and, as needed, elective inpatient admissions to ensure that they meet clinical and financial admission criteria. The admitting department case

manager also assists with communication and collaboration between the payer and the physician to obtain authorizations for admission and other alternate care delivery services.

- The *social worker* typically carries a caseload and provides additional support to patients throughout multiple levels of care (inpatient and nonacute), focusing on crisis intervention and psychosocial counseling. In cases of suspected abuse/neglect, the social worker initiates referrals to protective services as required by law. The social worker also serves as a consultant for processing issues such as guardianship, power of attorney, health care surrogate, advance directives, and financial/health program coverage.
- A *resource center* serves as a support center for the clinical care coordination program, integrating the functions of denial and UM. The development of the resource center improves the efficiency of care coordination by reallocating time-consuming case management functions (e.g., communication to payers, arrangement of simple nonacute services, administrative/secretarial functions, data analysis, and denial management process) to a central support area. The resource center allows the outcomes managers, case managers, and social workers to focus on the care facilitation, patient/family issues, and concurrent UM components of these roles. The roles typically seen within the resource center include
  - *Denial management specialist* is responsible for the denial management and appeals writing process. The primary focus is on the "per diem" paid patients of the managed care populations.
  - *Payer specialist* effectively communicates clinical information and negotiates with payers to obtain authorization for necessary levels of care and LOS.
  - *Clerical* performs secretarial and administrative duties for the clinical care coordination department, serving as the clerical coordinator of clinical and/or nonclinical activities.

For a group of 100 patients, depending on the population (i.e., demographics, diagnoses, payer mix), a team will typically include one outcomes manager, four case managers, one social worker, and the resource center. The team manages the assigned patients 24 hours a day, 7 days a week. Coverage is organized to achieve the goals of effective LOS, resource utilization, and denial management.

Analysis of Models

Figures 1–2 and 1–3 both use the outcomes specialist/manager role. In each model, the role varies by its definition and intention. In either case, the organization's level of sophistication and readiness to invest in longer term returns on investment are key determinants to the effectiveness of the outcomes manager role. The danger in implementing the role as defined in Model 3 is the potential for the role to become unmanageable, based on caseload size, multiple handoffs, and unclear definition concerning what criteria are used to constitute the "high-risk" patient classification. In discussion with organizations that have implemented the outcomes manager role, these organizations articulate that substantial efforts are ongoing to fully define and clarify the role.

Table 1–1 outlines suggested staffing levels based on current leading practice and benchmarking in the industry. It is important to keep in mind that these are only suggested staffing levels, and that each organization must consider its own particulars in determining final staffing requirements. Case manager staffing levels must be based on an average. There will be some patient populations that lend themselves to a higher caseload size (i.e., uncomplicated maternal/child cases) and other patient populations that lend themselves to a smaller caseload size (i.e., trauma, burn).

The appendix to this chapter provides sample job descriptions for each of the positions described in the models outlined here. Although the job descriptions vary slightly, there are some common themes regarding the roles and responsibilities for each position in the model. It is important to recognize that job descriptions are developed using

Table 1–1 Staffing Recommendations for Case Management Models

Model	*Caseload*
Model 1	
Case manager	1:20–1:25 patients
Social worker	1:50–1:60 patients
Resource center	1 resource center staff person to support every 6 case managers and social workers
Model 2	
Case manager	1:20–1:25 patients
Social worker	1:50–1:60 patients
Resource center	1 resource center staff person to support every 6 case managers and social workers
Outcomes specialist	1 for every 250 active cases
Model 3	
Case manager	1:20–1:25 patients
Social worker	1:50–1:60 patients
Resource center	1 resource center staff person to support every 6 case managers and social workers
Outcomes care manager	1:20–1:25 patients

the same principle as model development, that is, "form follows function." It is unwise for an organization to adopt any job descriptions without defining the expectations of the roles and providing in the job descriptions the required level of authority to meet those performance expectations.

ORGANIZATIONAL STRUCTURE AND REPORTING

As with the selection of a model suited to the organization, organizational reporting structure is equally critical to program success. There is no single structure that works universally for all case management programs. However, there are some basic premises to be considered during the decision-making process.

- To promote an enterprisewide approach to care management, an organizational integration of care functions is optimal.
- To set strategy, accelerate decision making, and minimize duplication, a centralized reporting structure is optimal.
- To establish the accountability and responsibility for achieving results, a centralized reporting structure is optimal.
- To achieve the centralized supporting structure, select personnel and resources may need to be reallocated and/or realigned.
- Case management touches all levels in the organization; accordingly, the relationships and communication lines are linked from people to results.
- Physician alignment with case management and organizational goals is critical, and the structure must reflect reporting lines in which the physicians feel that their interests are protected.
- To realize cost savings and service improvement objectives, operations executives will need to be linked to case management in order to address capacity management, financial management, and quality improvement issues.

Because of the professional disciplines involved, there is often debate regarding the best reporting structure for the organization. The organization must position case management where it will have the greatest opportunity and likelihood of achieving organizational goals. Because case management has been associated most frequently with nursing, there is a strong preference to place case management under the direction of nursing leadership. In recent times, this has met with some resistance from the medical staff because of the following:

- Previous attempts by nursing to introduce the concept of case management did not sufficiently involve physicians in design and decision making.
- Critical pathway development was introduced by nursing and is often seen as strictly a nursing initiative.
- Physicians are disinclined to have issues related to their clinical practice, peer review, and personal conduct reported through nursing leadership. They see these reporting lines functioning outside the scope of the peer review process and have concerns about the confidentiality of the information as protected under peer review.
- Physicians perceive the nursing model to be "nurses telling physicians how to practice medicine."

When the structure aligns the case management function more closely to physician leaders in the organization, and to administration, the readiness of physicians to embrace the concept of case management increases incrementally. Figures 1–4 through 1–6 represent various reporting structures that have proven to be effective and that have received the endorsements of

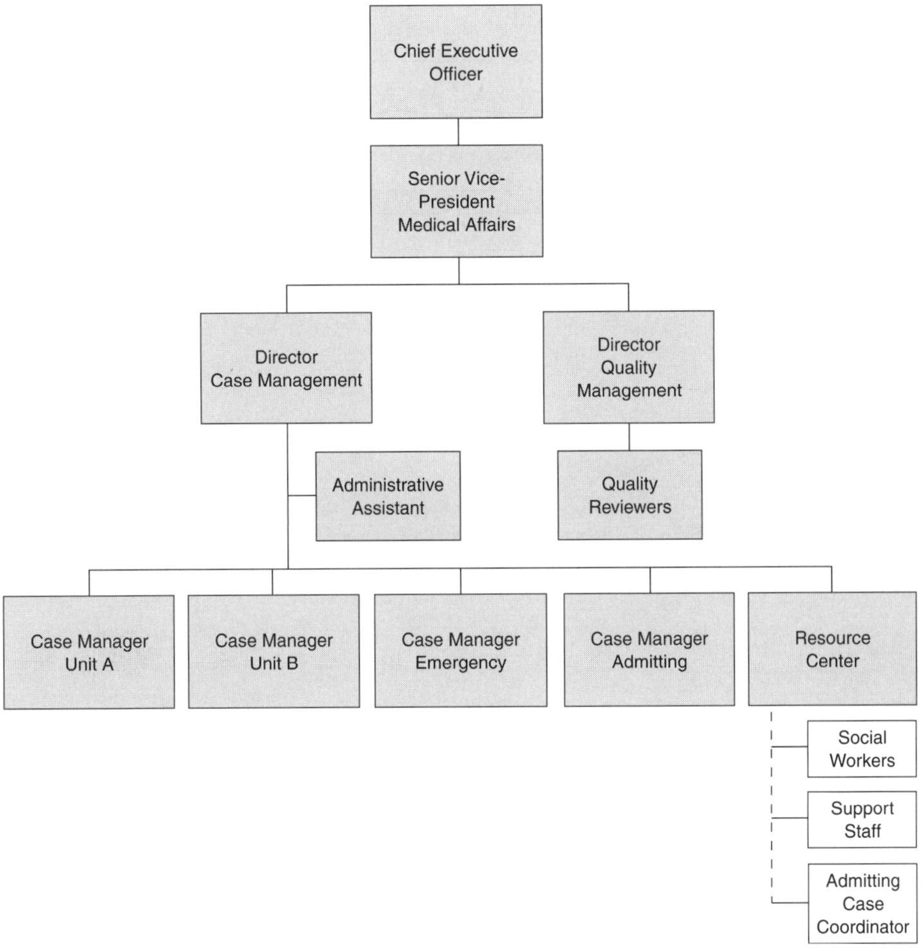

Figure 1–4 Organizational Reporting Structure

the respective medical staff organizations in which they have been implemented.

Figure 1–4 presents a case management department that reports directly to the senior vice-president of medical affairs, who reports to the chief executive officer (CEO). The quality management functions or performance improvement functions have been separated to allow the case managers to concentrate on care facilitation, discharge planning, and resource utilization. In this model, the case managers participate in some concurrent data collection that is then incorporated into the work being done by the quality management staff. Of note in this model is the significant importance placed on case management in the organization. Case management, through the senior vice-president of medical affairs, reports directly to the CEO. This alignment reflects recognition of the impact that well-implemented case management can have on an organization. It also reflects one of the key considerations for members of the medical staff. The CEO is paying attention not only to the financials associated with running the organization, but also to the clinical aspects of care, and is being provided with feedback regarding the interdependencies of clinical and financial operations.

Figure 1–5 represents a similar, but slightly different variation of Figure 1–4. In this representation, there is actually a physician medical group, which has come together for purposes of contracting and health plan management. Because of the strong interdependencies of inpatient activities linked to the health plan and, consequently, to members of the medical group, the medical group has assumed responsibility for

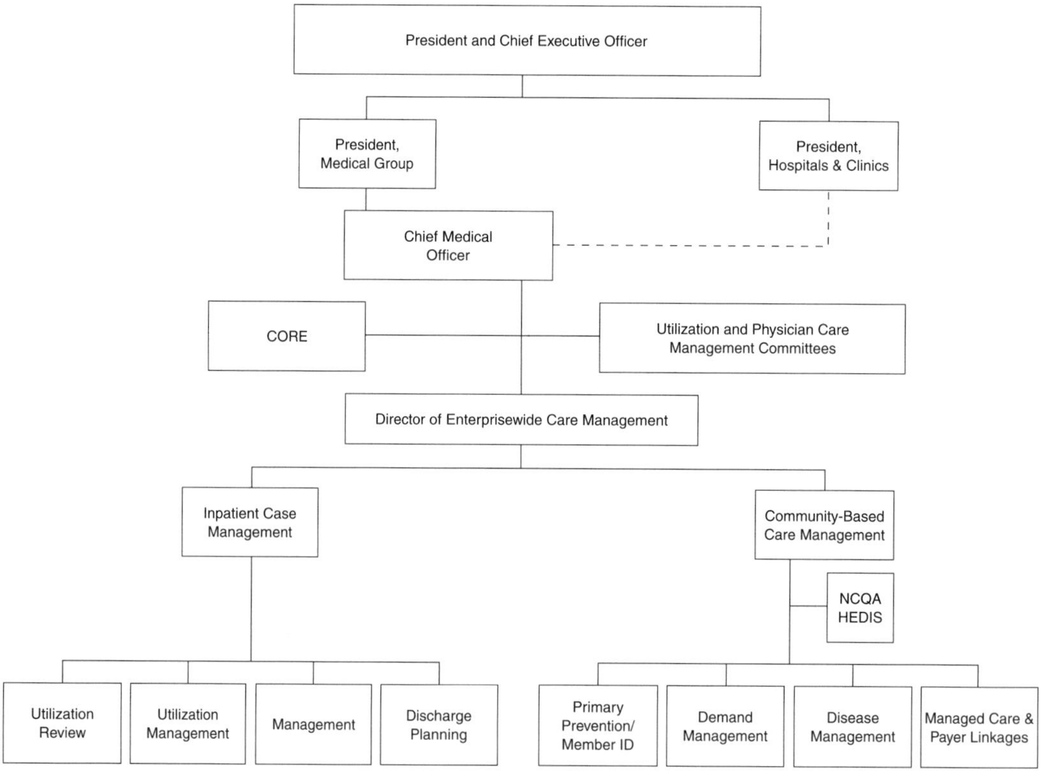

Figure 1–5 Organizational Reporting Structure Delineating Inpatient and Community-Based Case Management Operations

case management functions. In this case, as in Figure 1–4, the function of case management reports through a physician leader directly to the CEO. The rationale behind this reporting structure is similar to the rationale described for Figure 1–4.

Figure 1–6 is similar to that of Figures 1–4 and 1–5. Figure 1–6 reflects the strong working relationship between the vice-president of patient services and the chief medical officer. It also draws the working links between the directors of nursing and the director of case management. In this case, as in Figures 1–4 and 1–5, the function of case management reports through a physician leader directly to the CEO. The rationale behind this reporting structure is similar to the rationale described for Figures 1–4 and 1–5.

It should be noted that there are exceptions to case management reporting to the CEO either directly or indirectly through a chief medical officer. However, these cases are being seen with less frequency. A major reason for this shift is that organizations have begun to realize that, over the course of recent years, most cost savings opportunities associated with operations, productivity, staffing, and product standardization have been realized. The ability of an organization to realize any additional cost savings resides in the ability of the organization to impact clinical practice and those things that are directly related to the delivery and facilitation of care. With this in mind, CEOs have become more and more intimately aware of and involved in the work associated with case management.

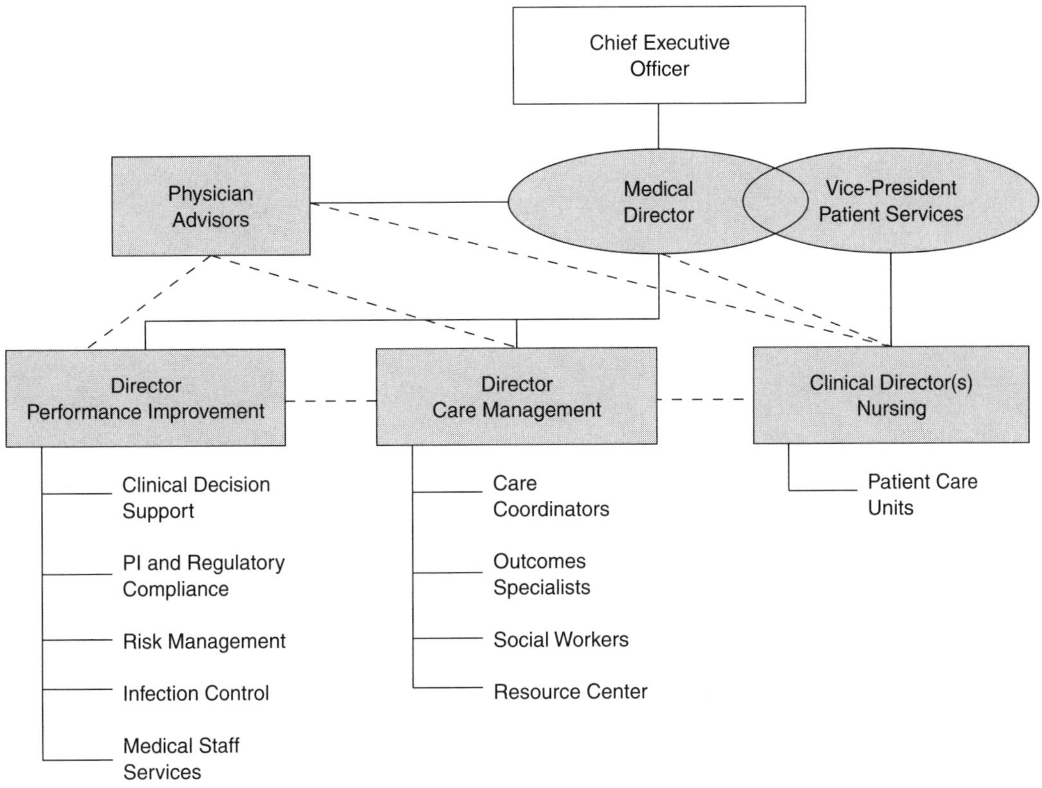

Figure 1–6 Organizational Reporting Structure Delineating Performance Improvement Functions

REFERENCE

1. NASW Clinical Indicators for Social Work and Psychosocial Services in the Acute Care Medical Hospital.

Appendix 1–A

Job Descriptions

JOB TITLE	***Director of Case Management***
DEPARTMENT	Case Management
REPORTS TO	Vice President Care Management

POSITION SUMMARY

The director of case management is responsible and accountable for the implementation of the case management program at the local level. The components/roles of the inpatient case management program consist of the following: care facilitation, utilization management, case management, and discharge planning.

The director is responsible for developing systems and processes for care/utilization management at the hospital level. In addition, the director is responsible for managing the department's activities related to discharge planning and clinical quality improvement. The director evaluates and ensures that hospital resources are used appropriately and effectively. The director oversees the collection, analysis, and reporting of financial and quality data related to utilization management, quality improvement, and performance improvement. The director promotes interdisciplinary collaboration, fosters teamwork, and champions service excellence.

REPORTING RELATIONSHIPS

The director of case management reports at the local level to the chief executive officer or to the chief medical officer, where one is in place and is matrixed to the executive director of medical management.

DUTIES AND RESPONSIBILITIES

1. Plans, directs, and supervises all aspects of the local level program.
2. Facilitates growth and development of the case management program consistent with enterprisewide philosophy and in response to the dynamic nature of the health care environment through benchmarking for best practices, networking, quality management, and other activities as needed.
3. Responsible for approving and managing the day-to-day local-level operational budget.
4. Responsible for identifying and achieving optimal targeted financial outcomes via the inpatient case management process.

5. Responsible for departmental personnel functions (e.g., hiring, firing, etc.) in conjunction with the executive director of medical management.
6. Writes and conducts annual and interim performance appraisal reviews for the professional and nonprofessional staff in the department.
7. Acts as liaison to facilitate communication and collaboration between all care partners (e.g., physicians, hospitalists, community care managers, nurses, community resources, etc.).
8. Responsible for leading a high-performance team of "system thinkers" who incorporate leadership principles and vision in performing the functions of case management.
9. Uses data to drive decisions, plan, and implement performance improvement strategies for case management.
10. Responsible for overseeing the education of physicians, managers, staff, patients, and families related to the case management process at the local level. Participates in this evolutionary process by constantly identifying future needs of current customers and/or identifying potential new customers.

POSITION REQUIREMENTS

- BSN or equivalent academic credit requirements for a BSN, clinical education, and experience required. Master's degree or equivalent experience preferred.
- Minimum five years experience in utilization management, case management, discharge planning, or other cost/quality management program.
- Three to five years experience in hospital-based nursing.
- Knowledge of leading practice in clinical care and payer requirements.
- Self-motivated, proven communication skills, assertive.
- Background in business planning and targeted outcomes.
- Working knowledge of managed care, inpatient, outpatient, and the home health continuum, as well as utilization management and case management.
- Working knowledge of the concepts associated with performance improvement.
- Demonstrated effective working relationship with physicians.
- Ability to work collaboratively with health care professionals at all levels to achieve established goals and improve quality outcomes.

JOB TITLE ***Case Manager***
DEPARTMENT Care Management
REPORTS TO Director of Case Management

POSITION SUMMARY

The purpose of the case manager position is to support the physician and interdisciplinary team in the provision of patient care, with the underlying objective of enhancing the quality of clinical outcomes and patient satisfaction while managing the cost of care and providing timely and accurate information to payers. The role integrates and coordinates utilization management, care facilitation, and discharge planning functions.

The case manager is accountable for a designated patient caseload and plans effectively in order to meet patient needs, manage the length of stay, and promote efficient utilization of resources. Specific functions within this role include

- facilitation of precertification and payer authorization processes
- facilitation of the collaborative management of patient care across the continuum, intervening as necessary to remove barriers to timely and efficient care delivery and reimbursement
- application of process improvement methodologies in evaluating outcomes of care
- support and coaching of clinical documentation efforts and serving as a clinical resource for coders, ensuring that documentation accurately reflects severity of illness and intensity of service
- coordinating communication with physicians

DUTIES AND RESPONSIBILITIES

1. Coordinates/facilitates patient care progression throughout the continuum.
    - Works collaboratively and maintains active communication with physicians, nursing, and other members of the multidisciplinary care team to effect timely, appropriate patient management.
    - Ensures appropriate clinical pathway assignment by staff nurses.
    - Addresses/resolves system problems impeding diagnostic or treatment progress.
    - Proactively identifies and resolves delays and obstacles to discharge.
    - Seeks consultation from appropriate disciplines/departments as required to expedite care and facilitate discharge.
    - Utilizes advanced conflict resolution skills as necessary to ensure timely resolution of issues.
    - Collaborates with the physician and all members of the multidisciplinary team to facilitate care for designated caseload; monitors the patient's progress, intervening as necessary and appropriate to ensure that the plan of care and services provided are patient focused, high quality, efficient, and cost effective; facilitates the following on a timely basis:
        - completion and reporting of diagnostic testing
        - completion of treatment plan and discharge plan
        - modification of plan of care, as necessary, to meet the ongoing needs of the patient
        - communication to third-party payers and other relevant information to the care team
        - assignment of appropriate levels of care
        - completion of all required documentation in TQ screens and patient records
2. Collaborates with medical staff, nursing staff, and ancillary staff to eliminate barriers to efficient delivery of care in the appropriate setting.
3. Completes utilization management and quality screening for assigned patients.

- Applies approved utilization acuity criteria to monitor appropriateness of admissions and continued stays and documents findings based on department standards.
- Identifies at-risk populations using approved screening tool and follows established reporting procedures.
- Monitors length of stay (LOS) and ancillary resource use on an ongoing basis. Takes actions to achieve continuous improvement in both areas.
- Refers cases and issues to physician advisor in compliance with department procedures and follows up as indicated.
- Communicates with resource center to facilitate covered day reimbursement certification for assigned patients. Discusses payer criteria and issues on a case-by-case basis with clinical staff and follows up to resolve problems with payers as needed.
- Uses quality screens to identify potential issues and forwards information to the quality review department.

4. Ensures that all elements critical to the plan of care and clinical path have been communicated to the patient/family and members of the health care team and are documented as necessary to ensure continuity of care.
5. Manages all aspects of discharge planning for assigned patients.
   - Meets directly with patient/family to assess needs and develop an individualized continuing care plan in collaboration with the physician.
   - Collaborates and communicates with multidisciplinary team in all phases of discharge planning process, including initial patient assessment, planning, implementation, interdisciplinary collaboration, teaching, and ongoing evaluation.
   - Ensures/maintains plan consensus from patient/family, physician, and payer.
   - Refers appropriate cases for social work intervention based on department criteria.
   - Collaborates/communicates with external case managers.
   - Initiates and facilitates referrals through the resource center for home health care, hospice, and medical equipment and supplies.
   - Documents relevant discharge planning information in the medical record according to department standards.
   - Facilitates transfer to other facilities for case management population.
6. Actively participates in clinical performance improvement activities.
   - Assists in the collection and reporting of financial indicators including case mix, LOS, cost per case, excess days, resource utilization, readmission rates, denials, and appeals.
   - Uses data to drive decisions and plan/implement performance improvement strategies related to case management for assigned patients, including fiscal, clinical, and patient satisfaction data.
   - Collects, analyzes, and addresses variances from the plan of care/care path with physician and/or other members of the health care team. Uses concurrent variance data to drive practice changes and positively impact outcomes.
   - Collects delay and other data for specific performance and/or outcome indicators as determined by the director of outcomes management.
   - Documents key clinical path variances and outcomes that relate to areas of direct responsibility (e.g., discharge planning). Uses pathway data in collaboration with other disciplines to ensure effective patient management concurrently.
   - Participates in the development, implementation, evaluation, and revision of clinical pathways and other case management tools as a member of the clinical resource/team. Assists in the compilation of physician profile data regarding LOS, resource utilization, denied days,

costs, case mix index, patient satisfaction, and quality indicators (e.g., readmission rates, unplanned return to OR, etc.).

EDUCATION AND EXPERIENCE

- Licensure to practice as a registered nurse in the state of ______________.
- BSN or BSN completion within three years and professional certification as a case manager required.
- Minimum three years clinical experience in clinical practice area to which assigned.
- Excellent interpersonal communication and negotiation skills.
- Strong analytical, data management, and PC skills.
- Current working knowledge of discharge planning, utilization management, case management, performance improvement, and managed care reimbursement.
- Understanding of preacute and postacute venues of care and postacute community resources.
- Strong organizational and time management skills, as evidenced by a capacity to prioritize multiple tasks and role components.
- Ability to work independently and exercise sound judgment in interactions with physicians, payers, and patients and their families.

JOB TITLE *Social Worker*
DEPARTMENT Medical Management
REPORTS TO Director of Case Management

POSITION DEFINITION

The social worker intervenes with patients who have complex psychosocial needs, require assistance with eligibility determination for social programs and funding sources, and qualify for community assistance from a variety of special funds and agencies. In addition, offers crisis intervention to patients and families with psychosocial needs and coordinates and facilitates the development of a discharge plan of care for high-risk patient populations. This role will receive referrals for individuals from at-risk populations from interdisciplinary team members (including physicians, case managers, staff nurses, and other members of the care team).

DUTIES AND RESPONSIBILITIES

Psychosocial Assessment and Interventions

- On the basis of preliminary risk screening, assesses patient's and family's psychosocial risk factors through evaluation of prior functioning levels, appropriateness and adequacy of support systems, reaction to illness, and ability to cope.
- Intervenes with patients and families regarding emotional, social, and financial consequences of illness and/or disability; accesses and mobilizes family/community resources to meet identified needs.
- Provides intervention in cases involving child abuse/neglect, domestic violence, elderly abuse, institutional abuse, and sexual assault.
- Serves as a resource person and provides counseling and intervention related to treatment decisions and end-of-life issues.
- Advocates for patient and family empowerment and independence to make autonomous health care decisions and access needed services within the health care system.

Complex Discharge Planning

- Participates in discharge planning activities for complex patients, in order to ensure a timely discharge and to provide appropriate linkage with postdischarge care providers.
- Deals with families exhibiting complex family dynamics that impact directly on patient care and discharge.
- Communicates with care coordinators regarding the discharge planning status of all patients referred by them.
- Assists case managers with discharge planning activities as requested.
- Provides consultation to case managers when coordination with significant or intensive community resources is necessary to achieve desired treatment outcomes.
- Receives referrals for complex patient problem resolution from case managers or care team members.
- Screens and coordinates all *new* skilled nursing facility (SNF) and rehab facility referrals. Referrals will be made to the resource center for determination of bed availability both in and out of the local area. Informs the resource center regarding trends and issues related to SNF and rehab

facility quality of care. When necessary, makes recommendations regarding facilities to be removed from the hospital's referral resources catalogue.
- Validates discharge criteria for patient and families and notifies case managers of newly identified resources or change in previously identified resources.
- Educates patient/family and physician regarding postacute options and addresses issues of choice.

Patient and Family Support in Legally Complex Cases

- Provides intervention in child abuse/neglect, domestic violence, guardianship (temporary/permanent), foster care, adoption, mental health placement, advance directives, adult/elderly abuse, child protection, and sexual assault.

POSITION REQUIREMENTS

Education and Experience

- MSW and certification as a clinical social worker or BSW who will function under the supervision of the director of case management.
- Three years hospital/health care field experience.
- Working knowledge/experience in utilization management, managed care, and payer issues.
- Experience in psychosocial and therapeutic counseling.

Other Position Qualifications

Strong interview, assessment, organizational, and problem-solving skills. Ability to identify appropriate community resources on assigned caseload and to work collaboratively with patients, families, multidisciplinary team, and community agencies to achieve desired patient outcomes.

Possesses excellent interpersonal communication and negotiation skills in interactions with patients, families, physicians, and health care team colleagues. Possesses strong analytical and PC skills. Exposure and/or experience in preacute and postacute care, as well as community resources. Ability to work independently as well as to develop collaborative relationships with physicians, families, patients, interdisciplinary team, and other community agencies. Demonstrates excellent communication and negotiation skills. Demonstrates ability to analyze, develop, and manage change and to integrate continuous quality improvement principles for service and organization work improvements.

Ability to work with people of all social, economic, and cultural backgrounds; be flexible, open-minded, and adaptable to change. Demonstrates the ability to connect patients and families with necessary services, both inside and outside the network. Maintains a current working knowledge of services available in the local community, particularly services available to patients with limited or nonexistent payment resources. Must demonstrate patience and tact when dealing with patients, families, and other staff.

CHAPTER 2

Recruiting Case Managers

Patricia L. Metzger

TAKE THIS TO WORK

1. Three major characteristics to look for when selecting case managers include (1) strong clinical expertise and critical thinking, (2) strong interpersonal communication skills, and (3) a mutual respect and trust with physicians and peers.
2. If a redesigned program is going to succeed, it is advisable to have staff reapply for their positions. It is important to acknowledge that roles and responsibilities have changed as a result of the redesign process, and all staff may not want to fulfill, or may not be capable of fulfilling, the requirements of the newly defined roles.
3. Interviewing each staff member to review the roles and responsibilities associated with newly defined positions is critical in determining the staff's level of commitment to the work at hand. Interviews provide a forum to discuss performance expectations, goal setting, and those things against which the performance of each case manager will be measured.

Many of the key responsibilities associated with the case manager's role were presented in Chapter 1, with the appendix to Chapter 1 providing sample job descriptions outlining these major responsibilities. Although the roles and responsibilities may vary slightly by organization, the overriding principles do not change. The ability of organizations to find individuals to fill these positions presents its own set of challenges. For many organizations, the transition to a redesigned case management model is a complete departure from the historical way that utilization management (UM) and resource utilization have been done. Historically, UM was approached retrospectively, and utilization staff spent their time justifying admissions or communicating with physicians about why their patients no longer met criteria for continued stay in the hospital. These communications were often difficult because physicians perceived that the staff's main focus was financially driven, and little consideration was given to the clinical needs of the patient. These perceptions strained relationships between physicians and UM staff and resulted in UM staff being viewed as ineffective and, more to the point, as the enemy.

CASE MANAGER ROLES AND RESPONSIBILITIES

When moving to case management, it is important to articulate goals clearly and define program objectives. The move to case management without clearly articulating goals and defining program objectives typically results in selecting staff who are not sufficiently prepared to move the organization toward meeting its long-term goals. We have all too frequently seen leadership in an organization determine the following:

- It needs to implement case management.
- There is no need to define program goals; they are already understood.
- Utilization review (UR) nurses can be redefined as case managers without determining that the staff can or are interested in assuming the additional responsibilities associated with case management.

A historical look at the stereotype of UR departments reveals that individuals moved into these departments for several reasons, including the following:

- UR departments were typically seen as Monday through Friday operations, requiring no staff time on holidays and weekends.
- Hours of operation were generally 8:00 AM to 4:30 PM and did not require overtime.
- UR was seen as a compliance-driven approach to managing care, and individuals whose strengths were rules, regulations, compliance, minimal negotiation, and interpersonal interaction saw this as more attractive than the staff nurse role, which required flexibility, creativity, and a significant degree of interpersonal negotiation.
- Nurses who could no longer function at the bedside were relegated to UM roles with minimal preparation and often minimal desire to function in that capacity.
- Individuals who were perceived to be controversial were often placed in these roles because organizations felt that these individuals could be more aggressive with payers, who were seen as the common enemy.

It is important to note that this stereotype does not apply universally, and that some departments and individuals have been extremely successful over time. But more importantly, we must recognize that, in redesigned case management models, the case manager selection process is critical to success.

KEY CHARACTERISTICS

As case management and the realization that case management is critical to organizational survival becomes more embedded in organizational culture, clinical disciplines begin to identify those characteristics of the discipline that make them suited to case manage patients. Three major disciplines see themselves as most likely to become case managers. They include nursing, social work, and rehabilitation services. Each discipline has its merits, but for purposes of this text, we will focus on the acute inpatient setting. Case managers in the acute environment need to focus on the physical assessment of patients. In addition, they must be prepared to develop a comprehensive plan of care that will help transition the patient into the alternative care setting that is best suited to meet the patient's needs. Acute care case managers must be capable of discussing the physiology of disease with physicians and must be prepared to discuss therapeutic interventions (i.e., medication, rehabilitative services, activities) as they relate to the patient's condition. Given the patient populations needing to be managed and the highly clinical focus that the inpatient environment requires, registered nurses seem to be the candidates of choice.

In reviewing roles, responsibilities, and job descriptions, there are several key characteristics that emerge as prerequisites to assuming the role of case manager. In the book, *Nursing Case Management: A Practical Guide to Success in Managed Care,*[1] Suzanne Powell lists the characteristics as follows:

- commitment and desire to be a case manager
- strong interpersonal communication skills
- ability to prioritize
- excellent assessment skills

- clinical expertise and critical thinking
- attention to detail
- understanding of insurance idiosyncrasies
- organizational skills
- ability to read poor penmanship
- management skills
- good follow-through
- knowledge of community resources
- respect and trust by peers
- resourcefulness
- team player
- knowledge of legal and quality issues and standards of practice
- self-esteem and confidence
- competency and adaptability
- ability to work with others
- self-directed and assertive
- diplomacy
- caring attitude and behavior
- adaptability, flexibility, and creativity
- negotiation skills

Many of the characteristics outlined by Powell can be captured in three major categories, without which a case manager cannot succeed.

1. clinical expertise and critical thinking
2. strong interpersonal communication skills
3. a mutual respect and trust with physicians and peers

The case manager must be viewed as an individual to whom physicians are willing to entrust the oversight of their patients. Physicians must see the case manager as an extension of themselves in facilitating and managing care. They must have a level of confidence that the case manager will recognize changes in patient condition, alert the physician to abnormal therapeutic findings, and work with the physician to find care alternatives that will meet patient need, all the while keeping in mind payer expectations and requirements. Case managers must be capable of discussing the clinical implications of treatment in real time in a way that demonstrates that they understand the disease process as well as leading industry practice in addressing the care requirements associated with the diagnosis. Case managers need to demonstrate their ability to problem solve and develop a well-integrated clinical approach to care and discharge.

Not only must case managers be clinically expert, but they must also be able to deliver the clinical and financial message to all members of the team in a way that prompts the team to action. The ability to communicate effectively relies heavily on clinical expertise, but also on a strong personal presence and self-confidence. A case manager's role is not one that lends itself to timidity. The interactions facing a case manager each day vary from the most sophisticated clinical discussions to the most basic explanations for patients and families about the plan of care. Communication also implies that interactions are not one sided, and that the care team, patient, and family all contribute to the work at hand. The art of listening and understanding the other's point of view before decisions are made and plans are developed and acted on is critical. Individuals who are not comfortable with active listening, negotiating, debate, and disagreement, and who cannot manage their personal reactions when faced with difficult situations, are not likely candidates to be case managers.

As presented in Chapter 1, the case manager's role gets redefined and clarified during the redesign of a case management program. Because there are many individuals vying for the role, it is imperative that the individuals selected to fill the role of case managers are individuals who have earned the respect of the medical staff and the care team. Change is difficult, and clinical change that affects patients and practitioners alike appears to carry a higher degree of difficulty. Practitioners are being asked to reevaluate practices that appear to have worked effectively for years. In order to have the kinds of discussions that often surround change in clinical practice, the individual broaching the discussion must be a person who is respected both personally and professionally. If the physicians or other members of the team perceive that their interests, as well as the interests of the patients, are not being considered, the level of cooperation in making the change goes down incrementally. Case managers are asked to confront crises on a daily basis and respond in ways that assure the care team that the situation can be managed. This requires that both the care team and physicians respect the case manager for his or her ability to effect change and trust that the case manager will provide information and alternatives that will meet the needs of all parties involved. Case managers also trust that, given sufficient information, the care team and physicians will respond in a way that achieves the clinical and financial goals needed to obtain desired outcomes.

TO GRANDFATHER OR NOT TO GRANDFATHER

It is important to acknowledge that roles and responsibilities have changed as a result of the redesign process, and that all staff may not want to fulfill, or be capable of fulfilling, the requirements of the newly defined roles. If a redesigned program is going to succeed, it is advisable to have staff reaffirm their interest in the redefined case manager role. This reaffirmation can take a number of different forms.

- Post all redefined positions to include a formal reapplication for the position of choice.
- Interview existing staff, reviewing and agreeing on the redefined roles, performance expectations, and accountabilities.
- Grandfather existing staff into the redefined roles.

Post All Redefined Positions

This is generally the most successful option from a long-range perspective. However, in the short term, this option creates a myriad of challenges that the organization must manage. Generally, staff do not respond favorably to the reapplication process. Most staff members perceive themselves as outstanding performers who should not be required to reapply for positions for which they feel they are qualified. They do not consider that, with the redesign of the case management program, roles, responsibilities, and performance expectations change, and, in fact, they may no longer have the qualifications needed to meet the performance expectations outlined for the new role. Additionally, some staff members are known to have "baggage" in their existing relationships with the medical staff. For this reason, it is essential that the physicians with whom the case managers will be working be involved in the interview process. Some individuals may not be able to overcome the historical relationships and perceptions.

The posting of all newly defined roles provides the staff with a graceful way to transition from positions for which they are no longer qualified, or from relationships where irreparable damage may have occurred. Despite an organization's best intentions, the self-preservation instinct surfaces. Staff members who will be expected to reapply for the redefined positions will often seek affirmation of their value by seeking out colleagues and physicians in the organization who they expect will champion the cause of not requiring the reapplication for positions. This creates a furor of activity and reactions throughout the organization, and many organizations are unwilling or unprepared to address the negative energy this can create among staff and physicians alike.

The downside of not requiring reapplication for redefined positions is that staff members who may be totally unqualified for the positions may be allowed to move into jobs where they cannot be successful, thereby delaying the ability of the organization to realize the clinical and financial goals associated with case management. It also conveys that, despite redesign, it is "business as usual," particularly if some staff members are not viewed positively by the organization. Generally, organizations that have been unwilling to require the reapplication process will also be reluctant to address a staff member's inconsistent or poor performance. In these circumstances, an organization will find itself unable to realize its clinical and financial goals, and will be positioned to have to take another attempt at case management implementation and be vulnerable to criticism from the medical staff concerning the inability of the organization to demonstrate the support and results that were expected.

Interview Existing Staff

This option is the next best option to the reapplication process. During the interview process, leadership in the organization has the opportunity to articulate the responsibilities, accountabilities, and performance expectations associated with the redefined roles. The interview process also affords the current staff members, after having a candid discussion regarding new performance expectations, the opportunity to decline the position, recognizing that their skills may not match well with position requirements. Exhibit 2–1 provides a sample discussion guide that can be used to generate discussions with existing staff around current experience, level of under-

Exhibit 2–1 Sample Discussion Guide for Interviewing Existing Staff

KNOWLEDGE AND EXPERIENCE

1. Criteria
   a. Interqual
   b. Milliman & Robertson
   c. MCAP
   d. Other (explain)
2. Federal and state regulations related to
   a. utilization review requirements
   b. quality assessment requirements
   c. discharge planning requirements
3. Managed care contract agreements related to
   a. utilization review requirements
   b. quality assessment requirements
   c. discharge planning requirements
4. Computer skills
   a. electronic utilization review tools
   b. word processing
   c. other (explain)
5. Describe a formal record review process.
6. Describe the case manager's role in Continuous Quality Improvement.
   a. training
   b. team participation
7. Describe the case manager's role in developing and monitoring clinical/critical pathways.
   a. development participation
   b. variance monitoring
   c. interventional participation
8. Describe the case manager's role in data collection.
   a. indicator monitoring
   b. data collection for outcome analysis
9. Describe the case manager's role in outcome analysis.
10. Describe your own case management experience.
11. Describe your own discharge planning experience.
    a. patient "needs assessment"
    b. levels of care
    c. community resources
    d. alternative care facilities
12. Describe your clinical experience and clinical skill set.
13. Additional comments

COMMUNICATION AND INTERPERSONAL SKILLS/ EXPERIENCE

1. Negotiation
2. Teaming
3. Managing conflict
4. Listens/understands and responds appropriately
5. Alters communication style based on "range" of people
6. Oral communication—clear/concise
7. Conversations/working relationship with payers? Can we reference them to assess your interpersonal communication skills?
8. Additional comments

LEADERSHIP POTENTIAL

1. Confidence
2. Motivated/inspired
3. Proactive
4. Assertive versus aggressive
5. Accountable
6. Problem solving
7. Goal oriented
8. Organization
9. Additional comments

continues

Exhibit 2–1 continued

COMMENTS

Highly Recommended: ______________________________

Recommend: ______________________________

Marginal: ______________________________

Do Not Recommend: ______________________________

Interviewer's Signature ______________________________ Date ______________

CASE MANAGEMENT INTERVIEW QUESTIONS (existing staff)

1. Explain the role of case manager, as you understand it.
2. Outline strengths you would bring to the program.
3. Describe the types of situations that are the most satisfying/rewarding for you.
4. Please provide an example of a situation that required less than straightforward problem solving. Explain the type of innovative/creative solution that you brought forward.
5. Outline those areas where you see you have opportunities for growth.
6. What types of situations are the most frustrating and stressful for you?
7. Describe one of those frustrating and/or stressful situations and how you went about dealing with it to reach conclusion/resolution.
8. Explain why you feel you are uniquely qualified to join the program.
9. Outline the depth of your experience/exposure related to discharge planning (i.e., LOC, community resources, managing care to facilitate patient discharge).
10. Describe the role of the case manager in quality measurement and monitoring (critical paths, data collection, analysis).
11. Describe your ideal third-party payer relationship (i.e., criteria sets, negotiation, communication).
12. Describe where you have your greatest clinical experience/expertise.
13. Why do you think you are qualified for this position?
14. What do you perceive will be your greatest challenge in the newly defined role?
15. Describe your dependability/attendance record.

standing of newly defined positions, and readiness/preparedness of staff to fill the position.

Prior to moving existing staff into the newly defined role, it is essential that the organization clearly outline whether a formal evaluation period will begin at the time of transition into the new role. It is highly advisable to put a formal 90-day evaluation period into place, just as one would do with any new hire, to begin on the first day of transition into the new role. The evaluation period provides some much needed time to determine that, in fact, the staff member has been successful in transitioning to the new role, or it provides the opportunity for a graceful transition to another role if the staff member is unable to meet performance expectations. Once the interview process has taken place, and interviewer and interviewee agree to proceed with transition to the newly defined role, the staff member should be provided with regular feedback at 30-day intervals regarding his or her performance.

Grandfather Existing Staff

This is the least desirable of the three options mentioned above. The downside of grandfathering staff into redefined positions is that staff members who may be totally unqualified for the positions may be moved into jobs where they may not be successful. Grandfathering staff conveys to the entire organization that, despite redesign, it is "business as usual." The "business as usual" mentality can create conflicting messages to the medical staff when, on the one hand, the organization openly states that "things will be different," and on the other hand, there is no change in personnel or the approaches to overall patient management. From the staff perspective, grandfathering can make transition to a newly defined model easy. From an organizational perspective, there are inherent risks, not the least of which is the organization's inability to realize targeted clinical and financial outcomes. Generally, organizations that have been unwilling to require the reapplication process will also be reluctant to address a staff member's inconsistent or poor performance. In these circumstances, an organization may find itself unable to realize its clinical and financial goals, will not be positioned for another attempt at case management implementation for at least a two- to three-year period of time, and will be vulnerable to criticism from the medical staff regarding the inability of the organization to demonstrate the support and results that were expected.

STAFF QUALIFICATIONS AND CREDENTIALS

The appendix for Chapter 1 provides sample job descriptions and, in each job description, the academic and clinical experience required for each job. The academic requirements and clinical experience requirements are both areas of significant debate and discussion in any organization. There are numerous things to consider, not the least of which is the availability of a sufficient number of credentialed individuals who meet position requirements. The first discussion in many organizations focuses around the academic preparation required to fulfill the requirements of the position. We go back again to the discussion in Chapter 1 around the need to have form follow function. Before academic credentials can be determined, roles and responsibilities must be clearly defined. In general, the minimum credential for a case manager's position is licensure as a registered nurse. Ideally, the candidate will be at least a bachelor's-prepared nurse who demonstrates an understanding and willingness to facilitate care, as well as to complete the requirements associated with UM. The number of bachelor's-prepared nurses available, however, disadvantages some areas of the country. In the absence of sufficient numbers of bachelor's-prepared nurses, an organization must be prepared to define the minimum qualifications required to fill case manager positions. The qualifications should include a minimum of five years of clinical experience and ability of the candidate to obtain certification as a case manager within a period of time specified by the organization.

It is imperative that no matter what credentials a case manager possesses, a comprehensive education program, geared specifically to preparing case managers to assume their new roles, should be provided prior to program implementation. Although this may seem redundant based on the educational preparation of the staff, transition into a newly designed, comprehensive case manager role is not something that is inherent in the makeup of the staff. When a staff member has a patient who is a health care provider, we remind the member to assume that the patient knows nothing, forget that the patient is a provider of care, and initiate a patient education program as with any other patient. This same basic principle applies to staff entering into new positions: Assume that they possess only basic knowledge, forget that they may be bachelor's- or master's-prepared individuals, and initiate a training program as with any new employee who is assuming the role of case manager for the first time.

It is advisable to have the case managers who will assume the newly defined positions take an initial competency evaluation exam prior to training, being certain to reassure staff that the competency exam is really intended to define the core knowledge that each of them possesses. Defining the core knowledge base will in turn help define the curriculum that needs to be provided to the staff prior to program implementation. Following education, you should repeat the competency evaluation to determine if any of the staff have remedial training requirements that will need to be addressed if they are to be successful. This baseline competency evaluation also serves to meet the Joint Commission on Accreditation of Healthcare Organizations competency requirements for staff. Exhibit 2–2 represents a sample curriculum based on competency evaluations done with the staff at Memorial Hermann Healthcare System.

One-time education is not sufficient, and plans should be put in place to provide ongoing education. It is most effective to attach continuing education credits to the ongoing education programs, particularly in those states where con-

Exhibit 2–2 Memorial Hermann Healthcare System Care Management Curriculum

Module 1:	Introduction to Care Management Education
Module 2:	Introduction to MHHS Care Management
Module 3:	Care Management Processes
Module 4:	The Changing Health Care Industry
Module 5:	Managed Care/Balancing and Managing Risks and Incentives
Module 6:	Introduction to Medicare, Medicaid, and the Balanced Budget Act
Module 7:	Utilization Management: A New Perspective
Module 8:	Interqual Criteria: An Overview
Module 9:	Interqual Criteria: Application Exercise
Module 10:	Case Management Integration with HealthNet Providers
Module 11:	Transition/Discharge Planning
Module 12:	Case Management Interface with Diagnosis-Related Groups/Pathways/Addressing the Target Length of Stay
Module 13:	Utilization of Postacute Services/Balanced Budget Act Implications
Module 14:	Care Management Processes: A Day in the Life of a Case Manager
Module 15:	Case Manager Interface with Nursing
Module 16:	Role of the Case Manager and the Care Management Medical Director
Module 17:	Negotiation and Conflict Management Skills
Module 18:	Documentation and Coding: Your Role as a Case Manager
Module 19:	Measures of Success: Data Collection and Outcomes Management
Module 20:	Managing Observation Status
Module 21:	Patient Rights, Organization, and Ethics/Legal Issues

tinuing education units are mandatory for licensure renewal.

PERFORMANCE EVALUATION

It is imperative that during the start-up of operations, performance evaluations be completed on the staff no less than once every 60 days. When organizations invest in the development of case management programs, they anticipate that they will see a return on their investment. Performance evaluations should be based not only on individual ability to perform the basic requirements of the job, but also on key indicators that directly reflect organizational performance. Some of these measures include

- length of stay/case mix index
- cost per case
- patient satisfaction
- physician satisfaction
- readmission rates within 31 days for the same diagnosis
- denials received
- successful appeals

If the case managers are working with their team, and in particular, with the medical staff, the organization should see positive results from their efforts. Organizations have high expectations of case management programs, and it is imperative that they invest in the selection and education of the best people for the position.

REFERENCE

1. S. Powell, *Nursing Case Management: A Practical Guide to Success in Managed Care* (Philadelphia: Lippincott Williams & Wilkins, 2000).

Part II

Guide to Utilization Management

CHAPTER 3

What Every Case Manager Should Know about Managed Care

Leslie A. McGregor

TAKE THIS TO WORK

1. In general, health maintenance organizations are losing market presence and preferred provider organizations are on a rapid rise.
2. Success with payers begins with optimal timing of discharge planning
   - before an elective admission
   - in the emergency department
   - on the first day of admission
3. Establishing and maintaining good relationships with payers can enhance the effectiveness of the case manager as a care coordinator, with emphasis on understanding payer criteria.
4. Consider including the payer case manager in the interdisciplinary team conference for the patient as a reference for available providers/services or as an intermediary to the medical director when options alternative to plan benefits might be offered.
5. The case manager can promote patient compliance by ensuring that referrals are made to the patient's in-network providers for postacute services and by identifying the patient's financial contribution up front.
6. As a hospital renegotiates its managed care contracts, its role as participating provider for many patients may also change. Ensure that a process is established to notify the case manager as changes in participation with managed care plans change.

THE RULES OF THE GAME

Case managers who approach managed care as the enemy will live in a battle zone. Instead, they should think of managed care as a game. All games have rules (e.g., the number of players, places to land on the game board, and items to acquire in order to reach the finish point). The health care game is not very different, but keeping abreast of the rules can be more complex. The rules change frequently, and at times, discretely. Game rules include terminology, the players, the order in which activities must be carried out, and coverage requirements.

Terminology

- *Risk*—the chance of losing money for the health care service.

- *Copayment*—the established fee the managed care member pays for a service received. This occurs most in health maintenance organizations (HMOs), with the member paying $5 to $20 each visit.
- *Coinsurance*—the percentage or dollar amount of the provider fee that the member pays for a service rendered. This occurs most commonly in preferred provider organizations (PPOs), with the health plan paying 80 percent and the member paying 20 percent.
- *Deductible*—the dollar portion the patient pays for services received yearly. This amount is capped. Once the member has paid the cap amount, the deductible has been met and the member pays a lesser amount for each service received. The deductible amount is generally inversely proportional to the amount of the established monthly premium. That is, as the monthly premium is reduced, the deductible generally increases.
- *Coverage or benefits*—those health care services that are paid for, fully or partially, by the payer.
- *In-network*—the providers, hospitals, physicians, or agencies that have accepted the payer's predetermined financial arrangement. These are the providers from which the members select to receive their health care services. Generally, in-network providers are listed in a health plan's directory, which is provided to the members and providers for reference.
- *Out-of-network*—providers who have not accepted the payer's predetermined financial arrangement and are not available for member selection. If a member selects an out-of-network provider, the consequences may include the member assuming financial responsibility for the service or the out-of-network provider receiving no payment for services provided.
- *Referral*—the permission and the document a member receives from the primary care provider (PCP) to obtain services from a specialist for specific service(s) (e.g., orthopedic surgeon for an evaluation or radiology center for a mammogram). Generally, referrals have either or both time limits for use and number of visits authorized. Some referrals are so restrictive that only listed tests or procedures can be carried out without financial penalty to the specialist or the member.
- *Per member per month (PMPM)*—the monthly stipend the provider receives under contract with the HMO in return for providing services to a set group of members.
- *Elective*—services that have no time urgency and could be optional. Some examples include tonsillectomy, breast reduction surgery, and bunion surgery.
- *Urgent*—services that must be carried out, but not immediately. Examples include closed reduction of a fracture or admission for simple pneumonia.
- *Emergent*—services that must be carried out immediately, where life or limb is at risk. Examples include compound fracture, major trauma, and status asthmaticus.
- *Precertification*—the member's permission to have a specific test or procedure, generally elective or urgent. This varies from a referral in that the payer is granting permission and not just the PCP. Additionally, these tests/procedures are more costly than a specialist visit and frequently include procedures such as magnetic resonance images, elective surgeries, or long-term therapies. A payer's list of tests/procedures requiring precertification is frequently updated yearly and is available to providers on request. The payer frequently requires receipt of clinical information prior to granting a precertification number for the test/procedure. This precertification number is crucial for reimbursement and is documented on the claim that is submitted to the payer for payment.

Types of Managed Care

There are three basic types of managed care that are differentiated from each other by the identity of the risk holder and the degree of choice given to the members (patients) of the plan. Before addressing these three types of managed care, let's review an important type of insurance that is not considered managed care—indemnity insurance.

Indemnity is that type of insurance for which the provider, that is, a hospital or physician, has no risk. The payer holds the risk and the member, or patient, has the greatest degree of choice. The patient chooses the provider and when to seek health care services, with no permission required from a PCP. The physician or hospital receives a usual and customary (UCR) payment for health care services provided.

Following are the three primary types of managed care plans for which there is reduced member choice and shared or shifted risk:

1. *PPO* is a plan wherein the provider holds some financial risk, generally in the form of predetermined, reduced fees. For example, the physician may charge $100 for the service but agree in advance to accept $80 or 80 percent of the UCR. The patient's choice is limited to the health plan's participating providers—those providers who agreed to accept the reduced fees in return for listing in the health plan provider directory as a preferred provider. The patient has no requirement for advance permission to seek services in a PPO. Impetus for a provider to accept this contract of reduced fees is the increased volume of patients entering the practice for treatment.
2. *HMO* is a plan wherein the provider holds the greatest degree of risk and the member or patient has the least degree of choice. Under this arrangement, the PCP agrees to provide all specified services for the member or patient in return for a fixed dollar payment. A PCP in an HMO receives a monthly fee (PMPM) based on the member's age and sex, no matter how frequently the patient uses health care services. If the patient never uses health care services, the PCP makes a profit. The financial risk to the PCP arises in that the patient may use more health care services than the PCP has been reimbursed. Additionally, a PCP may be financially responsible for a member's use of health care services outside of the provider's own. Thus, the plan requires the member to seek approval (referral) from the PCP in advance for specialty services such as surgery, radiology, and physical therapy. The PCP seeks to restrict health care services used by the member to those services that the PCP deems to be medically necessary. In return for this limited choice, the member is required to pay a small fee or copay for health care services received.
3. *Point of service (POS)* is a plan wherein the member has a blended health plan, sort of a combined PPO and HMO. If the member obtains a referral for services and obtains those services from a participating provider, the financial burden is the lowest copay, as in the HMO. If the member does not obtain a referral from the PCP, the financial burden is a fixed portion of the health care service fee, as in the PPO. The provider is paid according to his or her contract with the payer, as a provider in the PPO or HMO.

Players

- *Subscriber*—the person who purchases the health insurance and receives the health insurance benefits. There may be only one subscriber, but there may be several other people receiving health insurance benefits, called members.
- *Member*—a person who receives health insurance benefits from a health plan.
- *Provider*—the person or organization that delivers the health care services (e.g., physician, hospital).
- *Payer*—the health insurance company that pays for the services provided.

USING THE RULES TO FACILITATE PATIENT CARE

All planned health care services are determined base on the patient's identified needs. As case manager, the objective is to facilitate these health care services for the patient within the guidelines provided by the managed care organization (MCO). As a hospital case manager, the patient's health coverage and the facility's relationship with that payer determine which rules apply. The network or directory of preferred providers will vary according to the patient's plan. Rules include

- determining services the patient requires
- applying case manager's clinical expertise in conjunction with severity of illness/intensity of service criteria to determine the appropriateness of the service to be provided
- ensuring that the services to be provided meet the payer's criteria for medical necessity
- carrying out actions in a prescribed sequence
- ensuring that the patient's health plan covers the services to be rendered
- obtaining advance permission or authorization prior to carrying out certain services and developing an alternate plan if coverage/permission is not obtained

Sequencing—Order in Which Activities Are Carried Out

For the provider, success is measured by optimal patient outcome combined with full reimbursement for services rendered. For the patient and employer, success is prompt receipt of entitled health care services with no additional financial burden. And for the payer, satisfied employers, frequently the purchasers of health care insurance, indicate success. As in many games, correct sequencing is key to success at the finish line. For the provider to receive payment and the patient to avoid additional financial burden, actions must take place in a specific order. And, documentation must be available to support actions taken.

Data Collection

Correct sequencing requires accurate knowledge of the patient's health insurance; communication with the patient, provider(s), and payer; as well as current knowledge of the payer's requirements as they relate to the patient's diagnosis. For this discussion, the role of the hospital case manager is used, as it is within this arena that all the complexities come into play—multiple players, changing patient conditions, life and death, and related emotions.

The hospital entry point (emergency department [ED], admitting department, registration, and outpatient procedure area) is instrumental, as it is here that information is collected regarding the patient's demographics and insurance requirements. If at any point during the patient stay and during the reimbursement process, information is found to be inaccurate or incomplete, the case manager must seek immediate evaluation of the processes for data collection and documentation. Vital information collected at the entry point includes patient name, birth date, Social Security number, payer name, member number, subscriber name, PCP, admitting physician, and reason for seeking services. With this information, the facility is able to optimize the specifics of the patient's health coverage and benefits.

Verification of Eligibility

Using the information collected, staff in each hospital or provider agency verify the patient's insurance and eligibility to date. For example, a patient may indeed have XXX health insurance, but may not have coverage for psychiatric services. A patient may have an insurance card indicating coverage, but no longer be eligible for that insurance based on a change of employment. Investigation from the payer may reveal that the facility is not considered in-network for this patient, thus requiring transfer of the stable patient to an in-network provider prior to treatment in order to avoid denied payment.

The hospital entry may be emergent admission through the ED, urgent admission through the admissions department, or elective entry through the registration department. Note that elective treatment can be carried out as an inpatient or an outpatient. The sequencing rules vary depending on the level of urgency for services. Truly emergent conditions mandate medical stabilization, assessment, and initiation of treatment prior to payer concern. Clerical staff simultaneously collect data from family members or identification cards. Urgent medical conditions should provide time for verification of insurance coverage and patient eligibility prior to treatment. Elective treatment should never be carried out without meeting eligibility checks, as well as validating that precertification requirements have been met. Depending on the payer and contract, if the precertification requirements have not been met prior to rendering of services, reimbursement will be delayed or voided. In addition, the patient may be forced to assume financial responsibility for the procedure.

Most facilities provide a mechanism to easily validate that precertification requirements have been met. This often involves a field in the information system where the payer's precertification number is recorded along with the name and telephone number of the person from the payer or physician office that provided the information. Many providers extend documentation to include the statement and name of the payer representative advising that precertification is not required for a service in order to support provider appeal of denial based on lack of precertification. Pre-admitting case managers verify supportive documentation and ensure precertification has been obtained as required. It is wise to ensure that your resources include regularly updated precertification lists from payers. This payer compliance function may well be relegated to a resource center, freeing the case manager to attend to purely clinical disposition.

Coverage Requirements—Payer Criteria for Medical Necessity

There is an additional step that should take place for effective provider reimbursement and patient avoidance of financial burden with most managed care payers. Many payers have specific criteria developed indicating the presence of medical necessity for services to be provided. That is, the services to be provided are deemed by the payer to be necessary based on the patient's clinical presentation and history. When payers do not provide their own medical necessity guidelines, many facilities purchase or license criteria to ensure that the services to be provided are clinically supported for reimbursement. Use of medical necessity criteria is particularly applicable for urgent conditions, as elective conditions generally have been precertified and emergent conditions are supported by the risk to patient life or limb.

The process of applying criteria for medical necessity is discussed in more detail in Chapter 6. The key take away for the case manager at patient entry is the negative impact on reimbursement and patient financial burden when patient clinical presentation does not meet medical necessity criteria. If the condition is not emergent, ensuring the presence of medical necessity for inpatient treatment on entry will generally support appropriate reimbursement. Many facilities include the role of admitting case manager to collaborate with the physician at entry to ensure that patient medical necessity is present and that treatment is delivered at the appropriate level of care. In the absence of this role, the burden falls on the inpatient or acute case manager to validate appropriateness of the patient's level of care/status.

When the patient's documented clinical information and treatment plan do not meet payer medical necessity criteria for inpatient treatment, the case manager's knowledge of available services in the outpatient setting and patient health benefits enables an alternate plan of care to be developed. Here is an opportunity for direct communication with the payer to identify patient benefits that offer treatment options. Communication of available provider options and patient benefits to the physician is key to obtaining physician buy-in for an alternate treatment plan. Frequently, it is not possible to know all in-network options, but it is necessary to know where and how to identify options available to each patient. Again, case managers rely on accurate patient entry data and access to payer provider network directories to develop any plan of care.

Say, for example, that the patient is sent from the physician's office with orders for direct admission for pneumonia. However, a review of the patient's health coverage and available clinical information indicates that medical necessity criteria are not met for inpatient treatment. Further, discussion with the physician does not reveal additional data to support inpatient treatment. Admitting the patient for treatment, then, will most likely generate a denial for the inpatient stay and lost reimbursement for the hospital or patient financial responsibility for the inpatient stay.

In this instance, the case manager should contact the payer directly to discuss potential treatment options based on the patient's benefits and the payer's network of providers. The outcome may include managing the patient as an outpatient to initiate antibiotics and respiratory therapy, with discharge to home health services later in the day. Upon discussion, the payer may actually consider authorizing a one-day admission, followed by discharge to home health services. Initiating a collaborative relationship with the payer can result in more favorable options for the patient. Additionally, validating eligible home health benefits in advance of proposing the alternate plan to the physician supports the case manager's recommendation against a potentially denied inpatient stay. Ultimately, the decision to admit or not admit and the treatment plan are the physician's. However, experienced case managers describe agreement by physicians for alternate treatment plans increases as the relationship between the physician and case manager matures.

The benefits of ensuring accurate, complete patient data and evaluating medical necessity criteria prior to admission are a reduction of financial burden postdischarge, improved patient care coordination, and improved satisfaction. The outcome of validating home health coverage to meet the patient's postacute needs is a well-coordinated discharge plan and, more importantly, coordination of patient care without gaps in service. The patient benefits because there are no surprise financial charges and treatment is coordinated without gaps due to lack of coverage. Success is achieved because the steps were carried out in the appropriate sequence.

DISCHARGE PLANNING UPON ADMISSION

Because most payers in managed care require patients to meet criteria for medical necessity throughout the inpatient stay, the length of the acute care stay has decreased dramatically over the past 5 to 10 years. As the length of stay (LOS) decreases, the time available to arrange postacute services also diminishes. Managed care payers require that postacute services be provided by in-network providers. Sequencing includes the identification and selection of the postacute provider followed by arrangements for services to be delivered. Achieving the objective of discharging the patient to the postacute provider requires coordination and planning. Permission from the payer is frequently required prior to arranging these services. This permission may include a restricted number of postacute visits (e.g., home health visits) and type of service provided (e.g., registered nurse medication administration vs. patient instruction for self-administration of medications). Postacute care facilitation requires early understanding of the patient's postacute needs and health care benefits, knowledge of the payer's and provider's requirements, and communication with the patient, physician, payer, and postacute provider regarding the plan of care.

Most postacute providers initiate their own sequencing and verification processes to ensure their reimbursement once the patient is discharged or transferred to their care. Because many providers and payers are not fully operational on weekends or holidays, the importance of early planning cannot be overemphasized. If the patient cannot be discharged over a weekend, the inpatient facility can be burdened with several days deemed not medically necessary by the payer, waiting for placement into postacute services. Most days not meeting the payer's medical necessity criteria are not reimbursed.

Throughout this process, collaboration with the physician, the patient, and the family is required. The case manager alone cannot discharge the patient to home health or a skilled nursing facility (SNF). There must be initial and ongoing communication with the physician and patient regarding the target LOS, medical necessity criteria met, payer requirements, and plan of care to meet the patient's needs. The case manager can effectively communicate eligible treatment options under the patient's health plan to ensure that patient benefits are maximized. Many patients are not fully aware of their health care benefits or copays and deductibles. Communication of these costs may impact patient decisions regarding postacute options. Indeed, offering selections from the patient's in-network directory of home health providers will be key to successful arrangements and patient adherence to the discharge plan.

HEALTH CARE TEAM CONFERENCES

Health care team conferences can be effective in facilitating care coordination, particularly with more complex patient care needs or multiple physicians treating the patient. These conferences present the case manager with a unique opportunity to offer treatment options, inpatient and postacute, that are available to the patient based on covered benefits. The interdisciplinary approach offers the ability to determine the optimal treatment plan that meets payer requirements along the continuum. Including the payer in the interdisciplinary team conference can be an effective technique for discharge planning to receive immediate payer feedback on options discussed and receive required authorization for inpatient or postacute services.

Based on the number of people involved in a team conference, convening a conference on the day of discharge cannot be considered an effective tool. Initial patient assessment of complex discharge needs, multiple consulting physicians, or a changing patient condition offers the opportunity for effective use of an interdisciplinary team conference at early points in the admission. As the point person, the case manager facilitates the scheduling of key health care team members and the availability of information considered essential to development of a complete plan of care/discharge plan. The requirement for convening all necessary players at the same time begs for early planning. Ultimately, the effort spent on team conferences can be less than that spent by the case manager tracking down each physician for contribution to the plan.

ENSURING THAT COVERAGE REQUIREMENTS ARE MET

Certainly the game would be simpler if there were one point at which the case manager knew the payer's requirements had been met. Instead, this is an ongoing process; it occurs at multiple decision points during the hospital stay to ensure that patient benefits will be maximized and the hospital will be reimbursed fully.

INPATIENT DECISION POINTS

Most services provided during an inpatient stay are bundled, or included into the set fee that is contracted between the payer and the provider. Therefore, the hospital is usually not dependent on the payer for permission for individual tests, treatments, or procedures. These are the decision of the physician. In order for the hospital to avoid providing services that cost more than the reimbursement that is received, resources must be managed wisely.

The case manager plays a pivotal role during the inpatient stay, balancing the patient's needs, the facility's resources, and the physician's treatment plan in alignment with the reimbursement the facility will receive. The case manager is uniquely positioned to use clinical expertise along with payer knowledge to facilitate necessary patient care that ultimately ensures that the patient and the hospital are successful. Many facilities use objective criteria, such as InterQual Criteria or Milliman & Robertson guidelines to support recommendations for care. Questions must be raised regarding not only level of care, but also choice of medications and frequency of interventions. The case manager must be able to participate in evaluating whether the service is duplicative or necessary, or whether the $200 antibiotic is more efficacious than the $50 antibiotic. It is the case manager's job to ensure that the hospital provides necessary care while using clinical resources wisely. This requires knowledge related to leading practices of treatment as well as costs of care delivery.

Under a managed care contract, a provider is reimbursed a set dollar amount for services provided. Therefore, patient care decisions must be based on necessity and need in order to avoid either over- or underutilization of clinical resources. It is unacceptable to limit treatment or services to a patient who requires those services based on cost or reimbursement to the provider. For example, when critical care services are necessary to meet the patient's care needs, it is unacceptable to maintain a patient on a medical–surgical unit based on the cost of critical care services. However, managed care forces us to evaluate for all patients which services are required by every patient. Managed care contracts have forced hospitals to establish clear criteria for utilization of services such as critical care beds, specialty beds, high-cost medications, or the number of physical therapy visits.

CHANGING RULES

Most commonly, MCOs issue changes effective the first of the year. However, the case manager must ensure access to current payer bulletins on an ongoing basis. The most common information to change will be providers included in the payer's network and the patients' health insurance plan, including copayments, coinsurance, and deductibles. Additionally, as a case manager for a hospital or other provider, changes in reimbursement amount and processes may change on the anniversary of the payer/provider contract. It behooves the case manager, especially for a small provider, to maintain a record of these contract dates as an alert.

Most patients are unaware of their coverage limitations, making learning this information particularly key for the case manager.

What if You Did Not Follow a Rule?

Occasions will occur when you were provided with incorrect information or a time frame passed for reporting an admission to the payer. The best approach is to be straightforward and acknowledge the error to the payer. Deceit never pays here. Telephone the payer contact immediately with the correct information and the circumstances surrounding the error. Inquire what the next steps should be and document the communication, information relayed, contact name, and payer response, as well as date and time. Include in your documentation the explanation of the error for future reference. Financial penalties may be assigned, but many times they can be averted through immediate reporting. Many hospitals establish a process for internal reporting of errors. This may indeed be helpful to track a pattern of preventable errors.

WHAT MANAGED CARE HAS PROVIDED FOR US

Because of the financial constraints supplied by managed care, managed care has prompted health care restrictions. Contrary to popular belief, managed care has not stated that the physician or hospital cannot provide a service. Neither has it stated the patient cannot have surgery. It has, however, refused to pay for those services provided outside of the agreed-on guidelines. This is not a popular concept. What is really at issue is that the American consumer is not accustomed to any restrictions on health care choices. Within managed care, to receive full reimbursement or prevent additional financial penalty, care must be provided according to restrictive guidelines.

Managed care has prompted providers to evaluate patient information and condition prior to rendering services. As a result of sagging bottom lines, hospitals are reviewing and enforcing objective criteria for patient placement in critical areas or utilization of high-cost medications. Managed care has restricted the indiscriminate use of health care resources and prompted systematic approaches to decision making.

SUGGESTED READINGS

R. Herzlinger, *Market Driven Health Care* (Reading, MA: Addison-Wesley Publishing Co., Inc., 1997).

P. Kongstvedt, *Essentials of Managed Health Care* (Gaithersburg, MD: Aspen Publishers, Inc., 1997).

P. Kongstvedt and D. Plocher, *Best Practices in Medical Management* (Gaithersburg, MD: Aspen Publishers, Inc., 1998).

CHAPTER 4

Understanding Utilization Management

Cindy J. Urbancic and Leslie A. McGregor

TAKE THIS TO WORK

1. Utilization management is an ongoing, proactive process that serves to ensure that the patient receives the care that is necessary.
2. The patient is a key member of the health care team and must be involved in the care coordination process.
3. Collaborating with the physician regarding the target length of stay works toward developing a collegial relationship between the physician and the case manager.
4. Communicating the target discharge date upon admission provides the patient/family an opportunity to prepare for discharge.
5. Conducting the clinical review process enables the case manager to learn the patient's progress in the plan of care and identify barriers and variances that must be addressed.
6. The use of a tool, such as InterQual, provides the case manager with objective criteria for medical necessity against which the patient's status can be measured.

In the utilization management (UM) function, perhaps more than in any other aspect of the case management role, the case manager is challenged to reconcile the potentially conflicting interests of health care technology, patient and family expectations, physician practice patterns, and resource constraints. The capacity to function as an advocate for both patient and organizational interests while working collaboratively with physicians is one of the most distinctive competencies for success in managing patient care.

UM is the process involving the application of tools and techniques to identify and anticipate patient needs and to support proactive coordination and management of clinical resources to meet those needs. The misperception persists in some organizations that UM is focused solely on cost management and the restriction of payment for health care services. In reality, the UM process serves the interests of patients by identifying all reimbursement options and working to optimize these resources with the objective of achieving optimal health status outcomes. This chapter will define key terms related to UM, discuss essential UM processes, and identify the tools and interactions that enable the case manager to perform and document effective UM.

UTILIZATION REVIEW VERSUS UM

Prior to the widespread market penetration of managed care plans, most acute care hospitals in the United States identified utilization review (UR) as the primary point of contact with third-party payers (at that time, almost exclusively government payers and indemnity plans). In contrast to the definition of UM proposed in the introduction to this chapter, UR was most often a reactive, rather than proactive, process that had the objective of justifying the patient's hospital stay and level of care. There was often little physician participation in the UR process, and most routine UR activities were based on the documentation in the clinical record rather than on a comprehensive view of the patient's clinical needs and available treatment options. UR was typically performed in isolation from care facilitation and discharge planning (often retrospectively) and was fundamentally separate from the plan of care.

Retrospective UR, frequently performed in isolation from care facilitation, contributed to an adversarial climate between providers and patients when payers issued denials for services that had been provided in good faith and that patients and their families had believed would be covered. These conflicts were often compounded by the common practice of balance billing patients for denied balances, sometimes in violation of the provider's contractual arrangements with payers. The fundamental dilemma inherent in traditional UR arises at least partially from the fact that although services are ordered by physicians, the risk of payment denial and lost revenue remains with the hospital.

Based on these limitations, and in order to meet the changing needs in a managed care environment, traditional UR has largely been replaced by a focus on UM. Effective UM processes seek not simply to justify resource utilization, but rather to assess patients' clinical needs, evaluate available payment options, and plan proactively within the parameters of reimbursement possibilities. UM has the objective of meeting the patient's treatment needs while minimizing the provider's risk of exposure to unreimbursed services. Exhibit 4–1 summarizes the key distinctions between traditional UR and the modern concept of UM.

THE ROLE OF STANDARDS AND CLINICAL CRITERIA IN UM

In order to objectively assess patients' clinical treatment needs and evaluate the necessity of various treatment alternatives, external standards must be applied that can serve to support decisions made. Although some variability per-

Exhibit 4–1 Utilization Management versus Utilization Review

Utilization Management	Utilization Review
• Process designed to monitor, evaluate, and control resource use to a level that is optimal for a given event or situation • Activities incorporate and integrate several mechanisms, including referral policies and authorization; prospective and concurrent review of service use; case management; and discharge planning	• Formal review of patient utilization or of the necessity of health care services • Entirely retrospective • Compliance-focused • Oriented toward justifying need for services provided

sists among payers with respect to the criteria sets selected for this purpose, at least two specific criteria sets are used nationwide by large payers and are commonly regarded as industry standard for use by the case manager in performing UM activities: the InterQual criteria set and the Milliman & Robertson (M&R) *Health Management Guidelines*.

Both InterQual and M&R are proprietary licensed products and essential tools for performing effective UM; there is no substitute for proficiency in using these tools and documenting observations and findings in a clear and concise format. However, it must be noted that published clinical criteria must be employed in combination with, not as a substitute for, the clinical expertise and judgment of the case manager.

InterQual Criteria

InterQual is a set of objective, measurable criteria organized to assist in determining the necessity of health care services. InterQual provides diagnostic and therapeutic indicators that reflect patient need for hospitalization, indicators for specialized levels of care, medical necessity for continued stay, readiness for discharge, and parameters for transfer from the hospital to postacute venues of care. Consistent use of the InterQual criteria enables the case manager to identify and document clinical support for level-of-care decisions and the timing of transfer to more or less acute levels of care within the hospital. These criteria also provide guidance for discharge planning.

Within the InterQual set, clinical criteria are provided that support the use of alternative levels of care, including critical care, intermediate care, observation, general acute care, and alternate care settings. The *critical care* section is further subdivided into criteria for the use of critical care that relates to cardiac, medical, and surgical/trauma diagnoses. Criteria for the *intermediate level of care* are classified into cardiac/telemetry and medical/surgical sections. The necessity of inpatient versus outpatient settings for specific surgical procedures is also specified. The *general acute care* section is subdivided into criteria related to 14 body system categories, including cardiovascular, peripheral vascular, central nervous system, musculoskeletal, and infectious disease.

Each section and subsection of the InterQual acute care criteria set includes severity of illness and intensity of service (SI/IS) indicators and discharge screens with indicators for necessity of clinical services. The concepts of SI/IS must be considered together in determining medical necessity. As suggested in Figure 4–1, severity of illness focuses on the patient's clinical condition, whereas intensity of service reflects interventions provided in response to the patient's needs. The determination of medical necessity must be based on both indicators and must reflect the determination, based on objective criteria, that care is being delivered in the most appropriate venue of care, that is, the setting in which all required clinical services can be provided at the lowest possible cost.

In order to present a complete picture of the patient's clinical needs and response to treatment, the case manager should apply all relevant SI/IS criteria and document all criteria met. Discharge screens serve to identify not only readiness for discharge, but also key milestones in the progress of patients within specific diagnostic categories or patients having similar clinical profiles. A review of discharge screens and key milestones specific to the patient's condition will enable the case manager to identify a patient's lack of progress or failure to respond to treatment as anticipated.

The alternate levels of care section of the InterQual criteria set delineates indicators for placement of patients in each of the alternative postacute venues of care, including skilled nursing facilities, inpatient rehabilitation, and home health. These indicators include the patient's ability to progress toward independence, the potential to tolerate and respond to therapies, and the frequency with which physician assessment is required. By applying these criteria, the case manager can develop a realistic discharge plan early in the patient's hospitalization and update it as condition changes occur.

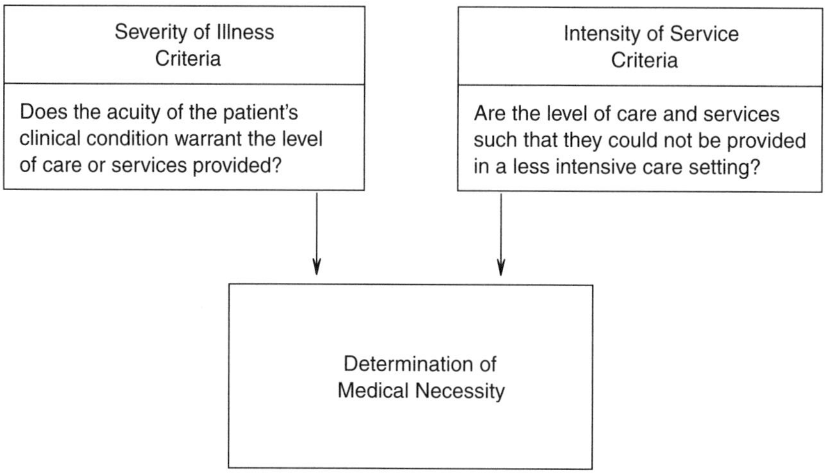

Figure 4–1 Use of Clinical Criteria in Utilization Management

Milliman & Robertson *Health Management Guidelines*

Widely used to determine target length of stay (LOS) specified by diagnosis-related group (DRG), the M&R *Health Management Guidelines* were developed in response to providers' desire to identify levels of performance that could be achieved in managing specific patient populations, benchmark their performance against comparable peer organizations, and initiate performance improvement activities. M&R LOS data were initially compiled in 1984 and have continuously expanded since that time to incorporate the performance of a large cross section of providers nationwide. Ambulatory care data were subsequently included, and the complete data set has been widely adopted as a performance benchmark by hospitals and managed care organizations.

The M&R guidelines are distinct from InterQual criteria; in addition to providing indicators for inpatient treatment and LOS, they can be used as a tool for developing a discharge-oriented plan of care. It should be noted that these guidelines are intended to reflect the management of "normal" patients within each DRG; that is, patients without multiple comorbidities. The M&R guidelines offer criteria and indicators to manage LOS and resource utilization in the form of practice guidelines, interventions, and patient progress milestones for patients within specific DRGs. Like the InterQual criteria, M&R guidelines provide indicators for alternate levels of care.

The M&R guidelines are targeted to specific patient populations, including

- inpatient and surgical care
- recovery facility and home care
- ambulatory care
- return-to-work planning and workers' compensation
- ambulatory surgery guidelines

The inpatient and surgical care guidelines, which will be used most frequently by inpatient case managers, include target LOS, case management guidelines, alternative treatment settings, utilization of inpatient resources by level of managed care control, and surgical guidelines. The guidelines are useful as a reference for developing clinical pathways or patient treatment guidelines to prospectively outline the anticipated course of treatment for a defined patient population.

Perhaps the most common use of the M&R guidelines is for the determination of targeted

LOS for patients within a specific DRG. These targets are differentiated for Medicare and commercial patient populations and are adjusted to reflect low, moderate, or high levels of managed care market penetration. M&R target LOS should be employed as a guideline rather than as an absolute standard for determining the necessity of a specific patient's LOS. DRG classification is by definition broad, and significant variability exists among the clinical needs and treatment response of patients within any given DRG. Moreover, although M&R's targets shorten in more highly managed markets, there are anecdotal reports of LOS rising as aggressive UM has resulted in only the sickest patients getting admitted.

M&R LOS guidelines can be used most productively when a provisional or working DRG is assigned to patients at the time of admission and a discharge plan is developed within the parameters of the target LOS for that DRG, taking into account the patient-specific variables that will inevitably impact the actual LOS. The DRG-specific patient management guidelines can be used as a standard for evaluating the accuracy and completeness of the plan of care, and the patient milestones suggested in the M&R guidelines can be employed to monitor variances in the treatment responses of individual patients. The following scenario illustrates how InterQual and M&R are used together by the case manager—InterQual for targeted SI/IS criteria and M&R for targeted LOS and patient management guidelines.

Case Study

Tom Jones, a 75-year-old, was admitted from the emergency department (ED) to a surgical unit after falling in his home. X-rays completed in the ED confirmed a fractured hip requiring surgical repair. Tom was accompanied by his son Jim, who had discovered his father on the floor at home. Tom has been living alone for the past five years since his wife's death and was unable to reach the telephone to call for assistance. Although he has been independent, he still relies on his son for some basic needs, such as transportation to the grocery store and doctors' appointments.

Tom's medical history is positive for congestive heart failure (CHF) and diet-controlled diabetes, both of which are monitored closely by his physician. Since Tom has been compliant with medications and daily weight, he has not required hospitalization for his CHF for the past three years. However, today Tom is distraught with pain and fear of losing his independence secondary to his fractured hip. His son, while reassuring him, is concerned about his father's safety and ability to continue living alone.

Upon admission to the surgical unit, the case manager reviews Tom's medical record, positive X-ray results, planned surgical intervention, and plan of care. The case manager introduces herself to Tom and Jim, explaining her role as a member of the care team. The case manager specifically focuses on evaluating Tom's level of understanding regarding the surgery and his needs postoperatively, and clarifies his current benefits. She inquires if Tom has used or is currently using any postacute providers, such as home health services, or has required the use of any assistance-related devices, such as a cane or walker. The case manager applies the InterQual criteria to support medical necessity criteria for admission to the acute care setting.

To ensure that Tom's plan of care is complete, the case manager reviews M&R patient care guidelines for surgical repair of a fractured hip and identifies the recommended LOS. Even though Tom has comorbidities of CHF and diabetes, the case manager concurs with the defined targeted Medicare LOS because Tom's diabetes has been well controlled prior to this hospitalization. Tom was able to list all of his medications and stated that his weight and blood sugar had remained stable. Although his comorbidities bear close monitoring, the surgical repair dictates the LOS. Had Tom's CHF or diabetes not been well controlled prior to the fall or during his initial hospital presentation, the case manager would potentially need to modify M&R's suggested LOS. Because Tom lives alone and will require rehabilitation following surgery, the case manager also reviews the suggested indicators for postacute levels of care in the patient care guidelines. She will discuss these options with Tom's son later in the day.

Because Tom's surgery is scheduled for this afternoon, the case manager will conduct the continued stay review the next morning, applying the InterQual criteria. Discharge screens will also be assessed to identify Tom's progress toward discharge criteria.

Although many patients do not fall neatly into categories, this scenario exemplifies the use of both UM tools in concert with the case manager's clinical expertise.

INFRASTRUCTURE ELEMENTS TO SUPPORT UM ACTIVITIES

In addition to the availability of clinical criteria, three additional elements of organizational infrastructure must be in place in order for the UM process to function optimally: UM policies and procedures, the electronic UM worksheet, and the resource center.

UM Policies and Procedures

In the absence of a current and clearly delineated set of policies and operating procedures for UM, it is difficult, if not impossible, to achieve consistent high-quality performance in this key area. Policies are best developed in a consensus environment with the input of the organization's best UM content experts. The process of policy development can be arduous and time consuming, and it may be a wise investment of organizational resources to use a process facilitator in order to expedite policy and procedure development. Once policies and procedures have been established and approved, a fairly high level of accountability may initially be required in achieving consistent adherence to these guidelines. As in the case of all operating procedures, the UM policy and procedure manual should be reviewed at least every six months to ensure that it reflects the way UM processes are actually being performed.

Electronic UM Worksheet

Few organizations find that the use of a manual UM worksheet meets their needs in today's electronic information environment. The handoffs required in order to use manual documentation and the variability it promotes argue strongly in favor of adopting an electronic worksheet for the capture of patient demographics and payer information and the documentation of initial and continuing stay clinical reviews. Additionally, tracking and trending key UM indicators is hampered with the use of the manual UM worksheet. Several high-quality UM software packages are on the market that have interface capabilities with patient management and patient accounting systems, and a number of organizations and provider systems have successfully developed their own approaches to managing the information flow essential for effective UM. In some cases, an approach as simple as shared access to an electronic worksheet in a Lotus Notes environment has proven effective for UM documentation and information transfer.

Regardless of the format selected, the electronic worksheet should provide for the capture of essential demographic and payer information from the patient registration system, as well as documentation of the following information by case managers in the course of the UM process:

- initial application of clinical criteria and determination of medical necessity
- provisional DRG and target LOS
- comorbidities and clinical complications with a potential impact on LOS and resource utilization
- documentation of benefit verification, precertification, and certification for subsequent inpatient days
- continuing stay review information
- communication with the attending physician or physician advisor related to UM issues and concerns

The electronic worksheet should be designed to eliminate as much manual documentation as possible, in the interest of both ease of access and staff time required to complete documentation. *One essential point regarding UM documentation is that it should never, under any circumstances, be entered into or filed with the medical record.*

Resource Center

The final infrastructure element to support UM is the resource center, a centralized point within the organization that is designed to provide clerical and administrative support, facilitate routine payer communication, and assist in managing denials. By using a centralized resource center, the organization is better able to leverage telephone and fax communication to designated staff and devote a higher percentage of the case manager's time and attention to care facilitation, clinical review completion, and interactions with attending physicians and the care team.

The critical success factor in designing and implementing an organizational resource center is ensuring that information can be handed off to resource center staff with minimal effort and complexity, and that their availability to make routine payer contacts is perceived as a benefit, rather than an additional burden, by case managers. Although efficient information transfer can be effected using manual documentation, this process is simplified and expedited through the use of the electronic UM worksheet. For instance, when an electronic worksheet is used for completing initial clinical reviews, these reviews can be accessed by the resource center payer liaison and transmitted directly to the payer by telephone or fax. Only in unusual or marginal cases is interaction between the payer and the inpatient case manager necessary.

THE UM PROCESS IN THE INPATIENT SETTING

By definition, UM spans the continuum of care and includes level-of-care and resource utilization issues in ambulatory and postacute venues of care. However, because the focus of this chapter is on the inpatient case manager's role in UM, the following discussion of UM processes will focus primarily on UM in the acute hospital setting.

In order to achieve the central objective of providing necessary treatment within the constraints of available payment resources, a systematic process must be developed and refined that facilitates the application of criteria at key points throughout a patient's hospitalization, validation of medical necessity for services provided, and documentation and communication of these observations to payers. Collectively, these assessment, interpretation, documentation, and communication activities make up the UM process.

Although this process must be tailored to the specific needs and structure of each organization, the key steps discussed here must be included in the development of any effective inpatient UM process. In addition to optimizing payment and minimizing the organization's risk of revenue loss, a well-designed UM process also provides for compliance with regulatory requirements, minimizes payer-issued denials, and enhances payers' perceptions of the provider's ability to manage patient care. A high-level overview of the inpatient UM process is presented in Figure 4–2.

The foundation for effective UM is established by the processes of benefit verification, notification, and precertification, which are typically performed by preadmission staff in the hospital's patient access area or the ED. The purposes of these activities are to determine the patient's benefit plan and coverage, to notify the payer of the admission, and to obtain initial certification or payment authorization for the services to be provided. Failure to complete these activities will increase the risk of payer-issued administrative and technical denials and compound the effort required for the appeal and reversal of denials. Noncompliance with administrative contract terms, such as that requiring precertification, frequently results in denials that cannot be successfully appealed by the provider and therefore are considered nonrecoverable revenue. Chapter 6 of this book provides an in-depth discussion of the categories of denials and the processes for managing them in order to maximize revenue recovery.

Initial Clinical Review

Initial clinical review is performed at the point of patient entry to the inpatient care setting, most often the patient registration or admitting office or the ED. In many organizations, substantial revenue loss can be averted by designing and

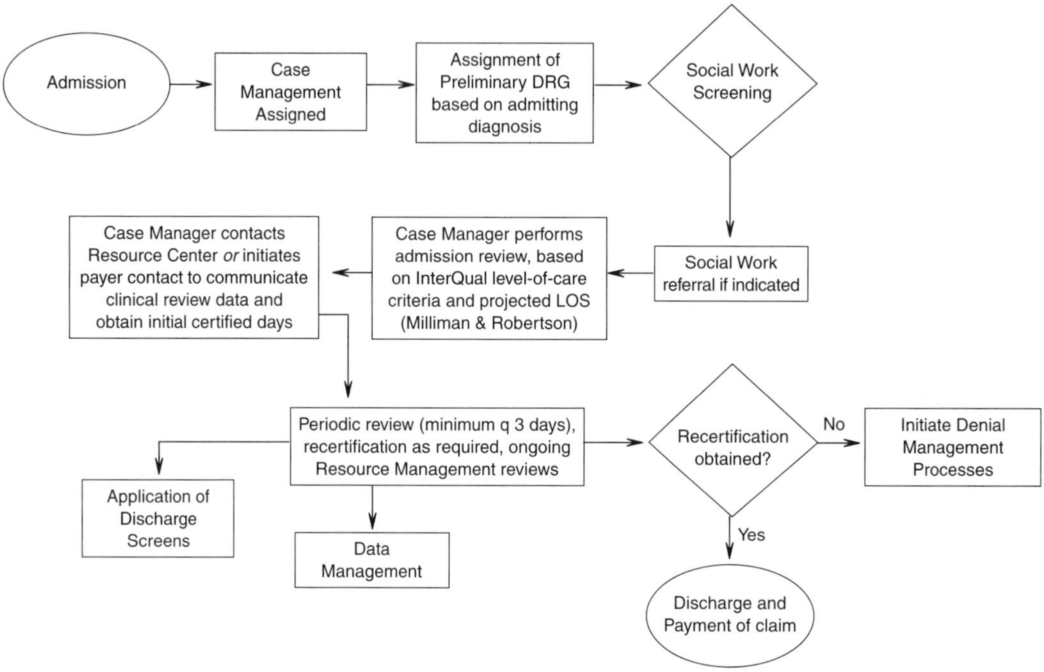

Note: DRG, diagnosis-related group; LOS, length of stay.

Figure 4–2 High-Level View of the Inpatient Utilization Management Process

implementing a structure that provides for the application of clinical necessity criteria for services at the point of entry. By assessing the patient's presenting problem, applying clinical criteria for the level of care or services ordered, and assigning a provisional DRG, the case manager can estimate a target LOS, communicate this to the admitting physician, and initiate the discharge planning process promptly. Target LOS and discharge planning needs must be adjusted to reflect patient variables, such as general state of health, comorbidities, and family or social support resources. The initial clinical review serves to answer three key questions:

1. Is the level of care or service ordered essential for the clinical needs documented?
2. What is the typical LOS for patients with similar clinical profiles?
3. What are the patient's anticipated discharge needs and what settings are likely to be required for postacute care?

Exhibit 4–2 suggests key data elements related to SI/IS that should be assessed and documented in the course of both the initial and the continuing stay clinical reviews.

The primary data sources for performing the initial clinical review include the admission note or ED treatment record, history and physical, laboratory and radiology reports, physician orders, and multidisciplinary progress notes. In cases where documentation is incomplete or inadequate to support the services ordered, the case manager may need to initiate personal contact with the physician in order to obtain and document additional clinical data or discuss the need for alternative treatment plans. The skill

Exhibit 4–2 Data Elements for Initial and Continuing Stay Clinical Reviews

Severity of Illness	Intensity of Service
• Presenting symptoms/reason for admission • Recent history supporting admission • Outpatient tests and treatments completed • Physical examination findings • Health history related to admitting diagnosis • Diagnostic results prior to and since admission • Baseline functional status • Response to treatment • Special circumstances that may support admission when criteria are not clearly met	• Admitting orders intended for treatment of presenting diagnosis • Treatments and procedures identified in the clinical pathway or plan of care • Data to support that ordered services cannot be appropriately provided in a lower acuity setting of care

gained and enhanced by performing frequent initial clinical reviews will enable the case manager to distinguish between a lack of medical necessity and missing documentation elements. In cases where the documentation in the clinical record does not clearly support medical necessity, a personal assessment by the case manager may provide the necessary insight prior to initiating contact with the physician.

The specifics of documenting the initial clinical review will depend on the organization's UM information system platform. The documentation protocol should be designed to minimize rework and capture essential clinical data in as concise a format as possible. Efforts should be made to eliminate the practice of documenting the review manually and subsequently transcribing the review data into an electronic worksheet. Electronic tools have been developed by some organizations that allow direct documentation into the criteria tool that specific SI/IS criteria have been met.

Following completion of the clinical review, essential information should be communicated to the payer via telephone, fax, or, in some cases, electronic transmission, in order to secure approval or certification for the services to be provided. This documentation should be transcribed on the UM worksheet and should include the certification or approval number, the name and telephone number of the payer contact issuing approval, and the number of initial days approved. Subsequent clinical reviews can be scheduled on the basis of the initial certification in order to ensure that updated clinical information is available and can be communicated to the payer in advance of the last certified day.

Continued Stay Review

A continued stay review applies the same tools and process as the initial review and is performed to identify the need for continuing the inpatient stay or level of care. SI/IS criteria are applied as in the initial review in order to confirm medical necessity for continued stay and/or modification in level of care within the acute care setting, as in a transfer from critical care to a general care unit. As noted above, when approval for admission to acute care is received from the payer, a specific number of days are generally approved or certified by the payer. Assuming that no unanticipated condition changes are identified in the meantime, and that no variances from the anticipated response to treatment are noted, the first formal continuing stay review should be conducted the day prior to the last certified day and communicated to the payer on the last certified day with the request that additional days be certified, if supported by clinical review data. A brief informal review should be performed (not necessarily documented) on the intervening previously certified days to confirm that the patient is progressing toward discharge as anticipated. Early identification of a lack of progress can generate a change in the plan of care and the targeted LOS. Conversely, if the patient is progressing more rapidly than anticipated, the potential exists that medical necessity may not be met on the last approved day, in which payment for that day may be denied, even though it may have been certified.

When the patient's stay is not governed by a per diem payer contract and reimbursement is DRG based, it is essential for the case manager to establish a schedule of clinical review that effectively facilitates LOS and clinical resource UM. In these cases, the case manager should still perform and document initial and continued stay clinical reviews, even though the information documented may not be communicated to the payer. Patients should be managed in a consistent manner regardless of payment source, both for ethical reasons and in order to minimize the risk of allegations that standards of care provided by the organization are variable for patients with differing payment sources. In the case of government payers, including traditional Medicare and Medicaid, the governmental oversight agency (i.e., Health Care Financing Administration in the case of Medicare and each state in the case of Medicaid) may require the use of specific clinical criteria sets for covered patients.

For per diem reimbursement, the clinical review process provides the same incentive—documented support of medical necessity for the admission or continued stay. The payer may review medical records and require retrospective repayment of per diem reimbursement when documentation does not support medical necessity for all or part of the admission or for specific services provided; this determination is referred to as an *inlier denial*. Unless required more frequently by payer contractual terms, a formal continued stay review should be performed and documented at least every third day throughout the patient's hospitalization.

Another factor in support of consistent, well-documented continuing stay reviews relates to the risk of incurring payer-issued denials. As the organization consistently submits claims to payers for services based on clearly documented medical necessity, and the frequency with which claims can be denied decreases, payers perceive the provider to be managing patient care and the reimbursement resources responsibly. This reputation for managing patient care responsibly results from effective UM, and experience suggests that it consistently leads to reduced levels of scrutiny by payers and increased willingness on their part to negotiate coverage in marginal cases.

Two additional benefits of frequent continuing stay reviews are that (1) they provide the case manager with information on which a timely discharge plan can be developed and modified throughout the patient's hospitalization, and (2) they provide a mechanism for tracking variances in anticipated clinical results that have been documented in the plan of care or clinical pathway. These clinical reviews incorporate the objectives of the fully integrated case management role: discharge planning, UM, and care facilitation. The interdependence of these functions is suggested in Figure 4–3.

COLLABORATION WITH THE PHYSICIAN

Effective UM cannot be performed without ongoing communication and collaboration with the attending physician. The case manager cannot order tests, modify the medical plan of treatment, or transfer the patient independent of the physician.

Inevitably, the case manager's initial and continuing stay reviews will occasionally indicate that a patient's clinical conditions do not support medical necessity for services provided, and that a high probability exists for a payer-issued denial. In this case, it is critical that clinical review findings be communicated promptly to the physician. In many instances, the physician may have knowledge of patient-specific factors that are not adequately documented in the patient's record, but that would serve to support the determination of medical necessity; such factors would include family history, prior medical treatment for the same or similar clinical conditions, and comorbidities and risk factors that are not typical of patients admitted with the same primary diagnosis. Clearly, it is essential that the

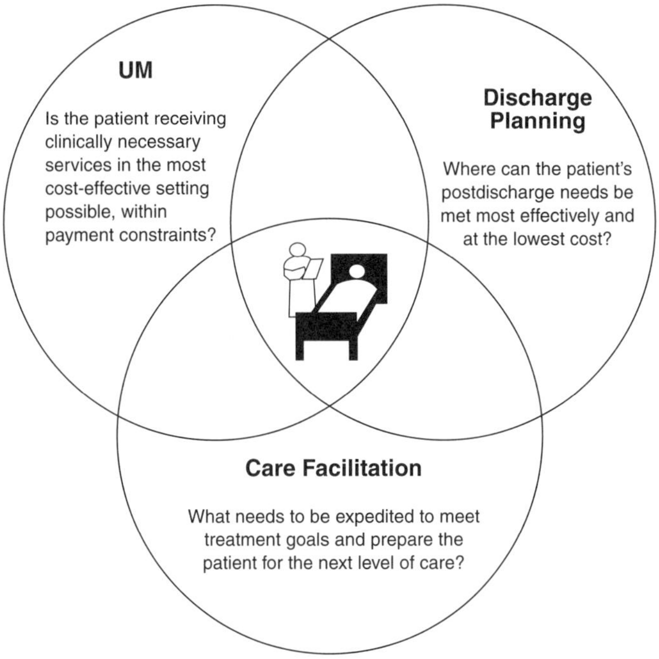

Figure 4–3 Interdependence of Utilization Management (UM), Discharge Planning, and Care Facilitation

case manager's clinical review be based on measurable and objective criteria, and it may be advisable to request that a colleague skilled in UM functions validate the case manager's impressions when lack of medical necessity requires that specific cases be referred to the attending physician for resolution.

One negative consequence of traditional UR that has lingered in some organizations is the perception among physicians that UM staff and case managers essentially serve the function of "LOS police" whose primary interest is in discharging patients as promptly as possible, rather than in facilitating necessary care in the most cost-effective manner possible. This consequence of separating care facilitation from UM functions argues strongly for an integrated role in which the case manager is engaged in collaborative practice with physicians and the care team to facilitate care as well as perform UM activities.

By forming strong collaborative relationships with physicians and demonstrating sound clinical judgment, case managers can gain the confidence of physicians with whom they work and establish a climate within which medical-necessity and level-of-care decisions can be discussed and resolved objectively, rather than representing a threat to the physician's judgment and professional autonomy. For a more detailed discussion of issues related to physician partnering and conflict resolution in the case manager role, refer to Chapter 7.

THE PHYSICIAN ADVISOR ROLE

However positive the relationships between physicians and case managers, circumstances occasionally arise in the UM process in which the patient's clinical condition does not adequately support medical necessity for continuing stay or for the specific level of care ordered. In these instances, a key resource for the case manager is found in the physician advisor or physician liaison role.

The physician advisor role has two central objectives: (1) to serve as a clinical resource and consultant to the case manager and (2) to facilitate resolution of level-of-care and utilization issues when direct communication between the case manager and the patient's attending physician is ineffective. Specifically, the physician advisor provides support to the case managers in problem resolution involving

- necessity of admission and level of care (based on clinical criteria)
- level-of-care requirements during the patient's hospitalization
- discharge planning
- reimbursement and quality issues
- physician education related to care management and payer issues

Prior to initiating a referral to the physician advisor, the case manager should make every attempt to resolve the identified issue or problem directly with the individual physician involved. *Under no circumstances should the physician advisor be consulted until after the case manager has had a face-to-face or telephone conversation with the patient's attending physician.* In situations where no resolution is reached following the case manager's interaction with the attending physician, the physician advisor should be contacted and informed fully of the circumstances of the case and the specific level-of-care or utilization issues that are unresolved; in most organizations, policies have been developed that require that physician advisor consultations be requested in writing and communicated to the physician advisor by fax or e-mail.

Following a review of the case and, if indicated, a personal assessment of the patient, it is the responsibility of the physician advisor to contact the patient's attending physician to discuss alternative courses of action or modifications to the treatment plan that will resolve the utilization issues in question. It may occasionally be necessary for the physician advisor to intervene directly with payers in cases where a denial has been or may be issued, and the case manager and physician advisor can provide adequate support for medical necessity; in these cases, the most productive approach is typically a dialogue between the physician advisor and the payer's medical director. As in the case of all UM activities, physician advisor interventions should be documented clearly and concisely, preferably in an electronic worksheet, but in any case in a location that is entirely separate from the medical record.

In order to provide in-depth clinical expertise in the management of specific high-risk patient populations and as a resource to the primary physician advisor, the organization may elect to use a panel of physician specialists in clinical areas where physician advisor intervention is required on a regular basis. For example, in cases where the primary physician advisor is an internist, it may prove beneficial to maintain contractual relationships with one or more surgical specialists who can be requested to review complex or problematic surgical cases and to facilitate discussions with surgeons.

INTEGRATION OF UM AND CARE FACILITATION

An additional component of the case manager's role includes care facilitation. Using the principles of UM, the case manager, in collaboration with the attending physician and care team, ensures that the patient is progressing correctly through the health care system. The case manager works to expedite care, follow up on diagnostic studies and reports, and track the patient's progress toward discharge.

SUGGESTED READINGS

B. Bean, "A Moving Target: Case Management Models Evolve as More Risk Is Assumed," *New Definition 13*, no. 1 (1999).

P. Kongstvedt and D. Plocher, *Best Practices in Medical Management* (Gaithersburg, MD: Aspen Publishers, Inc., 1998).

K. Zander, "Rethinking Discharge Planning," *New Definition 12*, no. 3 (1998).

CHAPTER 5

Understanding Chart Review

Patricia L. Metzger and Dale H. Metzger II

TAKE THIS TO WORK

1. Review of the medical record is an essential component of case management and requires a thoughtful, deliberate process that includes analysis, planning, and problem solving.
2. The initial review should find documentation of the plan of care associated with the episode of illness. The plan of care should include an acute and postacute treatment plan, physician orders that are consistent with the treatment plan, and discharge plans that reflect ongoing consistent treatment following discharge.
3. Concurrent review of the Medicare patient population is often overlooked or put last on the list. Where Medicare patients take least priority in the concurrent review process, the risk of eroding reimbursement without sufficient attention being placed on length of stay and resource utilization is high.
4. Retrospective reviews may be needed for several purposes, such as quality evaluations or denial management.

Review of the medical record is an essential component of case management and requires a thoughtful, deliberate process that includes analysis, planning, and problem solving. Specifically, the case manager should review the record for documentation on a history of the presenting illness that includes a summary of onset, duration, intensity, symptoms, and clinical findings.

The initial review should find documentation of the plan of care associated with the episode of illness. The plan of care should include an acute and postacute treatment plan, physician orders that are consistent with the treatment plan, and discharge plans that reflect ongoing consistent treatment following discharge. It is important that during the initial review and all subsequent reviews, the case manager review all diagnostic testing and procedures that have been ordered. They should be evaluated for their relationship to patient status as well as patient diagnosis. Each diagnostic test and procedure should be viewed from the context of medical necessity to arrive at a diagnosis or to make determinations about additional treatment required. For example, what is the benefit achieved by performing an ultrasound of the gallbladder when the admitting condition is status post fall, rule out left hip fracture?

During the initial review, the case manager should evaluate the patient's response to initial treatment in order to assist with determinations concerning severity of illness as well as intensity of services required (SI/IS). This will assist the care team in gauging a projected length of stay (LOS). Some questions to consider when performing an initial review include the following:

- Has there been a relief of symptoms associated with treatment?
- Has there been improvement in the patient's condition?
- Have abnormal diagnostic values begun to return to normal?

All of the above should be well documented in the record. Without this information, progress toward discharge or transfer can be delayed. It becomes the responsibility of the case manager to assist in the education and coaching of physicians and other members of the care team regarding adequate medical record documentation.

INITIAL REVIEW

An initial comprehensive review must be completed on all admitted patients. The initial review is one that serves as the baseline against which case managers and payers measure clinical improvement. The patient record should reflect the patient's presenting illness, past history that may be impacting the current illness, and anticipated course of treatment to resolve the patient's condition. If the case manager is unable to find the clinical information needed to complete a comprehensive review in the record, it is incumbent upon the case manager to communicate with the attending physician and secure the information needed to complete the review. During the initial review, the case manager should also apply the criteria used to define SI/IS. Application of these criteria helps determine both level-of-care requirements and projected resource utilization. During the initial review, the case manager will work with the physicians to identify a primary diagnosis and a commensurate targeted LOS. This assists in the development of the plan of care and helps progress toward actual implementation of the discharge plan.

During the initial review, the case manager should also determine the accuracy of payer information. The intent here is not to invalidate the work that was done during the preregistration and registration phases of the patient's hospital stay. However, during the stressful time of admission to the hospital, the accuracy of preliminary information documentation is known to be suspect. Validation of information in resource management is essential, as each payer source may have idiosyncratic requirements regarding initial notification, certification of care, precertification of specific procedures, and written or telephonic review requirements.

Historically, case management departments have not been involved in contract negotiations, and consequently are unaware of the payer-specific requirements for approval of services unless they have actively sought out the information. The validation of information should also include seeking out information pertinent to postacute services. Case managers are better served if they are able to determine, at the time of admission, the resources and funding available to the patient for postacute services. This minimizes the risk of the case manager committing to postacute services for which the patient has no coverage or funding. Exhibit 5–1 is a sample of an initial review checklist that case managers have found helpful in making certain they have met patient needs and their own performance expectations.

Case Manager's Clinical Summary

The case manager has the responsibility to make certain that the clinical record accurately reflects patient status. In the absence of documentation, the expectation should be that the case manager will document case management findings in a comprehensive summary that reflects the following:

- a principal or working diagnosis and a secondary diagnosis
- synopsis of the reason for admission (may include comorbidities, history of past illnesses)

Exhibit 5–1 Initial Review Checklist

Initial Review	*Complete*
Apply intensity of service criteria.	
Apply severity of illness criteria.	
Identify options if the patient does not meet intensity of service/severity of illness criteria.	
If patient meets intensity of service/severity of illness criteria:	
Identify working diagnosis and targeted length of stay.	
Determine if patient is to be placed on a clinical protocol/pathway.	
Identify plan of care recommendations.	
Consult with health care team members: Patient's special needs Plan to ensure that patient moves toward targeted discharge date	
Document activities and recommendations.	
Ensure that patient and family are included in discharge plan and are aware of the plan of care.	
Communicate findings to payer per coverage requirements.	

- documentation of interventions and procedures related to the present diagnosis
- documentation of treatment plan to reflect the SI/IS in concise chronological order

A comprehensive initial review will allow the care team to initiate anticipatory planning and provide patients and families with information to prompt decision making around discharge planning. Anticipatory planning minimizes the potential for avoidable days, denials, and an increased cost per case. Expected outcomes should be discussed with the family as early as possible following the initial review to arrive at realistic expectations surrounding the plan of care and anticipated discharge.

CONCURRENT, CONTINUED STAY REVIEW

Concurrent review is a real-time assessment of patient status, level-of-care requirements, and patient needs throughout the course of the hospital stay. It should be completed on the first business day following the initial review and should be done no less than three times per week during the time the patient remains in the hospital. Concurrent chart review establishes and records the ongoing care requirements of the patient. It is intended to support the coordination of the health care team efforts to expedite care and facilitate the use of resources. It serves as the basis for identification and trending of treatment barriers and delays.

The plan of care needs to be updated at least every other day and definitely each time the patient experiences a change in clinical condition. During the concurrent review process, the case manager applies the criteria to make determinations about the issues mentioned above and documents findings in the patient record. The case manager is expected to document clinical findings on a case management worksheet or in an automated program that allows him or her to track and trend the use of resources, delays in care, and progress toward the goal of discharge. This is information that must be communicated in a systematic, timely way to third-party payers in order to secure payment for services rendered.

Concurrent review for the Medicare patient population is overlooked or prioritized to last on the list. This occurs because there is no real-time active intervention demanded between the hospital and the payer. Case managers are not required to submit any formal review updates to Medicare, and there is no need to secure certification for additional days. Although we recognize that other third-party payers routinely place demands on the case manager's time and resources, it is also important to recognize that the hospital is at risk for the management of Medicare patients. Because traditional Medicare cases are paid on the basis of diagnosis-related group (DRG), once the patient has been admitted to the hospital, the hospital assumes the risk for managing the patient and for the efficient use of resources. The hospital will get reimbursed the DRG rate for the Medicare patient, regardless of the resources used. Where Medicare patients take least priority in the concurrent review process, the risk of eroding reimbursement without sufficient attention being placed on LOS and resource utilization is high.

During the continued stay review, the case manager needs to be cognizant of assigning a certification level of care that most accurately reflects the patient's condition. The levels of care include

- acute care
- intermediate care
- intensive care
- subacute care
- transitional care
- skilled care
- long-term care
- home care
- outpatient services
- nonacute care

Regardless of which level of care is assigned, the case manager's documentation in the patient record and on the review sheets that are shared with the payers must reflect the clinical picture that best compares to the patient's level-of-care requirements.

Exhibit 5–2 provides a quick checklist for case managers as they complete their concurrent review processes.

Discharge Screens

During the concurrent review process, it is also imperative to review the discharge screens for patients. Should a patient not meet discharge screens, and should this not be acknowledged in the record at the time of discharge, the hospital

Exhibit 5–2 Concurrent Review Checklist

Concurrent Review	*Complete*
Apply intensity of service criteria.	
Questions to consider:	
Is the patient sufficiently ill to remain in the acute care setting?	
Are the criteria met for intensity of service?	
Is continuation of stay in acute care supported by documentation in the record?	
Apply severity of illness criteria.	
Questions to consider:	
What is being done for the patient?	
Are the criteria met for severity of illness?	
Is continuation of stay in acute care supported?	
Document activities and recommendations.	
Consult with team members to track the plan of care and discharge plan.	
Communicate findings to payer per coverage requirements.	

can be subject to a quality review for prematurely discharging patients.

In reviewing discharge screens, the case manager needs to be cognizant of those things that need to occur in order for the patient to reach the targeted discharge date. Goals for discharge need to be clinically specific (i.e., able to ambulate to the bathroom independently, able to take oral medication, etc.). The case manager also needs to identify what modifications need to occur with the plan of care in order to facilitate discharge on the targeted date (i.e., dietary consult, physical therapy consult, etc.). Discussions and ongoing documentation of progress toward discharge must be evident in the record. To minimize the risk of premature discharge, concerns and modifications to the discharge plan need to be discussed with the attending physician and be reflected in the record.

During the concurrent review process, the case manager assesses the patient and substantiates any variance between the documented clinical picture and the assessment. If there are variances, these variances should be resolved directly with the attending physician and resolution of the variances should be documented in the patient record.

Concurrent review may lead to a determination that the patient no longer meets the acute level of care. Prior to pending the day, and considering this an avoidable day, the case manager should interact with the nurse, the attending physician, and other members of the team to determine that his or her findings are accurate. Unfortunately, accurate documentation in the patient record continues to be an ongoing problem in most facilities. A case manager, unable to find substantiating documentation in the patient record for continued stay, may pend a day as an avoidable day, when in fact diagnostic interventions are taking place but have been poorly documented. That is why the daily, personal contact between the case manager and other members of the care team is so vital.

Avoidable Days of Service

An avoidable day is defined as a patient day at a level of care that is higher than treatment needs require. There are multiple reasons for avoidable days, but some of the more common include the following:

- *Inability to deliver treatment or provide testing when required*—This is a facility-caused delay and payers feel no obligation to pay for days in the acute care setting when no intervention or diagnostic testing occurs. The general feeling is that if a hospital espouses itself as a full-service facility, then the services that a patient requires should be available seven days per week. An example of this type of delay includes the decision not to provide therapy services or stress testing on Saturdays and Sundays. Organizations must evaluate the cost/benefit of incurring the lost day's charges against the cost of providing services. However, organizations must also consider the profile they represent when they are unable or unwilling to provide the services required by the patient without delay.
- *Lack of information or equipment required in order to carry out the treatment or service*—This is a facility-caused delay and payers feel no obligation to pay for days in the acute care setting where delays occur because of the absence of operating equipment. An example of this type of delay is the inability to complete a computed tomography (CAT) scan because the equipment was not operational. Organizations need to attempt to mitigate these types of delays by considering transport of the patient to an alternative site where testing can be done.
- *No availability of a required bed at a lower level of care*—This type of delay can be an internal or external problem. Case managers encounter this delay when they are unable to move a patient out of the intensive care unit into another level of care within the hospital or when they are unable to transfer the patient to another level of care outside of the hospital. When working with the external environment, this type of delay needs to be evaluated in the context of available beds versus beds to

which the physician or family will not accept a transfer.

- *Patient not discharged or transferred*—This delay relates to a discharge or transfer that was scheduled but did not occur as planned. This can occur for a number of reasons and will need to be evaluated for root cause to determine why the transfer did not occur as scheduled.
- *Less than optimal coordination or planning for discharge*—This delay relates to days within the stay or added on to the stay that are directly related to inadequate coordination or planning for discharge. The days can be associated with the need for patient teaching or can relate to changes in decisions concerning the level of care to which the patient should be transferred (i.e., home care vs. skilled nursing). As described earlier, the case manager is responsible to see that discharge planning efforts are coordinated and that discharge planning efforts are pursuing more than one alternative when determination has been made that the patient/family is/are unable to provide care at home.
- *Patient/family or attending physician disagreement with the plan to transfer or discharge*—This delay is the most difficult to manage and is highly contingent on the patient, family, and physician. The case manager's role is to facilitate resolution as quickly as possible.

Most avoidable patient days can be prevented with communication and education. Staff and physician education regarding alternative treatment options is essential. In many instances, staff and physicians have minimal understanding about the concept of avoidable days and their impact on the organization. Providing insight into the impact on the organization from a fiscal and profiling perspective has been received positively by physicians and staff.

Education of the health care team and patients and families is essential in managing avoidable days. The great majority of patients and families have not been informed about targeted LOS. Most have also not had discussions about their responsibilities in managing their own health and plans of care. Families will, for the most part, react favorably to accurate information and planning. One of the most effective ways to manage this process is to establish prior to, or at the time of admission, a targeted discharge date, and to initiate discussions around the posthospitalization level-of-care requirements that can be anticipated. This prompts family discussion and can surface areas of difficulty that the case manager and care team can work to overcome.

Most avoidable days can be prevented with discharge planning and coordination of care seven days per week. It requires proactive care management and early identification of patterns of delays in care. Concurrent reviews need to be focused on the progression of care toward discharge.

RETROSPECTIVE REVIEW

The third type of chart review is retrospective review. This is the least desirable and most time consuming of the chart review processes. Retrospective review is initiated for several reasons.

- payer-requested reviews to validate services
- quality reviews
- audits

Payer-Requested Reviews

If the case manager is functioning effectively, the number of payer-requested retrospective reviews should be minimal. Payer-requested reviews are generally the result of inadequate or incomplete clinical information, making it difficult for the payer to make a determination about ongoing certification to provide treatment. The most effective way to minimize the number of payer-requested reviews is to develop a methodical, systematic approach for conducting and documenting chart review and use a consistent format to present review information to the payer. One organization with whom we worked invested the time to meet with each payer and have them outline precisely the information each expected to receive during initial and concurrent review update. Then, the organization developed a comprehensive worksheet that would be automated and used universally for all payer reviews. By implementing the consistent format for review, the case managers were able to reduce their number of retrospective reviews by 60 percent. Exhibit 5–3 provides a sample worksheet that can be used by case managers as

Exhibit 5–3 Concurrent Review Worksheet

Patient Name ______________________________ Social Security Number ____________________

Type of Admission ______________________ ER ________ Direct _______ Scheduled ________

Date of Admission ______________________ Time of Admission ______________________

Reason for Admission ____

Failed Outpatient Treatment: Yes______ No______

Date	**Diagnosis/Comorbidity**	**Date**	**Procedure**

Initial Vital Signs: __________________________

Activity	Day_____ Date______	Day_____ Date______	Day_____ Date______
Consults			
Vital Signs			
Diet/Activity			
Foley Catheter			
Last BM			
IV Meds			
PO Meds			
Lab Work			
C&S			
X-rays			
Therapy Activities			
Cardiopulmonary Diagnostics			
Treatments			
Discharge Plan			

a reference point to make certain they have considered all aspects required for a comprehensive review.

Quality Reviews

Quality reviews are a more intense type of retrospective review. A quality review is usually precipitated by a payer's notification that a quality concern exists and the organization is being put on notice that an investigation is underway. The notification gives the provider an opportunity to pull the patient record, review it specifically for the quality issues identified by the payer, and make a response to the quality concern. Once quality concerns are raised, the challenge that such notifications present to the provider is the increased potential for intensified review. In the case of intensified review comes the potential for payers to find other discrepancies, be they real or perceived, regarding the way care is provided in the organization. The best way to avoid such scrutiny is to ensure, from the inception of the patient's record, that documentation is complete and comprehensive and that it accurately reflects the diagnosis, plan of care, patient's response to treatment, and discharge plan.

Audits

Audits are another type of retrospective review. Audits are conducted to reconcile that the services charged for were in fact provided. Audits can prove to be challenging because, as discussed throughout the course of this chapter, as well as in the chapter on documentation, the medical record does not consistently reflect the care provided. Many of us can recall any number of times that, as staff nurses, in the frenzy to complete the activities of care, we overlooked documentation of medication administration, treatments provided, vital signs taken, glucose fingerstick levels checked, and so forth. Unfortunately, when medications are charged to the patient's account through the automated pharmacy distribution process and the audit process identifies that the patient record does not reflect actual administration of the dose, in the eyes of the payer, this constitutes billing fraud. Several organizations have elected to develop their own internal audit process to mitigate the potential risk of a third-party audit and the associated ramifications.

Retrospective audits are completed to respond to third-party payer denials. These audits are time consuming, require an intense level of effort on the part of the case manager, and may or may not be effective in successfully overturning the denial. The appeal process can be a lengthy one, particularly if the case manager exercises all levels of appeal available. The most effective way to address the denial process is to put mechanisms like concurrent review and effective clinical documentation in place so as to avoid denial from admission through discharge. Proactive case management will never eliminate the need to complete some retrospective review. Organizations have found, however, that with comprehensive, accurate clinical documentation, the level of effort associated with the retrospective review process is substantially decreased.

CHAPTER 6

Denial Management and Related Care Coordination

Cindy J. Urbancic and James D. Witt

TAKE THIS TO WORK

1. Denials are decisions by third-party payers that reject full or partial payment and result in a discrepancy between expected and received dollars for the provider.
2. The goal of denial management is to minimize exposure to revenue loss based on payer-issued denials. Case managers play a critical role in the success of an organization's efforts to minimize and manage denials.
3. Effective case management interventions throughout the patient's episode can reduce to a minimum the number of denials incurred, as well as optimize revenue recovery from subsequent appeals.
4. Clinical or medical necessity denials are based on the absence of documented medical necessity or failure to meet severity of illness and intensity of service criteria that would justify the services provided; these denials typically represent the bulk of an organization's denial management opportunity, and case managers can have a major impact in preventing and managing them through focused utilization management and care facilitation activities.
5. Health care providers typically identify several distinct needs related to denial management.
   - poorly defined systems for monitoring denials and identifying the current days of care/dollars denied and under appeal
   - lack of a clearly defined system of procedures and accountabilities for denial management
   - the absent feedback loop necessary to reduce denials and improve appeal success

Denials can be defined as decisions by third-party payers that reject full or partial payment and result in a discrepancy between expected and received dollars. It is important to note that this definition encompasses payer decisions to reassign the diagnosis-related group (DRG) under which a claim is submitted; such decisions are referred to as *downcoding*. This distinctive type of denial will be discussed later in this chapter.

The goal of a systematic approach to denial management is to minimize the health care organization's exposure to revenue loss based on payer-issued denials. In order to achieve this goal, it is critical to address both aspects of revenue loss resulting from denials by (1) reducing the number of denials and (2) maximizing the organization's success rate in appeals. The case manager's responsibilities in care facilitation and utilization management (UM) are central to realizing both of these objectives. In order to develop a comprehensive approach to denial management, it is essential to understand the factors that most often contribute to payer-issued denials and to design an infrastructure that facilitates accurate initial submissions, prompt follow-up, and appeal of denials that are incurred.

Based on their root causes, denials must be accurately classified and processed in order to maximize revenue recovery. In many organizations, it has been noted that case managers lack adequate training to determine why denials are incurred and how to manage the appeal process most effectively. Before case managers can contribute effectively to the organization's denial management efforts, they must develop a clear understanding of the categories of payer-issued denials and the factors that contribute to each type of denial.

TYPES OF DENIALS

It is helpful to classify denials into one of three specific categories based on the payer's reason for denying payment to the provider. An accurate understanding of these denial types will guide the organization in designing and implementing effective approaches for managing denials and will enable case managers to support effective denial management.

Administrative and Technical Denials

Administrative and technical denials are issued by payers on the basis of noncompliance with administrative or technical contract requirements that are unrelated to patient care. Root causes of this type of denial include clerical errors in registration or claim submission, incorrect information provided by patients, and failure to comply with contract conditions related to precertification. In conducting a current state assessment of the organization's denial management competencies, accurate information regarding the frequency and amount of these denials can most often be obtained from designated staff members in the billing department or central business office. Additionally, a detailed denial analysis should be performed in order to assess and quantify the extent of denials that have been realized by the facility over a predefined time frame. Administrative or technical denials can be subcategorized into three broad categories as listed below. The goals for recovery of the initial denials are also included as reference points.

1. *Technical:* Accounts that have been denied for preexisting condition, lack of eligibility, or coordination of benefits. **Recovery Goal:** 85%
2. *Documentation:* Accounts where the payer is requesting further documentation before payment of the claim can be made; these are often "borderline" medical necessity cases and require appeals. **Recovery Goal:** 75%
3. *Authorization:* Accounts that have been denied because no authorization number is on file with the insurance company or hospital system. **Recovery Goal:** 85%

External Factor Denials

External factor denials are typically the least common type of denial incurred by providers. They are based on factors that are either outside of the organization's control or that are difficult or impossible to control. Common root causes of external factor denials include maximum benefit levels that have been exceeded and services provided that are defined by the patient's benefit plan as noncovered benefits. For purposes of developing denial management protocols, denials in this category are most often included with administrative and technical denials. As stated above, frequency and amount of these denials can also be obtained from designated staff in the billing department or central business office.

Clinical and Medical Necessity Denials

Clinical or medical necessity denials are issued by the payer on the basis of the absence of documented medical necessity or failure to meet severity of illness and intensity of service (SI/IS) criteria that would justify the services provided, either for the entire hospital admission or for individual days within an otherwise covered admission. Denials stipulating noncoverage for part of an admission are referred to as *inlier denials.* Because they are based on the application of clinical criteria, payer downcodes or DRG reassignments are considered a subcategory of medical necessity denials. Medical necessity denials typically represent the bulk of an organization's denial management opportunity, in terms of both days of care denied and potential for revenue loss. In many organizations, quantifying the financial impact of medical necessity denials resides with the business office or patient accounts department. Based on their central involvement in UM and care facilitation processes, case managers can have a major impact in preventing and managing medical necessity denials. The role of the case manager in the care facilitation process will be addressed later in this chapter.

Other Key Definitions Related to Denial Management

In addition to the three types of payer-issued denials, it is essential for case managers to understand two additional terms: appeal and write-off. *Appeals,* also called redetermination requests, are defined as written or verbal requests by the provider for the payer to reconsider an earlier denial decision and issue payment for the claim. Specifically in the case of medical necessity denials, the case manager is most frequently in the best position to positively influence payer decisions and enhance the success of the organization's appeal efforts.

In cases where appeals are unsuccessful, a *write-off* ultimately results. A write-off is necessary when the appeal is unsuccessful in having the denied amount paid. When a write-off decision is made, typically by a designated senior member of the business office staff, the associated balance is determined to be uncollectible and a general ledger entry is made to remove it from the organization's accounts receivable. Policy decisions must be made by the organization regarding attempts to recover revenue by billing patients for denied claim balances prior to initiating write-off actions.

COMPONENTS OF AN EFFECTIVE DENIAL MANAGEMENT PROTOCOL

In implementing a new or redesigned approach to denial management, the organization should consider the processes and accountabilities that must be developed for managing each phase of the denial cycle. Core processes within each phase of the denial management cycle must be designed and tested with input from case managers, patient registration staff, and representatives of the organization's billing department or business office, in order to ensure that the complexities associated with denials and appeals are anticipated and addressed. Particularly in the case of multihospital systems with a central business office, which may be physically remote from care delivery sites, it is critical to develop communication processes that will effect smooth handoffs of information and reduced cycle time. As suggested by Figure 6–1, effective denial mitigation and management are contingent on the skills of multiple internal team members.

Establishing Denial Management Benchmarks

Prior to initiating a focused denial management program, it is important to have established performance benchmarks against which progress can be measured. Although these benchmarks will be influenced in some measure by current performance levels and organiza-

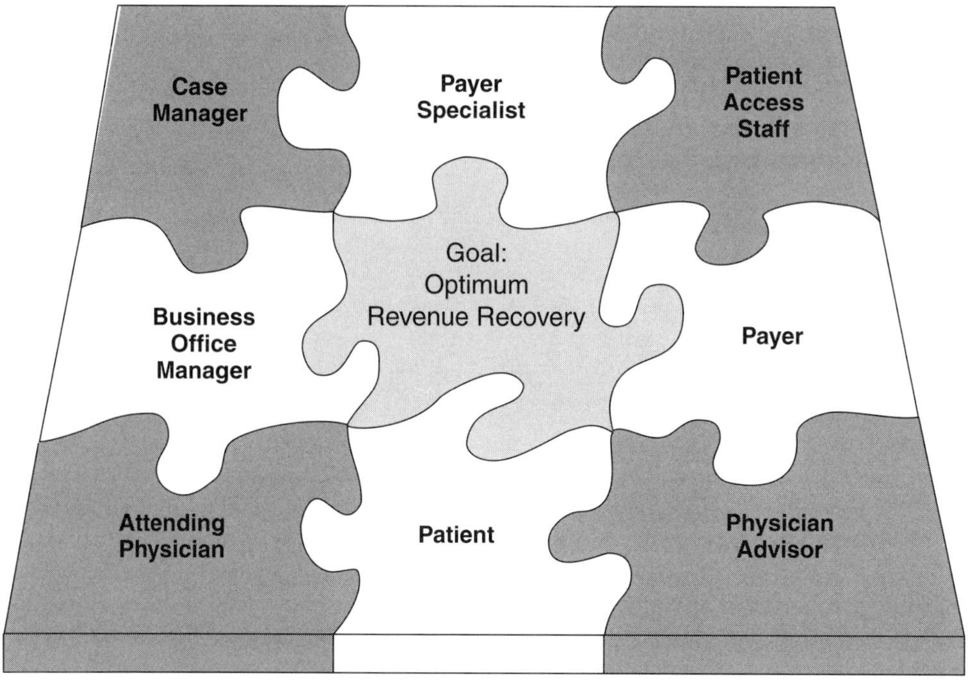

Figure 6–1 Key Roles in Denial Management

tional competencies in denial management, they should nevertheless reflect industry leading practice, even if this represents aggressive performance goals for the organization. Although the following targets may be aggressive, they can typically be achieved through a focused approach to minimizing denials and pursuing appeals in a systematic way:

- Total inpatient denials incurred should represent less than 1 percent of both days of care and net revenue, excluding contractual adjustment.
- All appeals should be submitted in writing within 21 days of receipt of the denial notification, or within a shorter time if required by specific payer requirements.
- Of those medical necessity denials appealed, an initial benchmark of 70 to 80 percent should be established for redetermination and payment of the claim. Paradoxically, as the organization's denial management processes improve, the recovery rate for appealed claims will actually *decrease,* because fewer cases will result in initial medical necessity denials. When medical necessity denials are minimized, most of the remaining cases will represent ineligible patients and noncovered benefits; fewer of these denials can be appealed successfully.

Receiving Denials

One of the initial sources of complexity in managing payer denials is that they typically enter the organization at a number of contact points, such as the business office, medical records department, case management department, and patient registration. In order to effectively track and respond to all denials, it is essential to develop a coordinated process to document that they have been received and then forward them to a single point for subsequent follow-up.

Denials may be received in the form of telephone notification by payers, denial letters addressed to multiple contacts within the hospital, or remittance advice documentation received by the business office or billing department. The central objective at this point is to ensure that all denials, regardless of type or point of entry, are forwarded to a designated central coordinator as promptly as possible.

The core process for receipt of denials should include date stamping the denial notification at the point of entry, initiating documentation in a shared database, and forwarding a hard copy of the denial notification to the designated denial coordinator during the same business day on which it was received. In order to facilitate prompt triage and routing, initial documentation in the database should include the date received, account number, claim submission date, dates of service, and reason for the denial as stated in the notification.

To expedite the denial management process, a single point to which all denial notifications should be forwarded after being date stamped and/or documented in the shared database should be designated. Many organizations have successfully developed a payer specialist role, which includes accountability for oversight and coordination of the denial management process. The payer specialist is typically responsible for the initial review of denial notification to confirm the denial type, assess the probability of successful appeal, and initiate a denial worksheet for documentation of all subsequent activities related to appeal and response.

In cases where the payer specialist determines that the probability of successful appeal is negligible, steps can be taken at this point to initiate write-off procedures in order to avoid expending time and resources on futile appeal activities. Prior to initiating a write-off of denied balances, the payer specialist should exhaust all other sources of payment, including identification of secondary benefits or collection of balances from patients in cases where the organization has determined that this step will be pursued. In these cases, an individual review of each case should be completed to determine whether the probability of collecting denied balances from the patient is sufficiently high to warrant the negative public relations consequences that may be incurred.

Triage and Routing of Denials

The objective in this phase of the denial management cycle is to ensure that all incoming denials are routed to the pertinent department for completion of research and submission of an accurate and timely response. Following review by the payer specialist to confirm that an appeal can be successfully pursued, and the completion of a denial worksheet for documentation and tracking, the case should be forwarded as promptly as possible to the pertinent department within the organization for research and response.

Administrative and technical denials, along with most external factor denials, should be researched by the business office or billing department, and medical necessity denials by case managers. Research related to payer downcodes and DRG reassignments will typically require a collaborative effort by case management and a medical records coding specialist to clarify whether the root cause of the denial is related to medical necessity or to documentation quality. In order to facilitate prompt appeal submission, the payer specialist should designate a due date for response by the department to which the case is forwarded for research, ideally not longer than seven days from initial receipt of the denial notification. Additionally, the appeal process needs to meet payer timing and resubmission requirements.

Researching Medical Necessity

The aspect of denial management in which case managers have the most central involvement is research related to medical necessity denials. The primary objectives of this activity are to (1) investigate factors contributing to the payer's decision that the services were medically unnecessary and (2) provide the documentation required to submit a timely appeal for reconsideration. After receiving denial notification and a worksheet that has been initiated by the payer specialist, the case manager will need to obtain the patient's record for more detailed review and response. If the denial has been issued retrospectively, which will most often be the case, an established requisition procedure should be followed for obtaining the closed record from the medical records department as promptly as possible.

The case manager's primary responsibility at this point is to perform a focused review of the record, *using the applicable clinical criteria set to determine whether documentation supports medical necessity for the services provided.* The findings of this review should be compared to the reasons for the denial decision as stated in the denial notification. At this point, the case manager may reach one of three conclusions.

1. Medical necessity criteria were adequately documented and an appeal should be pursued.
2. Documentation does not fully support medical necessity, but the patient's overall condition and presenting problem indicate that the services were medically necessary and a reconsideration should be requested.
3. The payer's denial is justified based on the lack of evidence supporting medical necessity and an appeal cannot be successfully pursued.

The case manager's determination regarding medical necessity must be documented clearly and concisely on the denial management worksheet in order to provide the necessary information for completion of an appeal letter. It is important to note that no documentation related to UM activities or denial/appeal activity should ever be entered into the clinical record.

In cases where chart documentation supports medical necessity on the basis of accepted clinical criteria, this should be documented and the corresponding criteria should be cited in the appeal documentation. In the interest of consistent style and format, it is advisable to use correspondence templates for all appeal letters; the payer specialist or a designated clerical staff member can prepare this correspondence, including the specific appeal factors documented by the case manager in the denial worksheet.

In cases where the payer's denial appears to be justified, the case should be reviewed with other members of the care management team for potential errors or omissions in the initial assessment prior to requesting that the payer specialist initiate a request for write-off. A mechanism should be developed for notifying attending physicians of all payer-issued denials and the stated reasons for these denials, regardless of whether an appeal is submitted. In cases where documentation fails to support medical necessity for the services provided, but the patient's clinical profile and diagnosis indicate that these services were nevertheless medically necessary, the case manager will need to seek additional input from the patient's attending physician or from the case management physician advisor.

Physician Collaboration in Medical Necessity Research

Payer contracts may require a physician's opinion as a condition for reconsideration of denied claims. Whether or not this requirement is imposed by specific payers, observation indicates that appeal success rates increase measurably with physician involvement in the appeal of medical necessity denials. In the interest of maximizing revenue recovery and reducing cycle times for appeal submission, specific procedures and timelines for physician review should be designed into denial management protocols. Physicians are frequently unaware of the significant revenue recovery potential represented by successful appeal of denied claims, and consistent communication of the organization's appeal success rate can reinforce the value of their participation in this process.

In negotiating their collaborative approaches to care facilitation, physicians and case managers need to address the communication channels for review of denials and completion of appeal documentation. Where feasible, it is always preferable to involve not only the physician advisor, but also the attending physician, in the denial management process. This involvement provides increased insight for physicians into the root causes of denials and the importance of consistently applying clinical criteria as a proactive measure to minimize the number of denials incurred.

In cases where a physician request is required by the payer, or where a medical opinion is requested by the case manager in clarifying whether medical necessity criteria were met, the request for review by the attending physician should be communicated as promptly as possible. These communications may be made by telephone, fax, or e-mail, and the denial worksheet and medical record should be made available. The case manager can expedite the review process by documenting and communicating clearly to the reviewing physician the specific factors in the case on which the payer's denial was based. As in the case of appeals submitted directly by the payer specialist, the use of correspondence templates will provide consistent style and format and minimize the time required for preparing appeal letters for the physician's signature.

When it is not feasible to obtain timely input from the attending physician in the appeal process, the review can be completed and the redetermination request signed by the care management physician advisor. In this case, it is vitally important that the attending physician be informed by the physician advisor that an appeal has been submitted in response to a payer-issued denial, that a copy of the appeal letter be provided, and that further information regarding the status of the appeal be provided as it becomes available. This communication is essential not only as a professional courtesy, but also to provide feedback to attending physicians regarding documentation, criteria, and utilization issues that may contribute to recurring denial patterns.

Submitting Appeals

In order to maintain a central point of accountability and to expedite the submission of appeals, it is generally most efficient for the case manager to return the completed denial worksheet to the payer specialist, who can assume responsibility for preparation, signature, and submission of all appeal letters. The payer specialist should initiate and maintain a central file containing the payer's denial notification, the completed denial worksheet, and copies of all documentation and correspondence related to the appeal process. The time parameters for receiving, routing, and researching denials should be designed to accommodate the appeal deadlines specified by payer contracts; the complete cycle time for researching and responding to denials typically should not exceed 21 days.

Monitoring the Status of Pending Appeals

After a redetermination request is submitted to the payer, the case should be monitored in order to ensure that the organization is aware of the status of all pending appeals. The payer specialist should monitor the status of all pending medical necessity appeals. Administrative, technical, and external factor denials may be monitored by a designated member of the business office staff in order to simplify subsequent communications with payers that may be required to resolve these denials. In cases where responses have not been received from payers within a designated time frame, typically 14 to 21 days, follow-up contact should be initiated by either the business office designee or the payer specialist.

Measuring and Trending Appeal Success Rates

As responses to pending appeal requests are received, the decision to reverse or uphold the denial decision should be documented in the denial worksheet by the payer specialist. By using the worksheet to document appeal resolution, it is possible to obtain real-time information on the organization's current appeal success rate by denial type, root cause, and specific payer. If possible, these worksheets should be designed as an input document to the electronic denial database. This information should be summarized in a concise format and included in the monthly reporting of care management performance metrics.

When trends in denials and appeals are reviewed frequently, proactive measures can be pur-

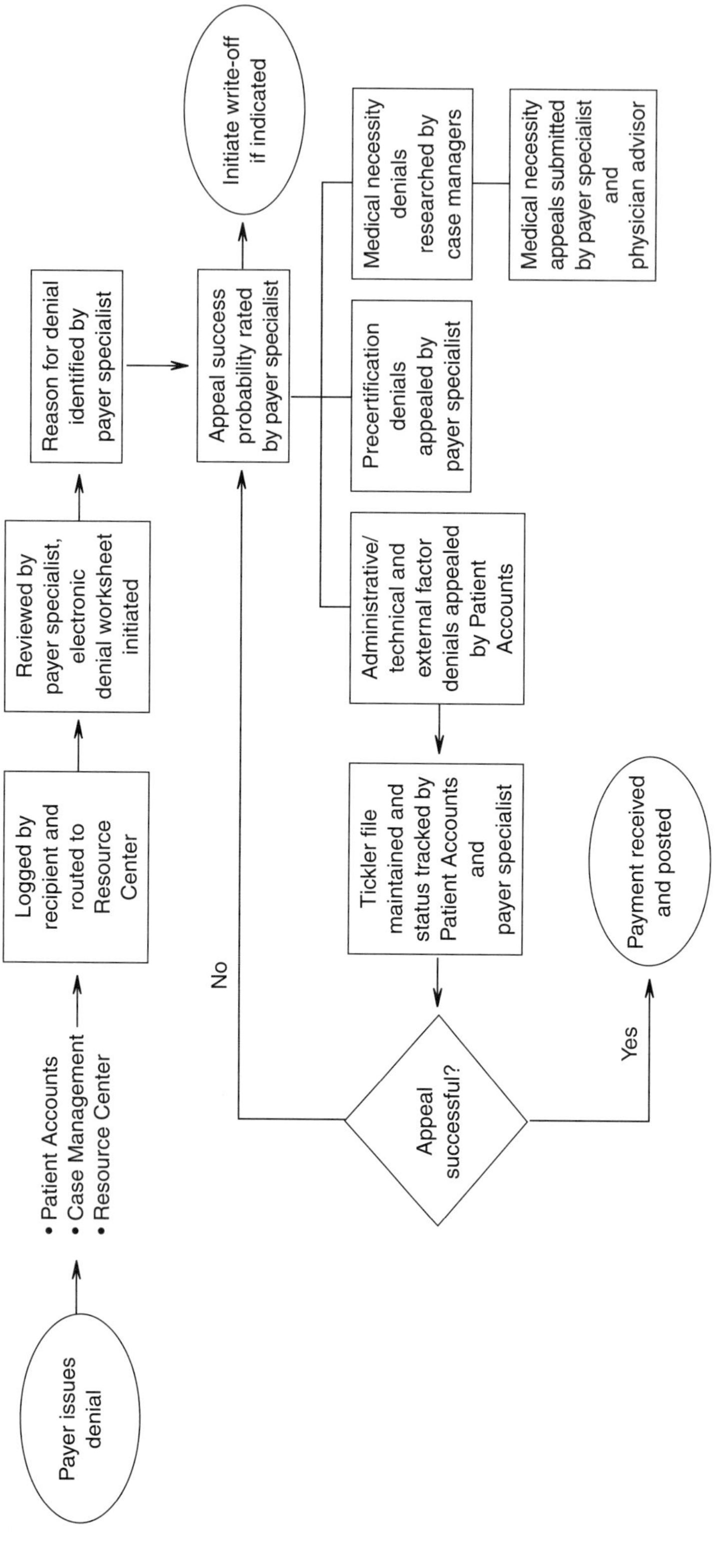

Figure 6–2 Sample High-Level Denial Management Process

sued to reverse negative trends early. By being aware of current denial trends, case managers can intervene during the patient's hospital admission to concurrently correct documentation and UM gaps that are likely to result in payer-issued denials. As illustrated in Figure 6–2, each phase in the denial management cycle builds on the competencies required for success in the preceding phase. It is important to note that the critical final step in effective denial management requires consistent monitoring of results and utilization of outcome data for ongoing process improvement.

Many organizations have found it useful to implement an interdisciplinary denial management task force made up of case managers, physician advisors, payer specialists, and representatives of the managed care department, business office, and/or patient financial services. This task force typically has accountability for reviewing denial and appeal statistics on a monthly basis and for revising processes for denial management and appeal submission. Regular review by an interdisciplinary team provides the feedback mechanism, which is frequently lacking, and prompts timely quality improvement actions. It is particularly important that a consistent communication mechanism be established for providing feedback to physicians regarding the rate and underlying causes of medical necessity denials and that issues of clinical documentation and level-of-care criteria be discussed with the medical staff concisely.

DENIAL MANAGEMENT AND THE CONTRACTING PROCESS

To efficiently and proactively minimize denials, the care management department and the managed care department must work closely through the payer contracting process. The care management leadership needs to review payer contractual terms focusing on UM requirements, including the denial and appeal process, prior to the organization signing off on these contracts. A collaborative approach to handling appeals will make the process run more efficiently. Additionally, an ongoing process between the managed care department and the care management department regarding modifications or changes to existing contracts must be established to ensure that case managers have the most current payer terms to support their proactive role in managing denials and appeals.

THE ROLE OF THE CASE MANAGER IN THE DENIAL MANAGEMENT PROCESS

The case manager plays a critical role in the denial management process, in particular with minimizing and *concurrently* mitigating clinical and medical necessity denials. Through their role in care facilitation and UM, case managers work closely with the physician and multidisciplinary team to ensure that the patient's plan of care and documentation support the SI/IS the patient is receiving. By being knowledgeable of payer's requirements, the case manager tailors the telephonic or faxed review to efficiently and effectively communicate the patient's hospital course against the payer's criteria and the transition plan in place. Given the time and costs incurred in appeals, even when a well-designed denial management plan is in place, the proactive aspect of the case manager's role in denial prevention and concurrent denial management is perhaps the most significant contribution that can be made to revenue recovery.

SUGGESTED READINGS

B. Bean, "A Moving Target: Case Management Models Evolve as More Risk Is Assumed," *New Definition 13*, no. 1 (1999).

L. Galvin and D. Baudendistel, "Case Management—A Team Approach," *Nursing Management*, January 1998, 28–31.

P. Kongstvedt and D. Plocher, *Best Practices in Medical Management* (Gaithersburg, MD: Aspen Publishers, Inc., 1998).

S.B. Perkins and M. Kassel, "Acute Care Case Management," *Inside Case Management 6,* no. 6 (1999): 1–4.

K. Zander, "Rethinking Discharge Planning," *New Definition 12,* no. 3 (1998).

Chapter 7

Physician Partnering and the Case Manager's Role in Conflict Mediation

David W. Plocher and James D. Witt

TAKE THIS TO WORK

1. Conflict in the work life of a case manager arises from the complex dynamics in professional relationships and the subjectivity that is inherent in making decisions that influence patient outcomes and organizational performance.
2. Unresolved conflict delays decision making; fosters inefficient resource utilization; compromises the satisfaction of patients, case managers, and physicians; and may even jeopardize the quality of patient care.
3. When effectively managed, conflict serves to challenge the status quo, expand perspectives, and add creativity to the problem-solving process in managing the care of patients.
4. When team members establish "ground rules" in advance for making decisions and resolving conflicts, consensus decisions can be reached in 70 to 80 percent of all exchanges between physicians and case managers.
5. Case managers and other members of the care delivery team need to clearly understand the difference between *compromise* and *consensus*, and understand that it is possible to reach mutually satisfactory resolution to conflict without "giving in."
6. A key first step in managing conflict positively is to understand typical physician expectations of the case manager role, including communication of patient status, input into the discharge planning process, and timely, focused outcome information.
7. Several specific action steps can consistently enhance the quality of physician–case manager partnerships: involving physicians in the case manager selection and assignment process, establishing ground rules for care facilitation, participating in interdisciplinary care conferences, and developing the role of the case manager as a clinical expert and staff mentor.

Central to any care management initiative is the ability of physicians and case managers to work collaboratively, each using distinctive clinical and interpersonal skills to achieve optimum results for patients and to meet desired organizational targets in length of stay (LOS), cost per case, and other performance metrics. Effective case manager/physician partnering and the capacity to resolve conflicts promptly and objectively are core competencies that must be developed in order to derive maximum value from care management processes. This chapter presents basic concepts and approaches for partnering with physicians and constructively managing conflict among members of the interdisciplinary care team. This chapter also provides specific steps for building functional partnerships between case managers and physicians.

BUILDING SKILLS TO MANAGE CONFLICT

Understanding Potential Sources of Conflict

Some degree of conflict is inherent in all professional relationships and interactions. Frequently identified as a source of stress and anxiety, conflict actually serves several constructive purposes in the case manager's interactions with colleagues, physicians, and payers. The well-worn axiom, "no friction, no traction," seems to apply here. When effectively managed, conflict serves to challenge the status quo, expand perspectives, and add creativity to the problem-solving process in managing the care of patients. Conflict in the work life of the case manager arises from several sources.

- the intrinsic challenge of working with multiple stakeholders who may have differing needs and priorities
- the highly subjective position of making determinations of what actions are in the best interests of patients
- the dynamics of interactions between professionals who bring high levels of both knowledge and personal investment to their roles in the health care system
- the usually unspoken question in the mind of the rounding physician, "What's in it for me or my patient if I cooperate with your recommendation?"

Multiple Stakeholder Needs and Priorities

The challenge of bringing together and meeting the needs and wants of patients, physicians, payers, and hospitals defines the case manager's role. In any health care delivery exchange, the patient's expectation of optimum health and functional status may be at least partially incompatible with the payer's expectation of reduced health care expenditures and the hospital's expectations of shortened LOS and more prompt discharge to postacute care. The case manager's objective is to facilitate the health care delivery process to satisfy the expectations of each of these key stakeholders as closely as possible.

Subjective Decision Making

Typical of professional service encounters, there is an underlying consumer-oriented expectation in health care delivery that providers and payers will act in a manner that is consistent with the best interests of the patient. This expectation and the professional ethic on which it is based are the key distinctions between professional and purely commercial/economic relationships. This ethical foundation frequently necessitates a decision concerning which of several possible courses of action is truly in the patient's best interest, and such decisions are always made on the basis of subjective criteria. The complexity-of-care decision is compounded when the patient is not fully competent, but even when patients can participate in decisions related to their care, subjectivity is inherent in the case manager's role and is a potential source of conflict.

The Role of Knowledge and Personal Investment

Physicians, nurses, social workers, and other members of the health care team all bring years of educational preparation and high levels of specialized expertise to their roles. In addition to academic preparation for these roles, there is a strong socialization process and accompanying values, autonomy, and professional judgment that can only be acquired over time. Health care professionals, in particular, have a strong sense of personal investment in their work life. Challenges to their professional autonomy and decision-making capacity often have the potential to elicit defensive responses and interpersonal conflict because of this high level of personal investment.

Negative Consequences When Conflict Is Not Managed Effectively

Conflict in the case manager role can arise from any one of a number of sources, and, frequently, from a combination of the complex factors underlying health care delivery and professional relationships. When conflict is managed effectively, working relationships and collegiality are strengthened, and, over time, a culture of collaboration emerges. The underlying goal of conflict management is to promote this culture within which consensus decisions become the norm.

Ineffectively managed, conflict generates dysfunctional interactions among members of the health care team, strains interpersonal relationships, and compromises the success of even a strong care management initiative. Unresolved conflict delays decision making and may jeopardize the quality of patient care, as well as contribute to medically unnecessary utilization and excess costs. Additionally, team members often retreat to narrowly proscribed "safety zones" in the interest of avoiding confrontation and are reluctant to explore new solutions and approaches to care facilitation. Finally, the interpersonal dynamics resulting from poorly managed conflict inevitably obstruct communication and compromise the satisfaction of patients, case managers, and physicians.

Understanding Consensus and Compromise

In managing conflict, it is essential to understand the distinctions between consensus and compromise. Although closely related, these terms are not interchangeable, and understanding the difference between them is a key insight in developing conflict resolution skills. Case managers and other members of the care delivery team may be guarded and defensive in response to conflict simply because they see *compromise* and "giving in" as the only option when *consensus,* not compromise, should be the objective of conflict management.

In compromise, one party in an interaction acquiesces his or her interests and expectations to those of the other party; this assumes one weak and one strong participant in the exchange. One participant's gain must be achieved at the expense of the other. In the short term, the party who "wins" in a compromise may achieve the desired outcome, and in one-time commercial exchanges, the compromise approach may be a valid solution to resolving conflict. However, in ongoing professional relationships, the dynamics of this win/lose exchange are invariably negative, and it becomes more and more difficult to achieve a collaborative practice environment in this climate. In addition to the negative dynamics fostered by the compromise, the quality of patient care often suffers because the input of some team members is inhibited or devalued and the full range of treatment perspectives is not considered.

Consensus implies a dialogue in which both parties are open to evaluating and adjusting their expectations during the course of the exchange. Rather than being forfeited, expectations are voluntarily moved toward a center point where a mutually acceptable outcome can be achieved. When consensus is achieved, it is unlikely that either party to the transaction will have his or her original expectations fulfilled, but both parties will agree to support the conclusion reached. Rather than adding to interpersonal tension, the process of negotiating expectations and building consensus actually enhances the quality of professional relationships when it is practiced consistently over time.

There is a common misconception that conflict resolution and the ability to facilitate consensus are intrinsic qualities that an individual either has or does not have. However, experience suggests that these skills, like many aspects of effective interpersonal and organizational behavior, can be acquired and improved over time. Assuming a basic level of motivation, individuals and teams can learn to approach conflict from a different perspective and can reduce the potentially destructive consequences related to ineffective conflict resolution. In the end, each party may be 80 percent satisfied and in agreement, and 100 percent committed to the same overall care management goals. The matrix in Exhibit 7–1 suggests the potential outcomes in compromise and consensus approaches to conflict resolution.

Exhibit 7–1 Consensus versus Compromise

Your Outcome

The Other Party's Outcome	WIN	LOSE
WIN	Both Parties Win 1	2 You Lose and the Other Party Wins
LOSE	3 You Win and the Other Party Loses	4 Both Parties Lose

Quadrant 1: Consensus
Quadrants 2, 3, and 4: Compromise

IDENTIFYING EACH STAKEHOLDER'S HIGH-PRIORITY INTERESTS

One possible definition for the term conflict is *a situation in which two or more stakeholders have high-priority interests that cannot be achieved simultaneously.* In order to manage conflict successfully and reach consensus, it is often necessary to look one layer below the surface of apparently conflicting interests to identify the underlying expectations of each party in the exchange.

Many of the conflicts encountered by the case manager are based on a lack of clarity related to the high-priority interests of stakeholders. What professionals express as their expectations in a conflict-prone situation may not be their high-priority interests at all, but the only option they see for *achieving* their interests. High-priority interests typically represent an *end,* and the expressed expectation may be the only apparent means to *achieving* that end. In reality, there are frequently alternative means of achieving the same end that have not been explored. In this situation, unnecessary conflict can be avoided by recognizing that it is not high-priority interests that are in conflict, but rather the approaches to realizing those interests. Time and effort are frequently wasted in resolving a nonexistent conflict when the distinction between strategy and tactical approaches is not recognized.

Physicians and case managers often identify level-of-care decisions as the source of conflict in their working relationships. Case managers express concern that unnecessary costs are incurred by using critical care beds for particular patients, and physicians respond that, in their judgment, it is not safe to transfer these patients to medical–surgical units because of the need for close observation by nurses with the clinical skills and nurse-to-patient ratios found only in the intensive care unit. In this case, both the physician and the case manager are focused on the best approach to achieving safe, cost-effective patient care; it is unlikely that a fundamental conflict in high-priority interests exists. Once common high-priority interests are identified, they can serve as a starting point for conflict resolution.

Common High-Priority Interests as a Starting Point

A fundamental principle in conflict management is to *begin the dialogue by confirming high-priority interests around which the parties in the interaction are in agreement.* In the case of level-of-care decisions that have the potential to generate conflict, a logical starting point is to confirm that the physician, case manager, and other care team members share the primary objective of providing necessary patient care at the lowest cost possible without compromising quality. Beyond that high-priority interest, each member of the team may bring differing secondary interests to the decision process, and it is frequently these secondary interests that generate conflict. The case manager will almost certainly be focused on organizational objectives related to LOS targets and minimizing the possibility of payer denials. The physician will have an interest in minimizing the risk of clinical complications that could be attributed to premature transfer to a lower level of care. Ancillary professionals, such as respiratory therapists, may find it more difficult to ensure compliance with treatment regimens after patients are transferred out of the critical care unit.

The secondary interests of care team members multiply in proportion to the number of professional disciplines that are involved in the patient's care. In the case of highly complex patients with multiple comorbidities, the sources of potential conflict may appear almost infinite. The most productive starting point in resolving conflicts is for the care management team to confirm their common high-priority interests in managing the case, and to ensure that these interests are reflected in the plan of care.

Addressing Competing Secondary Interests

The optimum starting point for conflict resolution in the care management process is clarifying the common high-priority interests and also secondary interests around which there is disagreement. After these issues are articulated, the most effective approach to resolving conflict is an objective, candid dialogue among team members in which consensus can be reached related to secondary interests. The success of this dialogue will be directly proportional to the respect of team members for the perspectives of their colleagues; the degree of comfort in dialogue and decision making increases over time and reflects the developmental stage of the team.

The difficulty in reaching consensus in complex care management decisions arises precisely because there are few hard and fast rules; if such rules could be applied, these decisions and issues would be far less prone to conflict. Each patient's case must be evaluated individually, and competing interests should be evaluated as they contribute to the team's overall treatment objectives. In a climate where consensus decisions are the norm, team members will consider the perspectives of other stakeholders and voluntarily move their initial expectations closer together. As this process continues, a point will be reached where the parties in the exchange will identify a resolution that both (or all) can support.

It should be restated that consensus is fundamentally different from majority voting; the latter is seldom effective because many of these conflict situations involve only two team members and there is frequently a perceived power differential separating them, as in the case of conflict in which the primary parties are the physician and case manager. The care team must agree in advance to resolve conflict using consensus; consensus decision making cannot be forced on an unwilling participant. Majority voting may be identified in advance as a fallback position when consensus cannot be reached, but teams should resort to it only when other alternatives, including facilitation by a content expert, have been exhausted.

We have observed that when team members establish "ground rules" in advance for making decisions and resolving conflicts, consensus decisions can be made and conflicts resolved in 70 to 80 percent of all exchanges between physicians and case managers. In cases where this is not possible, one approach that is frequently effective is the use of a designated content expert to facilitate an appropriate resolution. This is one of the most significant areas in which a physician advisor can demonstrate value in the organization's care management processes. In order to provide content expertise in a wide range of clinical decision-making situations, many organizations have found it effective to contract with a panel of specialists to review cases where treatment plan or level-of-care conflicts have been identified so that they can facilitate timely resolution. The physician advisor role should be viewed as a facilitator, not an arbitrator, and physician advisor consults should be viewed as a resource for clinical decision making and conflict management rather than as the "court of last resort."

ASSESSING AND IMPROVING CONFLICT MANAGEMENT SKILLS

As stated in the introduction to this chapter, physician partnering and conflict management skills are two of the critical success factors in care management. In implementing a new or redesigned infrastructure for care management, it is valuable for the team to have a structured discussion in which they acknowledge that some conflict is inevitable in managing patient care decisions and ensuring that utilization management (UM) processes are optimized. Teams should establish ground rules for decision making and discuss the approaches they will use to resolve conflicts.

Several conflict management self-assessment tools are available for use by individuals in determining their current level of skill. It may be useful for the team to complete an assessment of their collective strengths and developmental needs related to this skill set. A team assessment should address how long team members have worked together, their prior experiences in care management, the organization's stated goals and objectives for care management, and members' individual interpersonal and decision-making styles. It is also helpful for teams in this "forming" stage to anticipate sources of conflict and to discuss guidelines and priorities they will consider in conflict management, including criteria for referral of cases to the physician advisor. Figure 7–1 summarizes some of the issues that should be addressed in the process of a team's self-assessment of its members' collective conflict resolution skills.

As is true of other core competencies, a developmental approach to conflict management skills should provide for the periodic review and assessment of progress. During the early stages of team development, it may be helpful to include an informal review and discussion in the agenda at each regular department meeting; as

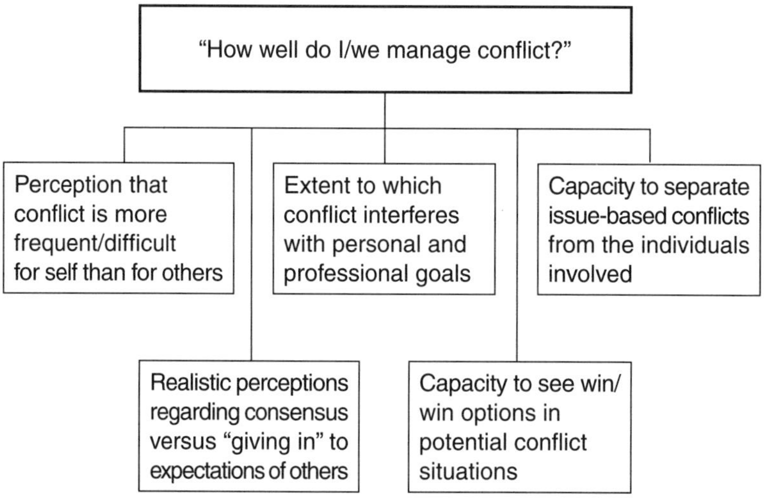

Figure 7–1 Conflict Management Self-Assessment Criteria

team members demonstrate success and gain confidence, it will be necessary to address conflict management less often. In addition to periodic review and reassessment, insight can be gained by debriefing specific cases where conflict situations arose and evaluating how these conflicts might have been managed more effectively. A formal module addressing conflict management skills should be provided as a part of the regular employee orientation program for new staff in the care management department. Directed role play with coaching and feedback is an effective means of identifying developmental needs and enhancing the conflict management skills of care management staff; the potential value of this activity is maximized if staff and key physicians can complete it together.

ESTABLISHING EFFECTIVE PARTNERSHIPS BETWEEN PHYSICIANS AND CASE MANAGERS

This section presents physician expectations of the case manager role, suggests specific ways in which case managers can increase the value they bring to their relationships with physicians, and identifies strategies for enhancing the quality of the working relationships between these key members of the care delivery team.

Physician Expectations of the Case Manager Role

Expectations of an integrated case manager role most frequently articulated by physicians fall into three general categories: real-time communication regarding patient status, identification of postacute resources, and trending and reporting of outcomes. In addressing each of these expectations, careful structuring of the case manager role and medical staff involvement determine the extent to which physicians identify case managers as valuable participants in the care management process.

Real-Time Communication

When questioned regarding their expectations of case managers, the most common response of physicians relates to real-time communication of patient status and response to treatment. Most physicians want "someone who can tell me at any time the exact status of my patient." Based on increasing patient complexity, expanded nurse-to-patient ratios, and the nurse retention challenges faced by many hospitals in recent years, physicians increasingly report difficulty in locating a single member of the care team who can provide them with a concise, timely status update on their hospitalized patients.

Despite the best efforts of nursing and other professional disciplines, fragmentation of care persists in many hospitals. This fragmentation manifests itself in incomplete communication loops, missing information, and the potential for error and rework, and it is a major source of frustration and dissatisfaction among physicians. Key clinical assessment findings, diagnostic studies pending and completed, and responses to medication are the issues around which physicians most often report difficulty in obtaining accurate and timely communication. The ability of the case manager to scan multiple information sources, synthesize patient data, and communicate concisely to physicians cannot be overstated as a high value-added competency from the perspective of physicians.

Identification of Postacute Resources

With the trend toward earlier discharge from the hospital and higher acuity on discharge, the appropriate placement of patients in postacute venues of care has become increasingly important in ensuring high quality across the continuum. Most physicians want "someone who can tell me about postacute options for my patients." This factor is also a key cost driver because physicians must have sufficient comfort with postacute plans to discharge patients within their targeted LOS.

Within the past few years, the options for postacute care have multiplied rapidly. Skilled nursing facilities are able to provide care for higher acuity patients than at any time in the past, long-term acute care hospitals are frequently able to care for even ventilator-dependent patients, and the range of services provided by home care agencies is more extensive than ever before. Simultaneous with this expanded range of options, the Balanced Budget Act of 1997 (BBA) imposed new reimbursement constraints that exert a major influence on the postacute care of patients within targeted diagnostic categories.[1]

Considering changes related to postacute care and the proliferation of new providers in many local markets, it has become increasingly difficult for physicians to maintain up-to-date information regarding all postacute venues of care, their admission criteria, and reimbursement options for each alternative care delivery setting. In order to evaluate postacute options realistically and provide sound guidance for patients and families, physicians must have access to complete and current information regarding both inpatient and ambulatory alternatives to which patients can be referred; they consistently express the expectation that case managers be able to provide this information.

In order to assist case managers in meeting this information need, the organization should maintain a catalogue of referral resources in the local service area that includes profiles of the patient population served, reimbursement options, and contacts at each facility or provider who can be contacted for further insight regarding the applicability of potential referrals. Typically, the hospital's social work staff will be the primary source of this information, and may in some cases serve as the organization's primary point of contact with community resources. Interdisciplinary collaboration and sharing of expertise are indispensable in capturing and maintaining this information in a format that is readily accessible to case managers and can be communicated to physicians as needed to facilitate prompt patient care decisions. Recently, Web-based solutions have appeared, with capabilities to electronically match patients' needs with postacute facilities, and even e-mail admission orders and treatment plans. Further, though beyond the scope of this chapter, physicians are especially well served when the case manager and hospital administration have established contracts with dedicated postacute providers who are willing to accept transfers on evenings, weekends, and holidays.

Trending and Reporting of Outcomes

Few physicians would challenge the value of an evidence-based approach to the care and treatment of patients with similar clinical profiles and needs, particularly those in high-risk and high-cost diagnostic categories. The difficulty in transition to this model of practice is obtaining the right information in a usable format and in a timely manner for clinical decision support. Provider organizations frequently find themselves "data rich but information poor," based on the tendency to invest piecemeal in information systems with less than functional interfaces and incomplete capabilities for transfer of information between clinical and financial operating platforms. Clinical and financial results are often captured and reported separately, requiring that relevant information be extracted from large volumes of data on an ad hoc basis when required. Seeking to base clinical decision making on outcome data, but unable to obtain these data in a concise, user-friendly format, physicians frequently cite outcome measurement and reporting as key components of the case manager role. Physicians want "someone who can provide me with meaningful outcome information."

Given the profusion of data available in most organizations, outcome measurement requires discipline and focus in order to ensure that only the most useful information is tracked and reported on a regular basis. The challenge is in identifying the critical few variables that will most accurately reflect the impact of care management interventions, and physicians must be involved in identifying parameters for the measurement of clinical treatment outcomes, resource utilization, and service quality/satisfaction. Considering that the value of outcome information is directly proportional to its timeliness, the organization's information system professionals should be involved in determining the approach and format for the reporting of selected outcome measures as close to real time as possible.

Approaches for Enhancing Physician/Case Manager Partnering

Strong positive relationships between physicians and case managers occasionally develop spontaneously, but we have observed that the probability of success in forging these relationships can be enhanced by clarifying mutual expectations and providing structure and support for case manager/physician teams as they work together. Recognizing that physicians consistently express expectations of the case manager role that fall into fairly predictable categories, specific approaches can be developed and implemented in order to promote an environment of collaborative practice and to solidify working relationships. These approaches relate to the selection and hiring process, methods of case manager assignment, and physician/case manager interactions related to care facilitation and UM.

Physician Involvement in the Selection and Hiring Process

In situations where a new or redesigned care management model is being implemented, there is a unique opportunity to integrate physicians into department operations, beginning with the selection and hiring of the case managers with whom they will be working. Physician involvement in the interview and selection process helps to create the optimum match in styles and approaches that is so necessary in successful case management. This observation has proven to be true regardless of the specific method used for assigning case managers. To the extent feasible, interviewing should be conducted in a panel format, and selection decisions should be based on consensus among physicians and department managers. In order for this involvement to be productive, physicians need clarity at the outset regarding the degree to which their input will influence hiring decisions.

Prior to beginning the interview process, physicians and other members of the interview panel should formulate specific questions and scenarios that can be posed to all candidates in order to build as much consistency as possible into the selection process. Open-ended questions related to the case manager role can be posed by physicians on the interview panel, and candidate responses to these questions will serve as reliable predictors of compatibility in style and approach with individual physicians. Recognizing that physicians have widely varying working styles and communication preferences, personality clashes can be minimized by striving for the best possible matches at the outset, without compromising the organization's established criteria for the case manager role. At this point, there should also be candid discussion with candidates regarding the extent to which they will be expected to accommodate and adapt to the individual preferences and styles of the physicians with whom they will work. Individuals selected to fill case manager roles have frequently held other positions in the organization, and sound judgment precludes matching case managers and physicians who have had a pattern of negative interactions in the past, regardless of their common areas of clinical expertise.

Partnering Implications of Case Manager Assignment

There are three fundamental approaches for the assignment of patients to a case manager: assignment based on attending physician, assignment based on clinical service, and assignment based on unit. (To the extent that patients with similar clinical needs are aggregated on the same hospital units, the distinctions between the last two assignment methods disappear.) There is no single "best approach" for case manager assignment; the distinctive attributes of each organization imply the need to adopt differing protocols for assignment. Each approach has its own implications for physician/case manager partnering, which should be considered in the selection process.

The assignment of case managers to individual admitting physicians or physician groups typically promotes the strongest collaborative working relationships, simply based on the percentage of time spent together managing clinically similar cases. In this model, the case manager tends to assume a role more closely resembling the physician extender than in either of the other two approaches, communication is more easily facilitated, and case managers become better able to anticipate physician preferences and practice patterns. One potential disadvantage in physician-based assignment is that conflict of interest may arise with respect to UM processes; it may become difficult for case managers whose role resembles that of a physician extender to question the physician's decisions regarding clinical appropriateness and LOS. There is a fairly high risk that case managers in this model may lapse into a physician advocate role, rather than actively pursuing the organization's resource utilization targets. A related risk arises when the physician delegates tasks to this case manager, such as arranging amenities, that are not related to case managing the patient.

The assignment of case managers on the basis of clinical service line has the advantage of limiting the number of case managers with whom most physicians interact; similarly, case managers must learn fewer physicians' practice patterns and communication styles in order to function optimally. This model also reinforces the role of the case manager as a clinical expert whose responsibilities include coaching and mentoring of nursing staff and other care team members in the management of patient care. The clinical service line approach has the potential disadvantages of inefficiency and lost time associated with an individual case manager covering multiple units; this disadvantage increases with less efficient patient aggregation. From the perspective of physician partnering, an additional disadvantage is that physicians may have difficulty interacting regularly with case managers who cover multiple units and may not consistently be available for rounding with physicians.

Case manager assignment on the basis of hospital unit is probably the most common method currently employed by health care organizations. This is the simplest and generally the most efficient approach for assigning case managers and lends itself to automation with the support of most available care management information systems. This method works best in cases where patients on a given unit have a common clinical profile and a limited number of physicians account for a high percentage of the admissions to the unit. If patient aggregation is not performed well, physician dissatisfaction results from infrequent interfaces with a large number of case managers who may lack specialized clinical expertise and are unlikely to be familiar with the individual physician's practice patterns and preferences. This service quality risk can be addressed by designating a specific case manager as the liaison to individual physicians and practices with high admission volumes.

The advantages and potential disadvantages of each method for case manager assignment, along with their implications for physician partnering, should be considered in determining which approach best fits the organization and will best facilitate positive collaborative working relationships. Efforts should generally be made to employ a single assignment method across an organization; occasionally, the option of employing more than one method in order to achieve specific physician partnering objectives can be justified. The caution is to incur the complexity of multiple assignment methods only if it has payoff in physician partnering that cannot be achieved in any other way. Regardless of the approach selected, the organization's case manager assignment methodology should be reviewed periodically and new approaches considered if important physician partnering goals are not being met.

Negotiating Approaches to Care Facilitation

In initiating new physician/case manager partnerships, it is helpful for case managers and the physicians with whom they will be working to discuss their roles and how they can best work together to facilitate patient care. Periodic scheduled meetings between physicians and case managers, preferably in the physician's office and away from the distractions of a patient care unit, can meet the need for this focused interaction. In this context, mutual expectations can be clarified and the physician's preferences for communicating patient information can be identified. Potential approaches to conflict resolution can also be discussed in an emotionally neutral environment that is not typically possible once a conflict is in process.

Interactions between physicians and case managers are considerably more productive and less time is consumed by routine information transfer when communication preferences have been identified and efforts are made to consistently communicate in the agreed-on format. Options here might include a scheduled call placed to the physician's office by the case manager near the end of the work day, batching and faxing of diagnostic reports, and messages relayed via voice mail or digital pager. Given the unpredictable milieu in which physicians and case managers practice, it is important to maintain balance between the goal of consistent communication approaches and the need for flexibility.

In their individual meetings with physicians, case managers can negotiate how daily care management activities will be carried out to best meet each of their needs. Case managers may find it helpful to script their initial physician interactions in order to make the best possible use of the time available. These discussions should include specific operational issues, such as the physician's normal rounding preferences, the case manager's role in the use of standard order sets and guidelines, and approaches for communicating with the unit-based care team.

Periodic update meetings with physicians provide a format for follow-up discussion and renegotiation of care management processes that are not consistently meeting the needs of either physicians or case managers. In order to enhance communication with physicians' practices, it is worthwhile to include their office managers in discussions related to front-end case management processes, such as preregistration and the application of clinical criteria for inpatient admission. When members of the physicians' office staff understand case management processes, they can better support the case manager's efforts to provide smooth patient transitions into and out of the acute care setting.

Infrastructure and Case Manager Role Elements to Support Physician Partnering

In addition to systematic communication and negotiation around mutual expectations, several specific elements can be built into the organization's care management roles and infrastructure to enhance the collaborative relationships between physicians and case managers. These infrastructure supports include the interdisciplinary care planning conference, pathways and guidelines, and clinical documentation.

Regular care plan conferences and discharge planning rounds have proven to be effective means of synthesizing and documenting the perspectives of the interdisciplinary team. The physician's participation in interdisciplinary care conferences, or a means of communicating key information in conferences via the case manager, will need to be discussed and negotiated. Few physicians find it possible or valuable to participate in all scheduled care conferences, but it is important to have a mechanism in place for physicians to provide their input and perspectives when complex or problem cases are reviewed. This is particularly true when patient and family expectations regarding postacute care options are unrealistic, or when significant UM concerns have been identified.

In addition to participation in interdisciplinary care conferences, physician/case manager partnerships can be supported through the consistent use of clinical pathways and practice guidelines. In order to be effective, pathways and guidelines must be developed, not only with physician participation, but also under the sponsorship of thought leaders representing a cross section of the organization's medical staff. Pathways and guidelines have failed to gain widespread support in many organizations for three reasons.

1. They are frequently complex and awkward to use.

2. They are not consistently reviewed and revised to ensure that they reflect leading practice that can be supported by current medical literature and research.
3. They were originally conceived as "care maps" by nurses, without substantial physician participation.

Carefully drafted pathways and guidelines that reflect consensus among physician leaders and that are implemented with strong physician sponsorship can enhance physician/case manager partnerships by clarifying treatment expectations and allowing case managers to intervene proactively when variances are observed. When these tools are concise and user friendly in design, they also serve as a predictable source of patient status information and as a guide for discharge planning. Physicians should be involved not only in developing the content of pathways and guidelines, but also in evaluating the final documents for format and ease of use. Pathways and guidelines should reflect the normal course of treatment for 70 to 80 percent of patients within a specific diagnostic grouping or clinical profile. Well-designed inclusion and exclusion criteria serve to identify patients whose condition or comorbidities place them in outlier status and who are likely to require a higher level of intervention by case managers. These tools enable the physician and case manager to work together efficiently and to approach the management of atypical patients on an exception basis.

When pathways and protocols are correctly designed and used, they should serve as a guide for care planning, a standard against which patient progress can be evaluated, and a format for clinical documentation by all members of the care team. By addressing essential documentation requirements, the pathway or guidelines can potentially eliminate the need for documentation in multiple locations, which is cited as a recurrent source of physician dissatisfaction. The staff time and related expense required for documentation can be minimized, and the cycle time for diagnostic and treatment procedures can be reduced. Reductions in LOS and the elimination of duplicate testing can often be attributed directly to the use of these tools.

THE CASE MANAGER AS A CLINICAL EXPERT AND STAFF DEVELOPMENT RESOURCE

One of the primary areas in which case managers can demonstrate value in supporting high-quality patient care is their potential to serve as experts in the care of a defined patient population and as coaches in helping to develop the skills of unit nursing staff and other care team members. In this capacity, case managers fill a key patient advocacy role and support physicians' interest in ensuring that the staff caring for their patients have the highest skill level possible.

Early in the care management development cycle, LOS and level-of-care decisions are high-priority concerns. A frequent source of physician reluctance to transfer patients to lower levels of care is their lack of confidence that staff in lower acuity settings have the competencies or availability necessary to provide safe and necessary care. Protracted use of critical care beds for patients following cardiovascular surgical procedures is an example of this lack of confidence; physicians frequently express concern that nursing staff on medical–surgical units are not astute in observing and reporting potential postoperative complications.

In these situations, the case manager can leverage his or her clinical skill by providing both formal and informal staff education in the normal postoperative course of treatment and specific complications for which patients should be monitored. When staff demonstrate skill in making and reporting these observations, physicians are increasingly comfortable with earlier transfer from critical care to designated medical–surgical units. Unit nursing staff may demonstrate learning needs in a number of areas: the ability to identify and respond to clinical variances, application of discharge screens, postacute treatment options, and self-care education for patients and their families.

The importance of the staff development function emphasizes the need for case managers who are expert clinicians and who can provide mentoring and coaching to other care team members. The capacity to raise the overall standard of care for a designated patient population is in fact one of the most significant ways in which case managers can demonstrate their value in collaborative practice with physicians.

MEETING THE COLLABORATIVE PRACTICE CHALLENGE

This chapter has identified potential sources of conflict inherent in the case manager role and suggested specific approaches to developing conflict management skills. The dynamics of physician/case manager interactions are prone to conflict under the best of circumstances, and in order to meet their mutual objective of providing high-quality care in the most efficient manner possible, physicians and case managers must negotiate the specifics of their approach to care facilitation. The skills required to develop high-performing partnerships are refined and enhanced over time.

Productive, collaborative partnerships between physicians and case managers seldom occur without planning and focused effort, and the challenge of working together in a complex and constrained health care delivery environment can be formidable. The key to effective partnering is recognizing that physicians and case managers each bring unique skills to the delivery of patient care; diversity in expectations, approaches, and expertise is not a liability, but an asset. By involving physicians in case manager selection and development, structuring physician/case manager interactions around the common goal of providing the best possible patient care, and employing a consensus approach to conflict management, the collaborative practice challenge can be met.

REFERENCE

1. Ernst & Young, "Post-Acute Care Primer," (Ernst & Young, 1998), 1.

SUGGESTED READINGS

D. Borisoff and D. Victor, *Conflict Management: A Communication Skills Approach* (Needham Heights, MA: Allyn & Bacon, 1997).

C. Costantino and C. Merchant, *Designing Conflict Management Systems: A Guide to Creating Productive and Healthy Organizations* (San Francisco: Jossey-Bass Publishers, 1995).

L. Marcus et al., *Renegotiating Health Care: Resolving Conflict to Build Collaboration* (San Francisco: Jossey-Bass Publishers, 1999).

N. Shister, *Ten-Minute Guide to Negotiating* (New York: Alpha Books, 1997).

CHAPTER 8

Patient Rights and Effective Communication Techniques

Darlene D. Dymond

TAKE THIS TO WORK

1. Hospital case managers touch the patient throughout the health care process in all areas affecting patient rights: access, treatment, respect, and conduct.
2. It is critical for a case manager to understand his or her own professional licensure requirements and ethical standards and to have mature insight into his or her own values and ethics. As case managers fulfill the broad and demanding tasks inherent in the role, encounters with potential conflicts of interest and ethical dilemmas are inevitable. Knowing one's self is a cornerstone in resolving ethical issues.
3. Perhaps the most important area for case managers to be cognizant of confidentiality is in the everyday work environment.
   - Access to confidential medical records should be only on a "need to know" basis. Conversations, especially telephone conversations, and team conferences can be overheard.
   - Computer screens left active can be read by unauthorized personnel, including families and visitors.
   - The use of personal reminder notes has always been a potential source of breaches in confidentiality.
4. The case manager can further serve a role in legal risk minimization.

Recognizing that not all case managers work in a traditional hospital setting, it is still appropriate to reference the acute care hospital model as a basis for discussion because the developing environments using case managers can look to the traditional acute care hospital for basics in standards and interpretive guidelines. Hospitals have been formally licensed and surveyed by national agencies for many years, thus operating in compliance with nationally recognized standards regarding patient's rights.

THE ROLE OF THE CASE MANAGER IN ADDRESSING PATIENT RIGHTS

A vast majority of hospitals have opted for the voluntary Joint Commission on Accreditation of Healthcare Organizations (Joint Commission) surveys to renew operating licenses rather than to have the local (state) Medicare contractors survey them. The Health Care Financing Administration (HCFA) has long accepted the Joint Commission survey in lieu of a "Medicare" survey because there are few differences in the standards and survey process, with HCFA's requirements being slightly more stringent but comparable. HCFA validates a certain percentage of Joint Commission surveys annually to maintain a comfort level with this long-standing relationship. It is therefore appropriate to use Joint Commission accreditation standards and interpretative guidelines as the basis for this discussion of the interrelationship of case management and patient's rights.

Other health care entities employing case management are coming under the Joint Commission's accreditation umbrella both voluntarily as a recognized statement of quality and as a regulatory compliance option, much the same as hospitals. One need only look at the list of accreditation manuals published by the Joint Commission to gain a regard for the span of its influence.[1]

- *Comprehensive Accreditation Manual for Ambulatory Care*
- *Comprehensive Accreditation Manual for Behavioral Health Care*
- *Comprehensive Accreditation Manual for Health Care Networks*
- *Comprehensive Accreditation Manual for Home Care*
- *Comprehensive Accreditation Manual for Hospitals: The Official Book*
- *Comprehensive Accreditation Manual for Long Term Care*
- *Comprehensive Accreditation Manual for Long Term Care Pharmacies*
- *Comprehensive Accreditation Manual for Pathology and Clinical Laboratory Services*
- *Accreditation Manual for Preferred Provider Organizations*
- *Comprehensive Accreditation Manual for Managed Behavioral Health Care*

The Joint Commission's standards are comparable across their range of manuals and "deal with organizational quality of care issues and the safety of the environment in which care is provided."[1(p.31)]

The overview to the "Patient Rights and Organization Ethics" chapter of the *2000 Hospital Accreditation Standards* reads:*

> The goal of the patient rights and organization ethics function is to help improve patient outcomes by respecting each patient's rights and conducting business relationships with patients and families and the public in an ethical manner.
>
> Patients have a fundamental right to considerate care that safeguards their personal dignity and respects their cultural, psychosocial, and spiritual values. These values often influence patients' perceptions of care and illness. Understanding and respecting these values guides the provider in meeting the patient's care needs and preferences.
>
> A hospital's behavior toward its patients and its business practices has a significant impact on the patient's experience of and response to care. Thus, access, treatment, respect, and conduct affect patient rights.
>
> The standards in this chapter address the following processes and activities:
>
> - Promoting consideration of patient values and preferences, including the decision to discontinue treatment;
> - Recognizing the hospital's responsibilities under law;
> - Informing patients of their responsibilities in the care process; and

---

**Source:* © Joint Commission: *2001 Hospital Accreditation Standards.* Oakbrook Terrace, IL: Joint Commission on Accreditation of Healthcare Organizations, 2001, p. 69. Reprinted with permission.

- Managing the hospital's relationships with patients and the public in an ethical manner.[1(p.71)]

Hospital case managers as described in this book touch the patient throughout the health care process in all areas affecting patient rights: access, treatment, respect, and conduct. It is therefore also appropriate to use the acute care hospital case management environment as the model for this discussion, keeping in mind that adjustments peculiar to specific industry standards and regulations will need to be made for the nonhospital environment.

Patient Rights

It has been established that case managers are not direct clinical care providers, but function more in leadership roles as resources, facilitators, planners, mediators, communicators, and teachers. In addition to knowing the Joint Commission's standards regarding patient's rights and organizational ethics, it is critical for a case manager to understand his or her own professional licensure requirements and ethical standards and have mature insight into his or her own values and ethics. As case managers fulfill the broad and demanding tasks inherent in the role, encounters with potential conflicts of interest and ethical dilemmas are inevitable. Knowing one's self is a cornerstone in resolving such issues.

The next most important step is to know one's resources. It is vital that case managers understand and refer to policies and procedures for their respective health care entity as they interact with patient issues. To help do this, case managers should develop a personal master file reference or notebook with pertinent facility policies and procedures, Joint Commission standards, HCFA standards ("Conditions of Participation"), and any other learned treatise or reference that is on point or helpful with day-to-day issues. This personal reference should be a growing "work in progress," never reaching completion because new issues are rapidly emerging. This reference should be personally maintained and differs from a departmental policy and procedure manual. It may contain policies but should also contain other references, tools, and templates for the case manager such as care guides (clinical pathways), benchmarks, articles, and statutes.

Each case manager should clearly understand his or her management chain of command and use it whenever necessary. There should also be additional facility resources such as ethics committees, patient advocates, chaplains, and support groups who provide invaluable assistance with ethical or patient's rights issues.

Each accredited hospital is required to have, and to give to each patient, a written statement of patient's rights. Many hospitals ask the patient to sign an acknowledgment of receipt of rights that is then placed into the permanent patient record. A copy of the pertinent patient's rights would be an excellent first document in the reference source section on patient's rights. Case managers are expected to advocate on the patient's behalf regarding patient's rights.

The Joint Commission's delineated patient's rights comprise the bulk of this discussion, but should not be taken as comprehensive because one must also consider statutes and regulations such as Medicare compliance requirements and insurance contracts and their respective interface with each patient/case. Other chapters of this book address content areas that intertwine with patient's rights and organizational ethics.

Joint Commission chapter standard RI.1 is "The hospital addresses ethical issues in providing patient care."[1(p.75)] The Joint Commission acknowledges that mere words are no guarantee that rights are respected and surveys hospitals by coming on site with highly specialized teams who read local policies for compliance with standards and then observe staff adherence with both philosophy and policy. Joint Commission surveyors also talk with patients (after respecting the individual patient's rights to consent and privacy). The surveyors are trained in observation techniques and are content experts. They understand vested interests in responses and are cognizant of "performance anxiety," taking both human traits into consideration as they survey a facility. Case managers must develop many of the same observational skills and knowledge sets.

Access

Given that the first intent statement in the Joint Commission hospital manual for the above-referenced standard refers to the "patient's right to reasonable access to care," it is very important that surveyors have highly refined skills and experience. Otherwise, a surveyor could not make an accurate compliance assessment. One must synthesize policies with medical records, discussions, and observations in order to ascertain compliance. It is not expected that case managers will begin their careers with a surveyor's level of expertise regarding patient rights and organizational ethics; however, the case manager's level of expertise will become developed to an expert level very quickly. Case managers are in frontline positions, ensuring facility compliance with this, and many other standards, on virtually every case they manage.

So, exactly what is access? Access refers to the admissions process, emergency department presentation, outpatient services including day surgery, and all other services offered by a specific facility. But does this mean that every patient presenting should have unlimited, on-demand "access" to anything that that patient wants? The simple answer is no.

The key term in the intent statement is "reasonable." One must consider the totality of circumstances in order to know if a specific patient has the right to specific access at that moment. Inherent in the consideration is that the case manager knows and practices according to the rules, hospital policies, medical staff bylaws, rules and regulations, Joint Commission and HCFA standards, major laws such as the Emergent Medical Treatment and Active Labor Act (EMTALA), and the HCFA/Office of the Inspector General (OIG) Corporate Compliance Guidelines. It goes without saying that case managers must be clinically competent in their respective areas.

Depending on the third-party payer where applicable, the case manager may need to be familiar with or have access to contract terms in order to assist a patient with "access" to what the facility offers. For elective services, there is potentially a significant financial impact on the patient to be out of plan. Additionally, the facility will need to make special financial arrangements with the patient if the patient is out of plan. For "noncovered services," there are also direct financial ramifications for both the patient and the facility. It is a minimum requirement that a case manager recognizes that patients have the right to know how treatment will impact financially as well as clinically, and to refer the patient to a well-versed financial counselor, as necessary.

It is vital that the case manager ensures that this patient right is not abrogated. As the access process advances, there will be points wherein the case manager can ascertain and either document or facilitate documentation regarding financial impact and any planning that is done. Proper documentation enables the business office to make better decisions on collections efforts, including properly filing with the correct carrier(s) and timely balance billing if that is permitted.

It is an expectation that with case management as described in this book, all patients will be screened for appropriateness of admission (versus proper outpatient management) and level-of-care/bed assignment at the point of access. If a physician insists that a patient who does not meet criteria still be admitted, it is not within the scope of practice for a case manager to directly override the decision. However, the case manager should know and follow the facility's formal response to such a situation. For some hospitals, there are senior house staff physicians who can be notified/consulted; for smaller general community hospitals, there may be a section or department chairperson or committee chairperson to consult. In any case, there should be utilization management (UM) guidelines for reference. The case manager's most important role in this setting may be to provide options and to facilitate patient placement, once that placement is agreed to between the patient and the physician.

For emergency access, one must consider whether it is a true emergency or just a demand service. Since 1986, under the EMTALA, patients have had the right for an emergency screening examination in any emergency room. Some health maintenance organizations (HMOs) "refused to approve a visit" and tried to have patients seek care elsewhere; some hospitals may have transferred unstable patients to plan facilities based on reimbursement. There is a trend to enact statutes requiring HMOs to pay for members to seek true emergency care outside their plan (at the closest emergency provider). There are variations on who is financially responsible if the encounter is later determined by the carrier to be nonemergent. That discussion is beyond the scope of this chapter, but is mentioned as an area regarding access that case managers should follow in the media and in local regulations and statutes. Facility legal departments can provide local guidelines and legal interpretations and should review all policies for compliance.

The EMTALA law is clear: Patients with unstable emergency conditions (including active labor) must be provided a medical screening examination and may only be transferred if they need a higher level of care that is not provided locally and if the benefits of the transfer outweigh the risks of the transfer. This brief statement is a simplification of the federal law, yet imparts the rule. The rule exists to prevent "dumping" of patients—denial of care based on purely economic reasons. Violation of EMTALA can bring civil penalties up to $50,000 for both a hospital and a physician.

Once a patient is stable, the role of the case manager is to keep the carrier informed and to coordinate a transfer, if indicated. For true emergencies and with proper documentation, most carriers will now reimburse out of plan. They will then assist with a timely transfer, in keeping with the terms of the plan. Part of what a patient agreed to when contracting with an insurance plan was to follow the plan rules. Essential to case management is the ability to assist patients within their plans to meet the goals of the treatment plan that was developed at the facility. It may be necessary for a hospital case manager to enlist the assistance of a case manager working for the insurance carrier or patient's employer to jointly achieve the best clinical and economic outcome for the patient.

In an emergency room setting, stable patients, once screened, should be consulted regarding the need for continuing care and the possible economic ramifications of being out of plan versus in a member facility. Case managers should acquaint themselves with their local hospital policies regarding such transfers, using the appropriate chain of command at the time and reviewing quality indicator monitors on an ongoing basis as continuing performance improvement measures. Recalling that the decision to admit, discharge, transfer, or treat is made by a physician and the patient, the case manager's role is to facilitate, document, and educate the patient and the care team regarding plan terms and transfer requirements.

Concrete (visible) evidence of specific compliance with patient's rights standards should reside in a patient's medical and billing records. There should be proof of receipt of a statement of rights; signed consent forms (general and informed); properly completed memoranda of transfer, if applicable; evidence of clinical teaching; and other pertinent documents specific to the case, such as "referrals." The actual role of the case manager in complying with specific patient's rights will be facility specific.

The final thing a case manager at the point of access should do is to begin discharge planning as described in Part IV and to facilitate those active treatment or diagnostic measures that can be initiated.

Access also applies to the availability of specific services. Case managers must know how to assist patients in accessing protective services and client advocacy groups. Especially in an emergency setting, direct clinical care providers are frequently focused on the physical needs of patients. Case managers may be in the best position to address the psychological, sociological, and spiritual needs of patients. Case managers are expected to make the needed referrals (e.g., social services, chaplaincy, law enforcement, interpreters, etc.) and document interventions or referrals.

As previously discussed, hospitals have had voluntary Patient's Bills of Rights (American Hospital Association) and mandatory Patient's Bills of Rights (Joint Commission) for many years. Current popular and professional literature has frequent references to the need for a Patient's Bill of Rights,[2] as evidenced by the number of bills pending before Congress as this text is being authored. Those references are directed more toward what rights a patient has in being a member of an HMO than what rights a hospitalized patient has. However, the rights are not mutually exclusive, because access to services is at the heart of the pending legislation—that and what rights to redress a patient has for wrongful denial of access to care by an insurance plan. Some states, Texas being one of them, already have a state law concerning HMO liability. It remains to be seen what effect the federal legislation will have. Under preemption, if the federal government chooses to control an area of law that is not otherwise delegated to the states by the Constitution, then the federal law will control it. Case managers should be watchful for the emerging federal control over patient's rights as they interact with HMOs.

Case managers must stay current with national and local trends and statutes regarding patient's rights. It is not enough to master a knowledge base and fail to expand that knowledge base. Case managers must proactively participate in lifelong learning and in sharing knowledge in order to properly fulfill the requirements of this exciting role.

Treatment

Patients have the right to be informed about and participate in all decisions relating to their care and treatment. Some procedures, such as surgical procedures and radiation therapy, require informed consent (documented understanding of risks, benefits, and options). Patients have the right to considerate care that is respectful of their cultural or personal values and beliefs. Patients have the right to security, personal privacy, and confidentiality of information. Patients have the right to have family (or surrogates for family/decision makers) involved and informed as directed by the patient.

Case managers are expected to work with and through direct care personnel to ensure that patients' and families' questions are answered, informed consent is obtained (actually a physician responsibility), goals are set and communicated (pathways, care guides, maps), timely teaching is provided, and appropriate after care is identified and facilitated. Because case managers are not focused on the direct tasks associated with care, they are in an excellent position to look at the broader care environment and be vigilant for the personal privacy, cultural, and professional detail issues.

Depending on the organizational model, case managers may overlap with or function as outcomes coordinators. Case managers are in a position to directly reduce delays in care and in discharge by removing barriers. By gathering outcomes data and effecting changes in outcomes through championing timely interventions and delivery of care, customer satisfaction (patients, physicians, and staff) is improved.[3] Complying with a patient's rights to quality treatment is everyone's responsibility, but case managers are uniquely positioned to effect greater compliance.

The patient's right to communication appears repeatedly in Joint Commission standards. Effective informed consent is a form of communication, as is effective patient teaching. Before one can teach, one must assess and identify needs, then document and communicate those needs. Further, patients have the right to communicate freely unless there are extraordinary circumstances that are well documented.

Effective communication is critical and includes a component of confidentiality. The rule is that the patient owns the rights to and controls the exchange of confidential information regarding him- or herself. The facility owns the paper documents, but patients have the right to access them and to control the release of that information. Exceptions to the general rule will be facility specific.

Most states permit the disclosure of relevant health care information to third-party payers in order to facilitate reimbursement. Patients usually sign a specific consent to the release of this information at the time of access to the facility. Case managers relate pertinent information along the continuum of care in order to get treatment authorized and to facilitate reimbursement. Case managers should thoroughly understand and adhere to release of information policies for their facility, paying close attention to requests for information for "quality-of-care" issues made both verbally and in writing by carriers/third-party payers and even family members. Such requests are usually beyond the scope of the case manager's role and should be referred to the local release of information professional who is probably located in medical records.

The patient's right to expect confidentiality cannot be overemphasized. The case manager has an absolute duty to maintain the confidentiality of a patient's confidential health care information. What is confidential varies slightly among states. It is imperative that case managers familiarize themselves with federal, state, and local facility requirements and release-of-information policies (another section in the personal reference notebook). Of extraordinary privacy concern is information relating to substance abuse, psychiatric care, or psychological testing, as well as any information relating to human immunodeficiency status. Case managers must recognize their professional responsibility and liability when discussing these issues and commit to memory local confidentiality requirements for the listed topics.

The Health Insurance Portability and Accountability Act's (HIPAA) final rules have been published, but no one knows exactly how they will be implemented or what the impact on hospitals and case management will be. What is known is that the regulations are onerous. What initially appeared to be rules for electronically transferred health care data for billing and reimbursement has evolved into rules controlling the release of any health care information that was ever stored or transferred electronically. Release of information must be logged. There will be many implications for case management because the UM function requires systematic release of information. Case managers should be aware that changes are imminent.

Perhaps the most important area for case managers to be cognizant of confidentiality is in the everyday work environment. Access to confidential medical records should be only on a "need to know" basis, and case related. If a case manager is not directly involved in a case, then access to that patient's records should be prohibited. Conversations, especially telephone conversations (cell phones are a major information security risk), and team conferences can be overheard. Computer screens left active can be read by unauthorized people, including family and visitors. The use of personal reminder notes has always been a potential source of breaches in confidentiality. It is a case manager's responsibility to safeguard and properly use the highly personal and confidential information entrusted to him or her.

Case managers need to know state laws and local policies involving patient's rights regarding ethics issues, conflict resolution (including billing disputes and insurance claim grievances), withholding of resuscitative services, forgoing or withdrawing of life-sustaining treatment, end-of-life issues, and participation in investigational studies or clinical trials. Specific third-party insurance contracts may need to be reviewed in order to assist patients with complete care planning. Case managers can and should consult with hospital business office personnel, insurance carrier representatives, and social workers, referring the case as appropriate.

If a patient has an advance directive (living will or medical power of attorney), it should be noted on the treatment and care plans. A copy of the document should become part of the patient's permanent medical record. If treatment has been initiated that is not in compliance with the advance directive, a case manager should bring the issue to the attending physician and take whatever other steps are appropriate under the circumstances. This potential ethical dilemma is ripe for academic discussions and legal exposure. Advance directives are intended to be instructions from the patient to health care providers if, and when, the patient is not then able to personally communicate his or her wishes. Patients have the right to have their advance directives followed.

Surrogate decision makers (holders of medical powers of attorney and guardians) stand in the shoes of the patient as decision makers and have the same rights as the patient concerning release of information. Facilities should have specific policies regarding the hierarchy of surrogate decision makers, including emergency condition professional decision makers. Having a patient's spouse give permission for treatment is not generally accepted as true consent, especially if the patient is conscious and capable of giving consent, but is just not physically present. Parents consent for minors unless there are unusual circumstances such as in consenting for blood transfusions for children of Jehovah's Witnesses. In that case, there will be specific facility policies that track state law, usually directing contact with the local form of children's protective services.

Respect

Patients have the right to expect care in response to their requests and needs, to the extent that that care is within the hospital's capacity, stated mission and philosophy, and relevant laws and regulations. When a hospital cannot provide the care a patient requests, the patient has the right to be fully informed of his or her needs and the alternatives to care.[1] The case manager will not necessarily be the person who informs the patient, but may be the one who reminds the care team, including the physician, that a patient has this right.

It has been well documented that a patient's psychological, spiritual, and cultural values affect his or her response to care. The medical treatment plan and nursing care plan should respect an individual patient's clinical, psychological, spiritual, and cultural aspects. Barriers to learning and language barriers should also be addressed. Case managers who are planning for the continuum of care will need to consider all of these aspects in order to provide for a comprehensive, best practices case plan.

Treatment and care plans inherently contain physical and clinical information and goals. Case managers, as coordinators of care, should ensure that all pertinent patient's rights be addressed and documented. As the patient advances through the continuum of care from prehospital to posthospital, special needs and values should be communicated early. For instance, if a patient has special holy days, discharging a patient on that day and expecting the patient's home and family to admit or focus on home health equipment deliveries is inappropriate.

Case managers are in an excellent position to anticipate and facilitate regarding special needs because the case manager may be the only person who "sees" the entire patient.

Conduct

Patients have the right to expect the actual provision of care to be conducted in a manner that is as comfortable and safe as possible. If case managers note deviations from standards of practice, they should intervene appropriately. Newly enforced patient safety requirements (sentinel event/root cause analysis) are beyond the scope of this chapter, but are mentioned to alert case managers that they, too, are patient advocates, risk managers, and quality managers. Case managers should familiarize themselves with the patient safety policies in their facilities.

Complaints or questions from patients or their families should be investigated and referred or handled effectively. Careful and complete documentation is as important regarding case management issues, including payer contacts, as is clinical documentation. Complaints and dispute resolution should be documented according to facility policies. The need for and style of documentation is more fully described in Chapter 11.

Because case managers are expected to see and talk to patients and their families, they should be able to form longer term relationships than shift personnel can and more fully understand the patient's response to treatment and how the patient interacts with the environment. Patients have the right to a discharge plan that returns them to a safe and therapeutic environment. Case managers are responsible to facilitate that process. When unsafe or nontherapeutic conditions arise, case managers should document these issues and make appropriate referrals to social services and to law enforcement agencies as indicated.

Case managers should locate or develop high-risk screening tools to assist them in addressing this area of patient's rights. A library of these tools should be in the personal reference manual for immediate location and use.

Primary job expectations for case managers include knowing what rights patients have and ensuring that patients are not disenfranchised as they advance through the continuum of care.

Ethics

A discussion of patient's rights is incomplete without a reference to ethics. Ethics is a philosophy term referring to the branch of philosophy that deals with understanding approaches to morality. Ethics are based in values and provide guidance in decision making.[4] The Joint Commission RI.1 Standard previously quoted used the term "ethical issues." Every accredited hospital must have written statements of organizational philosophy, mission, values, and goals. Case managers should add these statements of corporate bases of decision making to their personal reference sourcebooks, and, more importantly, should interview the corporation before being hired to ensure personal matches. Ethics statements form the structure for the case manager's efforts. Patients have the right to expect that hospitals act in an ethical manner, in a business sphere, with clinically competent staffs, and with due respect to the individual patient.

Federal corporate compliance guidelines mandate minimal health care organizational business ethics and may be found in the OIG's Corporate Compliance Guidelines. Most case managers should have been exposed to formal corporate compliance training during hospital orientation because one preventative strategy against health care fraud and abuse allegations and penalties is to have a formal mandatory corporate program in place.

For case management students who are curious about the fascinating field of health care ethics, there is currently much discussion of this topic in the popular press and in professional literature. One can hardly pick up a professional journal without seeing an article such as "Ethical Decision Making in Healthcare Management"[4] or "Ethical Guidance in the Era of Managed Care: An Analysis of American College of Healthcare Executives' *Code of Ethics*."[5] Because ethics are based on personal values, one should not expect "one answer fits all" guidance, but should expect more structured questions and overlapping answers to issues as one studies health care ethics.

There are no hard answers to ethical issues. Case managers have broad backgrounds and can draw from their education and experience to address ethical issues. Many times, the role for the case manager is to recognize that an issue exists and to facilitate the proper referrals. Case managers cannot be "everyman," but should try to acknowledge and respect every patient's personal values and needs.

LEGAL IMPLICATIONS ASSOCIATED WITH CARE FACILITATION AND DISCHARGE PLANNING

Case managers should not be either panicked or cavalier concerning legal issues associated with case management. They should use their professional standards, basic knowledge of legal requirements associated with corporate compliance, sound clinical judgment and expertise, critical thinking skills, chain of command, local policies, and ethics to make decisions. If what is right for the patient is kept at the forefront, case managers should avoid needless concerns about possible legal exposure. That said, it is still pertinent to educate case managers as to what areas of legal exposure exist, especially because criminal sanctions as well as civil penalties and recoveries are potential ramifications of case management that violates the law or breaches standards of care.

One small chapter in a book on case management cannot thoroughly cover health care law. In the same vein, case managers are not expected to be lawyers, but should be able to recognize legal issues. For more extensive discussions of pertinent law in a case manager's jurisdiction, the case manager should consult with the facility's legal department. Laws differ among the states, and federal districts interpret laws differently from one another. Jurisdictional differences and rapidly emerging law related to HMOs make it impossible to provide definitive "black letter law." Identification of legal issues for case managers is the goal.

Who doesn't know someone who has been sued for professional malpractice? Who hasn't heard of the Medicare fraud and abuse criminal prosecutions? A brief overview of both types of potential exposure follows but is not intended to be a complete discussion. Case managers should engage in self-study and should consult with their respective facility departments for definitive guidance. Popular and professional literature is replete with information on what legal liabilities are associated with health care, but should be read with the caveat that jurisdictional differences may apply and that health care law is changing.

Professional Malpractice

What professionals know as "malpractice" are actually the civil causes of action (cases) based in negligence that concern liability for physical (sometimes emotional) harm. There are common law causes of actions and statutory ones. This distinction may only be of interest to the legal community, but to the health care professional, a list of causes of action related to their field is helpful. For case managers, the emerging actions related to managed care are pertinent. Although physicians are more at risk, case managers should be aware of negligent discharge issues, wrongful denial of care or access, breach of contract, breach of confidentiality, negligent referral, and failure to properly refer. The traditional negligence causes of action that are related to direct nursing tasks such as taking vital signs negligently or not at all are not at the forefront for case managers, but should not be forgotten. Case managers are still using basic professional skills that can result in actionable causes if they are done negligently and damages occur.

Rarely, health care professionals are involved with the intentional torts ("wrongs") of assault, battery (remember the patient's right to informed consent?), or intentional infliction of emotional harm. These causes of action may not be covered by professional liability policies because they are willful, requiring "intent" rather than "plain negligence."

What is important for case managers to know about generic negligence or malpractice requires the following elements. There must be a (professional) standard (of care) that is breached that leads to an injury with damages that are identifiable/quantifiable. Legal scholars argue if there are three, four, or five elements; however, the ones listed above are always there. The differences are punctuation and dependent clauses. If a case manager has attended a legal seminar that taught three elements, that individual should neither be alarmed nor throw away the materials, but should review the materials with the understanding that semantics do not elevate form over substance.

Breaches of standards may be errors of omission or commission; they may be mistakes. They may occur in a professional setting (on the job) or under good samaritan or emergency circumstances (i.e., at home or at an accident scene with a health care professional bystander who renders care).

Case managers can use the information discussed earlier in this chapter and throughout this book to provide a basis for practice that is designed to diminish legal and risk exposure. There are no guarantees. The key is to know one's job; to always do it thoroughly and properly, without shortcuts; to provide proper objectives and quantifiable and verifiable documentation avoiding subjective, judgmental, or conclusory statements; and to respect patient's rights.

Fraud and Abuse

Criminal causes of action in health care are of major concern because insurance and Medicare fraud and abuse have become of primary interest to the OIG. Case managers should seek the facility's corporate compliance plan and training. If one does not exist, that facility is at high risk for an investigation with potentially severe penalties.

Very specific common law (case made law), statutory, and contract laws related to case management are state and locally specific. Case managers should seek local expert resources and should add the important policies, guidelines, and legal interpretations affecting them to their personal reference book. Important areas for concern are the concepts of tortuous interference with contracts (like telling a patient his insurance plan is bad where that discussion causes that patient to change plans), negligent referral, wrongful denial of access, and negligent UM.

As previously discussed, if a case manager is following professional standards and local policies, risk exposure to that individual should be minimal. If all professional practice occurs within the employment setting (course and scope of the job), the case manager is considered to be the agent/"servant" of or under the control of the employer, making the employer the party responsible for damages under the law. This is called the doctrine of *respondeat superior*. Even though the employee (here, the case manager) may be named (sued individually), the employer will defend and pay any damages and costs of defense. It is an individual decision for a case manager whether to carry private malpractice insurance. This is a topic that should be discussed with one's personal legal counsel.

Criminal acts are not covered by malpractice insurance. Repeat, not covered. Whether an employer will cover legal expenses related to criminal defense of its employees is a gamble no professional wants to take. Criminal attorneys must be paid in advance, and good criminal defense does not come inexpensively (financially or emotionally). At the level in the organization where a case manager functions, facility coverage for criminal defense is unlikely unless many levels of management are involved (indicted) and the facility wants to protect itself. Even then, there is no guarantee that some level of management will not be sacrificed or "scapegoated." Again, this is an area of potential risk that one does not want. The message here is to avoid engaging in criminal behaviors and to avoid employment situations that are suspect.

State professional licensing defenses following civil or criminal actions are rarely covered by insurance, but will certainly follow even successful defenses. Again, if a case manager is using good judgment and common sense, following policies and treating people with respect and dignity, and communicating well, legal exposure should be at a minimum.

THE IMPACT OF SPECIFIC COMMUNICATION STYLES ON MANAGING AND FACILITATING CARE

At the point in a case manager's career wherein he or she has achieved the level of knowledge and practice sophistication necessary to tackle case management, one should have been exposed to and mastered the basics of communication. In no way intending to reduce the importance of the information in the first part of this chapter, an illustration from Winnie-the-Pooh on communication will be used to show the universality yet simplicity of the information. One can turn to communications texts and other professional literature and will not find much more than the rules attributed to Winnie-the-Pooh, according to Roger E. Allen in *Winnie-the-Pooh on Management*.[6]

In the book scenario, Piglet and Pooh are discussing what day of the week follows Tuesday. Pooh reasons that Wednesday follows Tuesday, but Piglet recalls that last year, Christmas followed Tuesday. As the conversation continues, Piglet and Pooh encounter Tigger and ask him what day it is, hoping that it is Christmas because yesterday was Tuesday, but fearing that they are unprepared if it is indeed Christmas. All the while, they are supposedly looking for a stranger in the woods; a stranger who has a picnic basket and lunchtime is approaching. They begin to remember that they should be "establishing objectives and organizing" and get further distracted from their subject, becoming inattentive listeners, as they separate to look for the stranger. Tigger soon returns, telling Pooh that he has found the stranger. Pooh fusses at Tigger, asking why Tigger has not brought the stranger with him and claiming that Tigger has now caused them to waste time. Tigger's response to why he has not brought the stranger back with him when he returned is:

> "You didn't say to find him and come right back. You said to find him and then we would meet here for lunch. Which is now. I remember distinctly you said that."
>
> "Bother! You misunderstood me," said Pooh.
>
> "If you didn't mean what you said," Tigger pointed out logically, "then you should say what you mean."[6(p.69)]

Pooh's earlier conversation had been, "our objective should be to find him. . . . After we have looked, we'll meet back here just before lunch."[6]

There followed discussion of what communication is. It was described as telling everyone working on a project what is happening. From the discussion, the group developed a list of five communication rules that serve well in any environment, including case management. Universal rules serve many disciplines well, and who is willing to dispute the wisdom of Winnie-the-Pooh? If it works for Winnie and his pals, it should certainly work for the rest of us.

Pooh's "Rules for Effective Communication"*

- To communicate, there must be an exchange of information.
- All information exchanged should be as clear and complete as possible.
- The information should be meaningful to the individual who is receiving it.
- Always get confirmation that the message you are communicating has been understood.
- Information can be given in many ways. The more ways you use, the clearer and more believable it will be. However, the message must be the same in all ways. It is vital to be consistent. Remember, actions speak louder than words.[6(p.81)]

Direct implications for case managers are in direct communication with patient and families, among the health care team members, with carriers' representatives, via the medical records, and with referral sources. Calm, businesslike demeanor and control will serve a case manager better than will reactive, hurried half thoughts. The person speaking knows what he or she wants to communicate and may start midthought. It is therefore important to validate understanding so that effective communication can occur.

Ineffective communication can have disastrous effects on patient care and one's success as a case manager. Communicating with difficult people is a challenging opportunity, but one that must be faced and conquered. One must remain in control and remember that effective communication is the goal. Some tips for communicating with difficult people follow:

- Think before speaking.
- Be patient and allow others to speak.
- Control one's own behavior.
- Do not argue or disagree but ask questions.
- Model control and tranquility.
- Acknowledge feelings but control behavior.
- Use deliberate movements and lowered tones of voice and remain focused.

Case managers should be adept communicators/communications facilitators, developing their communication skills, paying special attention to listening actively, and carefully participating in and validating the exchange of infor-

**Source:* "Rules for Effective Communication," from *Winnie-the-Pooh on Management* by Roger E. Allen, copyright © 1994 by Roger E. Allen. Used by permission of Dutton, a division of Penguin Putnam, Inc.

mation. Even shy people can learn how to be effective communicators. In a professional setting, it can be easier because the focus is on professional goals and not on the case manager, personally. If extraordinary assistance is desired, case managers should look to community resources such as Toastmasters or adult-learning speech classes for support.

Personal style can be an asset to communication style, or it can be a drawback. Mature professionals will seek feedback on their individual styles in order to enhance the communication and case management process. Preparing for structured communication can help to avoid becoming diverted from the subject and causing goals to be forgotten.

There are no magic formulas to successful communication all the time and with every encounter. Case managers must recognize when communication has stalled and return to that topic because progress toward goals may also have stalled.

Patient's rights are inextricably intertwined with all areas of case management. There are legal risks associated with improper job performance. Astute case managers will undoubtedly see more aspects of rights than have been discussed, and that is to be expected. The goal of this chapter was to raise an awareness of issues. Case managers should hone their skills and practice within their professional standards and policies, thereby ensuring good communication and excellent case management that respects patient's rights.

REFERENCES

1. *2000 Hospital Accreditation Standards (*Oakbrook Terrace, IL: Department of Publications, Joint Commission on Accreditation of Healthcare Organizations, 2000).
2. R. Sorian and J. Feder, "Why We Need a Patient's Bill of Rights," *Journal of Health Politics, Policy and Law 24,* no. 5 (1999): 1137.
3. K. Johnson and L. Schubring, "The Evolution of a Hospital-Based Decentralized Case Management Model," *Nursing Economics 17,* no.1 (1999): 29–48.
4. K. Peer and J. Rakich, "Ethical Decision Making in Healthcare Management," *Hospital Topics: Research and Perspectives on Healthcare 77,* no. 4 (1999): 7.
5. W. Higgins, "Ethical Guidance in the Era of Managed Care: An Analysis of the American College of Healthcare Executives' *Code of Ethics*," *Journal of Healthcare Management 45,* no. 1 (2000): 32–41.
6. R. Allen, *Winnie-the-Pooh on Management* (New York: Dutton, 1994).

CHAPTER 9

Regulator Impact on Daily Work Flow

Judith M. Wilczewski

TAKE THIS TO WORK

1. Government-sponsored health insurance programs such as Medicare and Medicaid are in a state of accelerating evolution.
2. Rigorous management of care delivery and utilization are as important for patients with Medicare and Medicaid as for patients with commercial insurance coverage.
3. Effective case management will become even more important as Medicare expands the use of prospective payment systems and providers assume greater financial risk for the delivery of health care services.
4. Medicare often "sets the standard" for rules that govern the use of health care services that other insurance payers are likely to emulate, either in full or in part.
5. The Health Care Financing Administration maintains a useful reference site (www.hcfa.gov) for government programs and regulatory updates.

A working knowledge of Medicare and Medicaid and specifically the rules and guidelines enacted under these two programs that impact the daily care of patients, is fundamental to effective case management in the preacute, acute, and postacute care settings. This baseline level of knowledge is important for at least three reasons:

1. Medicare and Medicaid programs provide health care coverage to a large proportion of individuals consuming health care services in the United States.[1]
2. The delivery of high-quality, cost-effective health care services to older adults, indigent clients, and/or individuals with disabilities (the primary recipients of Medicare and Medicaid benefits)[2] can create significant challenges for providers of health care services.
3. Medicare often "sets the standard" for rules that govern the use of health care dollars for the delivery of health care services that other insurance payers are likely to emulate, either in full or in part.

The Balanced Budget Act (BBA) of 1997 created dramatic changes in the way that Medicare

Acknowledgments: Special acknowledgment and gratitude is extended to E. Dirk Hoffman and Barbara Klees, U.S. Department of Health and Human Services, Health Care Financing Administration, Office of the Actuary, for their invaluable guidance in refining portions of this chapter.

and Medicaid programs operate, the most substantive changes since the two programs were established in 1965.[3] BBA legislation improved access to health care services for those individuals with the greatest need, but also established new rules for reimbursement that place an even larger proportion of the financial burden for delivery of health care services on hospitals, home care agencies, and other providers of health care services. This chapter is intended to provide case management staff with a "nuts-and-bolts" overview of the Medicare and Medicaid programs, and to convey a baseline level of knowledge about Medicare and Medicaid that will be useful in day-to-day case management activities. Additionally, information provided will serve to increase general awareness about the significant changes created by the BBA that will impact the way care is delivered and how providers are reimbursed for health care services.

Several aspects of Medicare and Medicaid that are particularly relevant to case managers during the course of their daily activities will be covered, including program eligibility, enrollment, and coverage; case review requirements; management of observation status; hospital-issued notice of noncoverage (HINN); denial and appeal processes; the Medicare Special Planned Readmission (MSPR) rule; government-sponsored health insurance program quality initiatives; and issues of fraud and abuse. Numerous provisions of the BBA that are equally relevant include increased availability of health care services, increased availability of preventive care services, the role of Medicare+Choice, expansion of prospective payment system (PPS) reimbursement plans, and the Hospital Transfer Rule.

Information presented in this chapter was derived primarily from the Health Care Financing Administration (HCFA) source documents (via the HCFA, Medicare, and Medicaid Web sites), as well as the Cap Gemini Ernst & Young Care Management Training core curriculum. Information is intended only as a high-level overview and introduction to Medicare and Medicaid programs for case management staff. Because government-sponsored programs tend to be complex and evolutionary, the actual implication or application of any Medicare or Medicaid program rule, requirement, or guideline should be reviewed regularly and applied within the context of each unique health care environment. Addresses for HCFA, Medicare, and Medicaid Web sites are provided at the end of the chapter.

MEDICARE AND MEDICAID

Medicare

Medicare was enacted under Title XVIII of the Social Security Act in 1965. It is a federally funded health insurance program that is regulated and overseen through the Department of Health and Human Services (DHHS) by HCFA. Medicare provides health insurance coverage for most older adults, many individuals with disabilities, or individuals with end-stage renal disease.[4,5] Eligible recipients of Medicare may enroll for coverage in three major categories.

1. *Medicare Part A*[6,7] (Table 9–1) or hospital insurance (HI) covers inpatient hospital, skilled nursing facility (SNF), home health, and hospice care services. Medicare Part A is financed primarily through mandatory Federal Insurance Contributions Act (FICA) payroll deductions. The program also receives income from other less substantive sources. Inpatient hospital services provided under Medicare Part A are limited by a "benefit period."[8,9] A benefit period starts when a patient enters the hospital and ends after a period of 60 days without provision of acute inpatient or skilled nursing care service. A patient is eligible for 90 days of hospital care and 100 days of skilled nursing care during a benefit period. There is no limit to the number of benefit periods during a recipient's lifetime as long as the recipient remains eligible for Medicare Part A coverage.

   In addition to the defined inpatient hospital benefit, Medicare recipients can elect to use "lifetime reserve" days.[10,11] The lifetime reserve day option provides Medicare coverage for additional inpatient hos-

Table 9–1 Medicare Part A Covered Services

Service Venue	*Covered Service*	*Limitations*	*Recipient Responsibilities**
Inpatient hospital care	• Bed and board • Nursing and nonphysician services • Drugs and biologicals • Supplies, appliances, and equipment • Diagnostic and therapeutic services • Physical, occupational, and respiratory therapy and speech pathology services	Pays for up to 90 days of inpatient hospital care in each benefit period and nothing beyond the 90th day**	For each benefit period: • A total of $776 for a hospital stay of 1–60 days • $194 per day for day 61–90 • $388 per day for days 91–150** (if the patient opts to use nonrenewable "lifetime reserve" days) • All costs for each day beyond 150 days
Skilled nursing facility care	• Similar to inpatient covered services • Inpatient rehabilitation services • Appliances	• Admission must occur within 30 days following 3-day inpatient hospital stay • Skilled nursing or rehabilitation services after a 3-day hospital stay for up to 100 days in a participating facility in each benefit period	For each benefit period: • Nothing for the first 20 days • Up to $97 per day for days 21–100 • All costs for each day beyond 100 days
Home health care	• Part-time or intermittent skilled nursing care • Part-time or intermittent home health aide • Physical and occupational therapy • Speech-language pathology services • Medical social services • Medical supplies (not drugs or biologicals) • Durable medical equipment (DME)	Requires documented plan of treatment and periodic physician review	• No deductible or copay • 20% of approved amount for DME
Blood	• Blood replacement		Payment for or replacement of first 3 units

continues

Table 9–1 continued

Service Venue	*Covered Service*	*Limitations*	*Recipient Responsibilities**
Hospice care	• Physician and nursing services • Medical equipment and supplies • Drugs for symptom control and pain relief • Short-term in-hospital respite care • Home health aide and homemaker • Physical, occupational, and speech therapy • Social work counseling and support • Dietary counseling • Treatment for illness not related to terminal illness	Available to terminally ill Medicare recipients with life expectancy less than 6 months who elect to forgo standard Medicare benefits	• A copayment of up to $5 for outpatient prescription drugs • 5% of the Medicare payment amount for inpatient respite care

*Deductibles and copayments in effect in 2000.

**Medicare may provide inpatient overage for days 91–150 if the patient elects to use "lifetime reserve" days. Lifetime reserve days create an option to extend Medicare inpatient coverage for an additional 60 days after covered inpatient days have been exhausted for a benefit period. Use of lifetime reserve days is nonrenewable/a one-time option and requires a copayment of $388 per lifetime reserve day used.

Note: Medicare & You 2001 has been released along with 2001 deductibles and coinsurance amounts, which are now in effect.

pital days when hospitalization extends beyond 90 days during a single benefit period. Each Medicare beneficiary may elect to use days of Medicare coverage from a nonrenewable lifetime reserve of up to 60 (total) additional days of inpatient hospital care. Individuals can make the decision to use the lifetime reserve provision either prior to hospital admission or concurrently during a hospital stay, but the Medicare beneficiary retains sole discretion as to whether he or she uses this option. Hospitals have the responsibility to notify patients when they are approaching lifetime reserve day eligibility and must also notify patients that they can elect *not* to invoke this provision. A copayment is associated with use of lifetime reserve days.

2. *Medicare Part B*[12,13] (Table 9–2) or supplementary medical insurance (SMI)

Table 9–2 Medicare Part B Covered Services

Covered Service	*Recipient Responsibilities**
Medical and other services not covered under Part A • Physician services • Outpatient medical and surgical services and supplies • Diagnostic tests • Ambulatory surgery center facility fees • Durable medical equipment (DME) • Ambulance services	• Monthly premium ($45.50)** • Annual deductible ($100) • 20% of approved amount after deductible, except in the outpatient setting
Preventive services	
1. Annual screening mammogram for all women over the age of 40	1. 20% of Medicare approved amount/no Part B deductible
2. Pap smear/pelvic examination/clinical breast exam once every 3 years or every year for those at high risk	2. No coinsurance/no Part B deductible for the Pap smear; 20% of Medicare approved amount for other services/no Part B deductible
3. Colorectal cancer screening a. Annual fecal occult blood test b. Flexible sigmoidoscopy every 4 years c. Colonoscopy every 2 years if at high risk d. Barium enema instead of sigmoidoscopy or colonoscopy	3. a. No coinsurance/no Part B deductible b–d. 20% of Medicare approved amount after annual Part B deductible
4. Diabetes monitoring (includes coverage for glucose monitors, test strips, lancets, and self-management training)	4. 20% of Medicare approved amount after annual Part B deductible
5. Bone mass measurement for those at risk for osteoporosis	5. 20% of Medicare approved amount after annual Part B deductible
6. Vaccinations a. Annual flu shot b. Pneumococcal vaccination c. Hepatitis B vaccination if at high risk	6 a. No coinsurance or Part B deductible b. No coinsurance or Part B deductible c. 20% of Medicare approved amount after annual Part B deductible
7. Prostate cancer screening a. annual digital rectal exam b. prostate specific antigen (PSA) test	7. a. 20% of Medicare approved deductible after annual Part B deductible b. No coinsurance/no Part B deductible

continues

Table 9–2 continued

Covered Service	*Recipient Responsibilities**
Physical/occupational/speech therapy services	20% of the first $1,500 for PT/OT services All charges above $1,500
Clinical laboratory services • Blood tests • Urinalysis	No copayment or deductible
Mental health services	50% of charges for most outpatient mental health services
Home health care services • Part-time skilled care • Home health aide services • DME supplied by HHA while receiving Medicare covered HHC • Supplies and services	No copayment or deductible for services 20% of approved amount for DME
Outpatient hospital services • Services for the diagnosis or treatment of an illness or injury	Set copayment amount based on outpatient prospective payment system ambulatory payment category schedule
Blood needed as an outpatient	First 3 units—payment or replacement Additional units—20% of the approved amount after deductible

*Deductibles and copayments in effect in 2000. (Deductibles and copayments may vary if the patient has chosen to enroll in Part C/Medicare+Choice.)

**In some cases, the cost of Part B monthly premiums may increase by 10% for each 12-month period that an individual could have had Part B but did not take it.

Note: Medicare & You 2001 has been released along with 2001 deductibles and coinsurance amounts, which are now in effect.

provides coverage for the professional component of inpatient and outpatient physician services, outpatient laboratory and X-ray services, durable medical equipment, and other services necessary for care but not covered by Part A. Part B is financed primarily through premium payments ($50 in 2001) and contributions from the U.S. Treasury General Fund.

3. *Medicare "Part C"*[14,15] or *Medicare+ Choice,* enacted through the BBA, allows eligible recipients enrolled in both Medicare Part A and Part B to opt for enrollment in private sector health plans including health maintenance organizations (HMOs), provider-sponsored organizations (PSOs), preferred provider organizations (PPOs), or other publicly or privately managed, risk-based health plans that meet specific government requirements for participation. Medicare+Choice is a more stringently administered Medicare risk program that replaces previously established Medicare risk products. Financing of Part C is more complex and is dependent on the type of plan chosen.

Many services are not covered under standard Medicare. Examples of services not covered include outpatient prescription drugs, custodial care, annual physicals, routine foot care and orthopaedic shoes, most dental care and dentures, hearing aids, routine eye care, cosmetic surgery, or health care obtained while traveling outside of the United States. Medicare+Choice programs may provide some traditionally excluded services, like prescription drug coverage, and other traditionally excluded services, such as custodial care, may be available to Medicare recipients who are also eligible for Medicaid.

Provider Reimbursement for Medicare Services

Since 1983, Medicare has employed a prospective payment mechanism for the reimbursement of hospital services called diagnosis-related groups (DRGs). Under the DRG PPS, Medicare provides hospitals with a predetermined payment for each inpatient admission based on the DRG classification "as long as the admission is medically necessary," although additional outlier payments may be available for cases of extraordinary inpatient duration and complexity.[16] Under the DRG PPS, hospitals make a profit on some cases and incur a loss on others.

PPSs are designed to encourage providers of health care services to deliver care to patients more prudently. Like DRGs, ambulatory payment classification (APC) is the outpatient prospective payment system (OPPS)[17] enacted through the BBA to guide payment for hospital-based services provided in the outpatient setting. More information about OPPS and APCs will be provided later in this chapter. Other PPSs have or will soon be used to reimburse providers for delivery of skilled nursing, rehabilitation, and home health services.

Medicaid[18,19]

Medicaid was created under Title XIX of the Social Security Act, also in 1965. Like Medicare, Medicaid is an entitlement program designed to provide health insurance coverage for a defined recipient population, in this case low-income individuals who would otherwise have little or no access to health care services. Unlike Medicare, Medicaid is financed through both state and federal matching funds and, although the program is overseen by HFCA, each state is charged with administering its own program.

Within federally defined parameters, individual states have discretion in deciding who is eligible for Medicaid assistance in their state, as well as the type, amount, duration, and scope of services provided to eligible recipients. For states to be eligible for federal matching funds, they must provide Medicaid assistance to specific groups of individuals and must make available a minimum set of basic health care services to eligible recipients. Mandatory basic services include[20(p.3)]

- inpatient and outpatient hospital, physician, laboratory, and X-ray services
- family planning, prenatal care, nurse–midwife, pediatric, and family nurse practitioner services
- vaccines for children
- nursing facility services for individuals age 21 or older and home health care services for those eligible for skilled nursing services
- rural health clinic and federally qualified health-center services

Additional federal matching funds may be available for states that choose to provide additional optional services or that opt to expand coverage to a broader population base.

States have discretion to limit the amount and duration of services provided by their Medicaid program, but only to the extent that the level of service provided is sufficient to achieve the purpose of the benefit, and that set limits do not discriminate by medical condition or diagnosis. The practical application of this information and an understanding of available services for your patients will require a thorough understanding of your own state's Medicaid program.

ELIGIBILITY, ENROLLMENT, AND SUPPLEMENTAL SECURITY INCOME (SSI) INFORMATION

Government-sponsored entitlement programs employ stringent criteria for enrollment and eligibility for covered services.

Medicare Eligibility[21,22]

In general, individuals become eligible for Medicare coverage if they or their spouse have worked for at least 10 years in Medicare-covered employment, are age 65 or older, and are a permanent resident of the United States. Younger persons may become eligible for Medicare if they have a disability or have been diagnosed with chronic renal failure requiring dialysis or transplant. Some otherwise ineligible individuals may opt to pay a premium to enroll in Medicare.[23]

Eligibility for Part A Benefits[24]

Individuals may begin receiving Part A Medicare benefits at age 65 without having to pay a premium if they (1) are already receiving retirement disability benefits from Social Security or the Railroad Retirement Board, (2) are eligible to receive Social Security or Railroad Retirement benefits but have not yet filed for them, or (3) have worked (or have a spouse who worked) in Medicare-covered employment. Persons under the age of 65 may be eligible for Part A benefits without having to pay a premium if they received Social Security or Railroad Retirement Board disability benefits for a period of 24 months or have end-stage renal disease requiring dialysis or transplant. Some individuals age 65 or older and certain individuals with disabilities who are earning too much to continue receiving premium-free Part A coverage are eligible to continue coverage by electing to pay a premium.

Eligibility for Part B Benefits[25]

All individuals eligible for Medicare Part A are also eligible for Medicare Part B. Enrollment in Medicare Part B is voluntary and requires payment of a monthly premium ($50 in 2001) that is automatically deducted from Social Security or Railroad Retirement checks.

Eligibility for Medicare+Choice (Part C)[26,27]

Individuals with both Medicare Part A and Part B may opt to enroll in Medicare+Choice. Enacted by the BBA, Medicare+Choice offers Medicare Part A and B recipients the option of enrolling in private sector health plans (HMOs, PPOs, or private unrestricted fee-for-service plans) for delivery of health care services. Organizations that provide coverage under Medicare+Choice must meet specific administrative and financial requirements in order to participate. Additionally, Medicare+Choice programs must provide the minimum current Medicare package of benefits, may offer additional nontraditional Medicare covered services, and often offer lower deductibles and/or copays to participants.

Medicaid Eligibility

Medicaid eligibility requirements and services provided vary from state to state and within individual states over time; however, federal government matching funds are provided to state Medicaid programs only if health care coverage is provided to the following "categorically needy" mandatory groups of individuals:[28,29]

- individuals meeting Adult Families with Dependent Children (AFDC) Program requirements that were in effect on July 16, 1996
- infants born to Medicaid-eligible pregnant women
- children under the age of six and pregnant women whose family income is at or below 133 percent of the federal poverty level
- Social Security income recipients in most states
- recipients of adoption or foster care assistance under Title IV of the Social Security Act
- special protected groups
- children born after September 30, 1983, under the age of 19 whose family income is at or below the federal poverty level
- certain other Medicare beneficiaries (Qualified Medicare Beneficiaries and Specified Low-Income Medicare Beneficiaries)

States are eligible to receive additional federal matching funds by providing Medicaid coverage to broader categories of individuals defined as "categorically or medically needy." Individuals defined as "categorically related optional"[30,31] are similar to the mandatory group with enrollment eligibility defined more broadly (Exhibit 9–1).

Individuals defined as "medically needy"[32,33] also emulate the mandatory group profile but have income and/or resources that exceed the maximum eligibility level set by the state. Matching funds are available to states that extend Medicaid coverage to the medically needy only if the state provides a minimal level of services and coverage to specifically defined groups of individuals.

Spend Down[34]

Spend down is a provision that enables an individual to qualify for Medicaid assistance even if his or her income or assets exceed state-defined income eligibility requirements. Each state defines the maximum income eligibility requirements for Medicaid. An individual whose income exceeds this threshold can spend down to meet eligibility on a monthly basis, or eligibility may be established by payment of a monthly premium to the state in an amount "equal to the difference between total income (reduced by unpaid medical expenses) and state-defined income eligibility requirements."[35(p.2)] Each month, when medical expenses equal or exceed the spend-down amount, Medicaid can help cover the remaining expenses. Medical expenses that count toward the monthly spend-down amount include doctor visits, inpatient or outpatient medical care, prescription drugs, medical supplies and equipment, laboratory and X-ray services, health insurance premiums (including Medicare premiums), and the cost of transportation to medical appointments. Married couples have a combined spend-down amount, with both sets of expenses counting toward meeting monthly spend-down amounts. The medical expenses of a parent count toward the monthly spend-down amount for children under the age of 18 or a student age 18 to 20.

State Children's Health Insurance Program (SCHIP)[36]

The State Children's Health Insurance Program (SCHIP) was created under the BBA. The goal of this program is to assist states in extend-

Exhibit 9–1 Categorically Related Optional and Medically Needy Medicaid Coverage

- Categorically related optional groups share characteristics similar to the mandatory recipient group, with eligibility criteria more generously defined.
- Medically needy meets most standard Medicaid eligibility requirements except that resources/income exceed state eligibility threshold.
- Federally defined groups that may be covered under categorically related optional include the following:
  - Infants up to age 1 and pregnant women not covered under mandatory rules whose family income is less than or equal to 185% of the federal poverty level (FPL) (percentage amount set by each state)
  - Children under age 21 who meet AFDC income and resource requirements in effect in their state as of 7/16/1996
  - Institutionalized individuals eligible under a special income level (set by each state, up to 300% of supplemental security income (SSI) federal benefit rate)
  - Individuals who would be eligible if institutionalized but are receiving care at home or in the community
  - Certain aged, blind, or disabled adults who have incomes above those requiring mandatory coverage but below the FPL
  - Recipients of state SSI
  - Certain working-and-disabled persons with family income less than 250% of the FPL who would qualify for SSI if they did not work
  - Tuberculosis-infected persons who would be financially eligible for Medicaid at the SSI level if they were within a Medicaid-covered category (limited to TB-related ambulatory services and drugs)
  - Optional targeted low-income children included within the State Children's Health Insurance Program (SCHIP) established by the BBA
  - Medically needy persons

ing health care coverage to previously uninsured, low-income children by developing a separate SCHIP or expanding coverage through existing Medicaid programs. Again, the federal government allows state autonomy in determining eligibility requirements and service availability within strictly defined parameters (Exhibit 9–2).

Medicare Enrollment[37,38]

Medicare enrollment is handled either automatically or by application. Medicare enrollment is automatic when a Medicare card is mailed directly to eligible recipients 3 months prior to their 65th birthday or eligibility date; for both Medicare Part A and Part B if the recipient is not age 65 but already receiving Social Security or Railroad Retirement benefits; and for both Medicare Part A and Part B, if the individual has a disability, with coverage beginning in the 25th month of the disability.

Application for Medicare enrollment is required if an individual is not receiving Social Security or Railroad Retirement benefits three months before turning age 65 or is diagnosed

Exhibit 9–2 State Children's Health Insurance Program

Program Requirements	Child Health Assistance Coverage Requirement

• Includes all current levels of coverage available to children as well as all state initiated programs targeting uninsured children
• Coordination with public and private children's health insurance programs
• Defined operational methods
  • To establish eligibility
  • For eligibility screening
  • For enrollment
  • For delivery
  • For ensuring quality
  • To ensure access to services
  • Of outreach to families of eligible children
• Description of cost-sharing arrangements that meet the following requirements:
  • Medicaid limits apply
  • Income-related sliding scale (lower costs for lower income individuals and higher costs for higher income individuals)
  • Annual aggregate cost for all children in a family cannot exceed 5% of family's annual income
  • Not permitted for well-baby or well-child care, including immunizations
	"Benchmark" coverage
	• Equivalent to standard BC/BS preferred provider option offered under federal employees health benefit program
	• Health benefit plan available to state employees
	• HMO plan with the largest commercial enrollment in the state
	
	"Benchmark-equivalent" coverage
	• Equivalent to the aggregate actuarial value of benchmark packages for and includes the following services
	  – Inpatient and outpatient hospital services
	  – Physicians' surgical and medical services
	  – Laboratory and radiology services
	  – Well-baby and well-child care
	  – Age-appropriate immunizations
	• 75% of aggregate actuarial value of the benchmark package for the following services:
	  – Prescription drugs
	  – Mental health
	  – Vision and hearing services
	
	Existing comprehensive state-based coverage defined as:
	• Administered by the state and receives state funds
	• Offered in New York, Florida, or Pennsylvania
	• Offered on the date of enactment of this title
	• Provides a range of benefits and has an actuarial value equal to or greater than its value on 8/5/1997 or the value of one of the benchmark benefit packages
	
	Eligibility cannot be denied based on preexisting illness

with end-stage renal disease requiring dialysis or a kidney transplant. General enrollment periods are held January 1 through March 31 of each year. Part B coverage begins the July following enrollment.

Medicaid Enrollment

Because the amount, duration, and eligibility requirements for Medicaid coverage vary from state to state and within a state over time, a succinct description of Medicaid enrollment guidelines is not possible. In general, individuals may become eligible immediately once they meet mandatory or categorically needy criteria or they may be required to spend down excess income on medical expenses to meet the threshold eligibility level established by each state. Individual eligibility may occur retroactively up to three months prior to a change in condition (making them eligible for coverage) and ends at the end of the month in which circumstances no longer match eligibility requirements.

Medicare and Medicaid Enrollment

Individuals may qualify for health care benefits under both Medicare and Medicaid programs.

> Medicare beneficiaries who have low income and limited resources may receive help paying for their out-of-pocket medical expenses from their state Medicaid program. Various benefits are available to "dual eligibles," those persons who are entitled to Medicare and are eligible for some type of Medicaid coverage.
>
> For persons who are eligible for full Medicaid coverage, the Medicaid program supplements Medicare coverage by providing services and supplies that are available under their state's Medicaid program. Services that are covered by both programs will be paid first by Medicare and the difference by Medicaid, up to the state's payment limit.[39(p.3)]

SSI[40]

SSI is a government-sponsored program administered by the Social Security Administration. SSI is provided to qualifying elderly, blind, or disabled individuals on a monthly basis. As of January 1, 2001, the government provides a monthly SSI check of $530 for individuals or $796 for couples (the same in all states) to which individual states may contribute additional amounts. In order to qualify for SSI, total income and assets cannot exceed a predefined level: $2,000 for an individual and $3,000 for a couple. Among other assets, available cash, bank accounts, stocks, and bonds, are included in the calculation of this threshold asset/income level. Qualifying for SSI also means that the individual or couple may qualify for food stamps and Medicaid.

DIFFERENTIATION OF TRADITIONAL VERSUS MANAGED MEDICARE/ MEDICAID[41]

Traditional Medicare generally employed a fee-for-service mechanism of payment with payment provided for all services consumed. Managed Medicare and managed Medicaid programs place greater emphasis on more coordinated care options through HMOs and other types of private health plan contracting. The goal of managed Medicare and managed Medicaid is to bring down the cost of health care by increasing the financial risk carried by providers of health care service, while improving care by imposing a more rigorous set of quality checks and balances. The emphasis on managed Medicare was expanded through the BBA with the creation of Medicare+Choice, a program that replaces previously established Medicare risk-based programs. Medicare+Choice is intended to provide consumers with the choice of participating in an even greater variety of private health plans that may offer a wider array of health care services (like prescription drugs) and/or lower deductibles and copayments than does traditional fee-for-service Medicare.

Health plan options available within managed Medicare and Medicare+Choice include HMOs, point-of service (POS) plans, PPOs, PSOs, private fee-for-service plans, and medical savings accounts (MSAs). Organizations that provide coverage under Medicare+Choice must meet specific administrative and financial requirements in order to participate, and the availability of Medicare+Choice plans varies by locality. Along with the expanded list of available plan options are a more comprehensive set of quality assurance requirements, more safeguards against fraud and abuse, and greater risk for plan liability and/or nonrenewal of contracts.

Traditional fee-for-service and managed Medicare programs both provide all basic Medicare services including Part A covered services and both preserve all basic Medicare rights and protections. The two programs may vary concerning availability and choice of plan or physician, referral requirements, choice around Part B service participation, coverage of patients with end-stage renal disease, amount of out-of-pocket expense, and the need for supplemental coverage and availability of additional service coverage, including coverage for outpatient prescription drugs. Table 9–3 provides a comparison of traditional versus managed Medicare.

REVIEW REQUIREMENTS[42,43]

Medicare does not require precertification or preauthorization for health care services unless the patient is enrolled in a managed Medicare plan, but entering into an agreement to become a Medicare provider implies assurance that care and services provided to recipients are both medically necessary and delivered without restriction or bias. Except in the case of SNFs, Medicare requires implementation of a formal utilization review (UR) program to ensure that medical necessity requirements are met. Providers may implement UR programs internally or may contract for these services, but once assuming this responsibility, become liable and responsible for ensuring responsible utilization management (UM), including ensuring appropriateness of admissions and delivery of medically necessary care. Because hospitals (and now SNFs, hospital services provided in the outpatient setting, and home health care services) are reimbursed on a PPS basis, it is in the hospitals' interest to monitor utilization regardless of the requirement. Disciplined UM is and will become more essential to ensure clinical appropriateness and optimal length of stay (LOS) and resource utilization for the Medicare population. Sound management of resource utilization can translate into increased financial stability for health care organizations.

Unlike Medicare, Medicaid UR requirements may vary from state to state, but like Medicare, a sound UM program[44] is essential to the delivery of cost-effective care to this high-risk population. Case management staff are invaluable to the UM process for Medicare and Medicaid populations by ensuring clinical appropriateness, facilitating the delivery of health care services, expediting early discharge planning, and supporting comprehensive documentation of the patient's clinical condition in the medical record.

Admission Review

Both Medicare and Medicaid programs provide coverage for services that are clinically necessary to diagnose and treat illness. Inpatient hospital care will be covered only if the patient meets defined inpatient admission criteria. Individual physicians and hospitals are responsible for deciding whether a patient meets inpatient admission criteria and for making the decision whether to admit the patient to the hospital for treatment. The determination of admission appropriateness should be based on consideration of the patient's medical history and current medical needs, including the severity of the presenting condition, current signs and symptoms, and available alternatives to inpatient care. State peer review organizations (PROs) determine standard clinical appropriateness criteria that will be used for Medicare and Medicaid populations within each state and make the final determination whether clinical appropriateness criteria were met through an audit of inpatient records. PROs were established under the Tax Equity and Fiscal Responsibility Act (TEFRA)

Table 9–3 Traditional Medicare versus Managed Medicare

	Traditional Medicare (Fee-for-Service)	*Managed Medicare*
Availability	Nationwide	Limited to defined service areas
Choice	Any Medicare-participating doctor, specialist, or hospital	Limited to plan participants
Referral for service	Not required	• Required for specialty services • Some increase choice through point-of-service plans
Part A services	Covered	Covered
Part B services	Optional	Mandatory
End-stage renal disease patients	Covered	Excluded unless ESRD develops while enrolled in managed Medicare plan
Out-of-pocket expense	Annual deductible Monthly Part B premium if applicable 20% copayment with each service visit	Monthly Part B premium Possible extra monthly premium in addition to Part B premium $5–$10 copayment with each service visit
Supplemental coverage	Employee coverage Retiree coverage MediGap insurance	Not required
Basic Medicare services	Covered	Covered
Additional service coverage	Not available	Depending on plan
Coverage for outpatient prescription drugs	Not available	May be available in some plans
Medicare rights and protections	Preserved	Preserved

in 1982 as a mechanism for monitoring health care service utilization and controlling quality of care delivered. Hospital/PRO agreements are a prerequisite to receiving Medicare payments under PPS.[45]

Medicare requires that all Medicare-covered inpatient admissions be reviewed for clinical appropriateness within 24 hours. Admission review entails application of PRO-defined clinical appropriateness criteria to ensure that admission is necessary and that placement for care occurs in the most appropriate venue and level of care. Clinical appropriateness criteria provide a measure of the severity of patient illness and the intensity of service required to diagnose or treat the patient's condition. Medicare assumes that physicians and hospitals admit only patients who meet clinical appropriateness criteria, bill only for services actually provided, and that billed services are clinically necessary to diagnose or treat the presenting illness. If a PRO-initiated medical record review is performed for any reason, and medical necessity or clinical appropriateness cannot be established, organizations are at risk of losing reimbursement and/or incurring a monetary penalty.

Concurrent Review

With the exception of managed Medicare, Medicare generally does not explicitly require additional or continuing care reviews; however, by virtue of their participation in the Medicare program, organizations assume the risk for managing the care of Medicare-covered patients and the costs associated with delivering that care. Concurrent review is considered good practice for all Medicare cases. Does the patient continue to meet criteria for inpatient care? Does the patient continue to meet criteria for the current level or venue of care? Does the patient meet discharge readiness criteria? Depending on the answer to these questions, case management staff must work with the attending physician and members of the multidisciplinary care team to clarify the patient's current status and determine the most appropriate alternatives for care. In some circumstances, it may be appropriate to involve physician advisors or physician liaisons in order to ensure that all available information is clarified, and that an appropriate plan of care is identified, implemented, and accurately documented in the medical record.

Retrospective Review

State PROs have the right to request any number of medical records for review for any reason (see the section on mandatory case review later in this chapter), and providers have an obligation to provide medical records for review on request.[46] Whatever the initial intent of the review, organizations become subject to intensified scrutiny by the PRO if, during those reviews, it is determined that cases have not been well managed or if there is a concern about quality. Intensified reviews commonly focus on the following:[47]

- quality of care concerns
- inappropriate admissions, continued stays, and discharges
- inappropriate transfers or readmissions
- DRG validation
- appropriateness of hospital-issued notices of noncoverage

MSPR Rule[48]

The MSPR Rule combines two admissions into one for purposes of billing if a patient is readmitted to the hospital on an elective basis for a procedure or treatment directly related to the prior admission. This rule was enacted to ward off financially driven fragmentation of health care services. The MSPR Rule is applied (1) unless the patient's medical condition prohibits therapy or treatment during the initial inpatient stay, (2) unless the patient is undergoing a staged procedure (e.g., chemotherapy), (3) unless the patient desires a second opinion or time to consider options, or (4) if an interim inpatient admission occurs between the first admission and the subsequent planned readmission. This rule applies primarily to Medicare patients, but other payers, including Medicaid in some states, have adopted this provision. Case management staff should be aware of the use of this rule in their locality and be sensitive to the possibility that patients returning to the hospital within 31 days could be subject to the planned readmission status, and that the hospital may not be reimbursed for a second admission. When the planned readmission is appropriate, case management staff can help to ensure appropriate reimbursement by coaching clinical staff on the importance of clearly documenting the indications and rationale for readmission.

HOSPITAL-ISSUED NOTICES OF NONCOVERAGE (HINN)[49]

It may be determined during preadmission review that a patient does not meet medical necessity or clinical appropriateness criteria for inpatient admission. In such cases, provider organizations may issue a formal notice of noncoverage. A hospital-issued notice of noncoverage is a formal mechanism of informing patients that they do not meet Medicare requirements for admission and so will be held financially liable for the cost of inpatient care. Preadmission notices of noncoverage can be issued by the hospital without concurrence of the admitting physician or PRO. When patients are issued a notice of noncoverage, they must be informed about their liability for the cost of care. Additionally, it is incumbent on hospital staff to work with and inform patients about alternative care resources, help to identify means of obtaining those services, and document all relevant interventions and interactions in the medical record.

Hospital-issued notices of noncoverage may also be indicated and issued after the patient has been admitted to the hospital during a concurrent review. For example, a patient or his or her family member may refuse discharge or placement to a clinically appropriate lower level of care. Medicare will not cover services that do not meet medical necessity criteria, and hospitals have the right to notify patients of impending financial liability in these circumstances. Unlike notices of noncoverage that are issued prior to admission, the hospital must seek concurrence from either the attending physician or the PRO when issuing this notice to a patient in the inpatient setting. Documentation must support that the patient and/or family had been informed of the planned discharge or placement within a period of time reasonable to prepare. Documentation must also support availability of and assistance with obtaining alternative resources, venues of care, or health care services. PROs determine each state's specific rules surrounding hospital-issued notices of noncoverage, but in general, patient liability begins the third day following receipt or issuance of the notice.

DENIAL AND APPEAL PROCESS[50,51]

Medicare issues denials through state PROs. Denials are issued for clinically inappropriate care and medically unnecessary inpatient and outpatient hospital services identified through retrospective chart reviews. In such circumstances, the PRO will issue a preliminary notice of denial, allowing the organization an opportunity to respond and request reconsideration of the denial in the form of an appeal prior to a final denial decision. Unless organizations respond to preliminary denials, the PRO will assume agreement and a formal confirmation of denial will be issued.

OBSERVATION STATUS

The term *observation status* is very specific. Observation is intended to specify a level of care associated with evaluation and decision making about a diagnosis that is more accelerated than inpatient care. Observation is an outpatient designation. Observation status is used to determine the need for possible inpatient admission.

The *Medicare Hospital Manual* defines outpatient observation services as "services furnished by a hospital on the hospital's premises, including use of a bed and periodic monitoring by a hospital's nursing or other staff, which are reasonable and necessary to evaluate an outpatient's condition, or to determine the need for a possible admission to the hospital as an inpatient. Such services are covered only when provided at the order of a physician or another person authorized by state licensure law and a hospital's bylaws to admit patients to the hospital or to order outpatient testing."[52]

Observation Management and Documentation Requirements[53,54]

Medicare and Medicaid guidelines for management and documentation of observation status are very similar. Generally, patients are placed in observation status only if their condition is expected to stabilize, or a determination about the need for inpatient admission can likely be made within 24 hours. Observation status may be extended for up to 48 hours if the patient is not stable enough for discharge but does not meet criteria for inpatient admission. Patients can be converted from observation status to inpatient admission if they meet inpatient criteria;

however, patients can never be converted from inpatient admission to observation status. Observation status is never to be used as a substitute for an appropriate inpatient admission nor for the convenience of the hospital, its physicians, their patients, or the patient's family.

Patients on observation status may be placed in observation units, in nonobservation units, or in rapid treatment units. Some states have become much more stringent in their definition of what is allowable for observation. For example, in the state of New York, patients must be placed in a bed and cannot remain on a stretcher. Case management staff should familiarize themselves with rules that apply locally.

Medicare-required documentation associated with observation status is also very specific. There must be an appropriately worded written order in the medical record clearly stating placement in observation status. Use of the term "placement in observation status" or simply "observation status" versus "admit to observation" may help to avoid confusion and errors in appropriate patient typing and the need for retrospective correction.

All documentation must be geared to the patient's diagnosis or condition. A progress note stating the specific clinical criteria and indications for observation status must be documented in the medical record on admission and again within two to eight hours of placement. Documentation must reflect that medical personnel, including the physician, were actively involved in observing, treating, and reassessing the patient's condition at a frequency greater than once or twice per shift. Physician involvement and supervision of the care of patients placed in observation status is expected and must be documented. In addition to the initial assessment outlining indication for placement in observation status, two personal evaluations (not including the initial evaluation, but possibly including the discharge evaluation) are required. All written orders, physician progress notes, and nursing notes must demonstrate consistency with regard to why the patient is being observed, the plan of treatment, the patient response to treatment, outcomes of interventions, and plans for discharge. Exhibit 9–3 provides guidelines for observation status medical record documentation.

Observation status is an outpatient service and is billed as such. Hospitals may never bill outpatient observation services in conjunction with another service or procedure that is already covered (diagnostic testing/ambulatory procedure) unless the patient becomes medically unstable or experiences complications as a result of the procedure and requires additional observation to stabilize or determine need for admission. Billing for a patient encounter that is inconsistent with the documentation of treatment provided in the medical record constitutes billing fraud. The issue of fraudulent billing has become a more substantive issue for Medicare because of negative experiences surrounding inappropriate use of observation status over the past several years. For this reason, HCFA has revitalized an interest in this area and has begun to perform intensified reviews, increasing the risk for organizations where inconsistency between documentation and coding exists or inappropriate use of observation status occurs.

The BBA created additional complexity to the management of observation status. As part of the OPPS Rule enacted through the BBA, HCFA not only reinforced its previously defined position that observation status cannot be reported separately from a scheduled procedure unless the patient experiences a complication or becomes medically unstable, but it also defined certain "inpatient only" procedures that will not be reimbursed if they are performed in an outpatient setting. Additionally, and until hospitals can demonstrate responsible use of the designation, the BBA eliminated separate payment for observation status overall. These new rules do not exempt providers from using observation status when appropriate based on clinical circumstances, but instead create incentive for greater vigilance and propriety use of this designation.

The intent of these rules reinforces HCFA concerns regarding the inappropriate use of observation status historically as well as the belief that certain procedures should not be performed on an outpatient basis. More detail regarding the BBA is presented at the end of the chapter; how-

Exhibit 9–3 Medicare Observation Status Documentation

Observation Status Documentation Guidelines

- Documentation must reflect the reason why patient requires observation status.
- Documentation must reflect that medical personnel were actively involved in observing, treating, and reassessing the patient's condition. This implies assessment and intervention with frequency greater than every 4 hours.
- Documentation must reflect that a physician is actively involved in the care of the observation status patient.
- Physician and nursing documentation outlining why the patient is being observed, the plan of treatment, and the patient response, including the following, should be consistent:
  - signs/symptoms, pertinent history, lab tests, assessment and rationale supporting the judgment to use observation status
  - changes in the patient's condition
  - pertinent clinical findings on reexamination
  - assessment/interpretation of lab and radiology findings
  - patient's response to treatment
  - changes in the therapy plan
  - change in the anticipated time the patient is to be kept in observation
  - services provided to the patient, dated and timed
  - changes in symptoms
  - changes in the anticipated status on discharge
  - discharge planning assessment
  - post hospital plan of care, including instructions to patient and family
  - patient's discharge disposition

Observation Status Documentation Requirements

- Written order to place patient in observation status including date, time, and signature of physician or another person authorized by state statute and medical staff bylaws to admit patients or order testing
- Initial progress note defining clinical indication for observation status placement, why patient is being observed, the plan of treatment, and patient response/outcome
- At minimum, two additional physician evaluations outlining patient status, diagnostic and treatment services provided, outcomes, and patient response (the second to occur 2–8 hours following initial placement)
- Discharge note outlining final status, response to treatment, and rationale for discharge or patient admission

ever, such changes reemphasize the importance of remaining up-to-date on evolving health care rules and create an added challenge for case management staff as they attempt to do what is in the best interest of the patient and ensure appropriate reimbursement for services delivered.

ENSURING QUALITY

Medicare Quality[55]

The DHHS, under the administration of HCFA, oversees a number of initiatives designed to ensure the quality of care that is provided to Medicare recipients. These quality improvement programs fall under the auspices of the Health Care Quality Improvement Program (HCQIP) and are implemented through state PROs. HCQIP initiatives target improvement efforts in four distinct categories defined as national health care priorities, state and local health care priorities, health care services provided in nonacute care settings, and managed care. Additionally, PROs provide quality improvement consultation to local providers.

Cooperative Quality Improvement Projects[56]

Working through state PROs, cooperative quality improvement projects are an effort by HCFA to actively improve the quality of care that is delivered to Medicare recipients by examining and improving health care delivery processes. PROs, working in partnership with providers, focus on improving care for conditions of high prevalence within the Medicare population and incorporate "performance-based contracts with PROs to improve patient outcomes nationwide"[13] based on performance goals set under the Government Performance and Results Act (GPRA). Improvement efforts are based on industry leading practice, and cooperative projects may be focused on inpatient or outpatient and based on provider, physician practice, payer, or community. In the year 2000, national quality improvement projects focused on acute myocardial infarction, breast cancer, diabetes, heart failure, pneumonia, stroke, and reducing health disparities within the Medicare population.

Medicare "Sixth Scope of Work"[57]

In addition to working with individual providers on cooperative quality improvement projects, HCFA has expanded its focus to achieve statewide improvement in seven areas of strategic importance to the Medicare population. This program, identified as the sixth scope of work, targets seven strategic areas for focused improvement:

1. decrease mortality rates for persons hospitalized with heart attack
2. increase mammography rates
3. increase influenza immunization rates
4. increase pneumococcal immunization rates
5. increase rate of dialysis for patients with chronic renal failure
6. improve care for patients with diabetes
7. improve assessment and care of patients with heart failure in 2001

The sixth scope of work is financed by HCFA and implemented through state PROs, which work with local partners to determine the most effective way to achieve statewide improvement results.

Payment Error Prevention Program (PEPP)[58]

The Payment Error Prevention Program (PEPP) is a plan that is designed to reduce payment errors and protect the Medicare trust fund by monitoring PPS hospital claims and educating providers about payment errors. First, a baseline state error rate is estimated and state-specific data are reviewed to determine problem areas. Then, corrective payment error prevention projects and intervention strategies are developed to prevent future errors. The initial focus of PEPP includes miscoded DRGs, medically unnecessary or inappropriate care, unnecessary admissions and inappropriate transfers, premature discharges resulting in readmission, and inadequate documentation. Each PRO has autonomy and responsibility for identifying state-specific problem areas, determining areas for focused review, reviewing data, requesting improvement plans, and monitoring the success of plans through profiling and further reviews. Phased implementation of PEPP began in August of 1999.

Ensuring Quality through Mandatory Case Review[59]

HCFA employs a mechanism of mandatory case review to ensure that the care provided to Medicare recipients is reasonable and necessary and that recipients are not being denied service on any basis other than medical necessity. Acting through state PROs, HCFA requires that certain case types undergo mandatory review. PROs are required to respond to all written complaints. Reviews can be conducted for care delivered in any setting. Once investigated, PROs provide detailed feedback to beneficiaries regarding quality-of-care or medical necessity issues. When an instance or pattern of substandard quality or inappropriate or unnecessary care is identified, PROs will work with providers in question (hospitals, individual physicians, etc.) to initiate a corrective action plan. Certain case types trigger mandatory case review. These case types include those most likely to create clinical quality, medical necessity, and/or fraud and abuse concerns.

Beneficiary Complaints/Referrals. PROs receive individual patient complaints as well as referrals from HCFA regional offices, Medicare intermediaries, carriers, and the Office of the Inspector General (OIG) requesting review for clinical quality and/or medical necessity issues. Such referrals trigger investigation into a possible event or pattern of fraud, waste, and abuse.

Dumping Violation. The Emergency Medical Treatment and Active Labor Act (EMTALA) was enacted to prevent designated providers of emergency services from turning away any patient requiring emergency medical treatment or in active labor. The law states that hospitals must post a sign in the emergency room specifying rights of the individual with respect to examination and treatment for emergency conditions and women in labor. Violation of this law constitutes "dumping" and will prompt a mandatory PRO hospital review.

Alleged Fraud and Abuse. PROs will perform a review of any case where fraud and/or abuse is alleged and will offer an opinion with regard to clinical quality, clinical appropriateness, and/or medical necessity.

Higher Weighted DRG Adjustments. PRO reviews are performed on all cases of hospital-requested claims adjustments that result in a higher weighted DRG assignment. The PRO will evaluate the diagnosis, procedures performed, and assigned codes to ensure that they are substantiated by documentation in the medical record.

Hospital-Issued Notices of Noncoverage. PROs will review any case of hospital-issued notices of noncoverage to ensure that the denial of admission or extension in LOS or service is based on clinical appropriateness and medical necessity and not on financial incentives.

Medicaid

Like Medicare, state Medicaid programs have an interest in ensuring that quality care is delivered to Medicaid recipients. In general, Medicaid quality screens tend to focus on patient mortality, and surgical and medical complications, the dimensions around which Medicaid programs typically assess the quality of services provided by acute care hospitals. These three dimensions are often included in Medicaid managed care plan reviews.

Medicaid has a particular interest in preventing financially driven premature hospital discharge. Medicaid uses specific parameters as "red flags" for potential premature discharge:

- defined vital sign thresholds and suspicious physical findings
- presence of unexplained abnormal test results
- sudden and unexplained discontinuation of high-intensity therapeutics
- significant alteration in treatment made immediately prior to discharge
- evidence of discharge situation inadequate for patient safety

If any of these conditions are present but do *not* represent a significant contraindication to discharge, the physician should document carefully the rationale behind the decision to discharge in the medical record. Case management staff can help to identify potential red flags, intervene in potentially inappropriate discharges, or help safeguard the organization against unfounded allegations of inappropriate discharge by helping clinical staff understand the need for comprehensive documentation that supports clinical decision making.

FRAUD AND ABUSE

Fraud is "intentional deception or misrepresentation that an individual knows to be false or does not believe to be true, and makes, knowing that the deception could result in some unauthorized benefit to him/herself or some other person."[60] Abuse includes "incidents or practices of physicians or other providers or suppliers of services, that are contrary to sound medical practices, that directly or indirectly result in some improper gain, unnecessary costs to the program, or program payment for services that fail to meet recognized standards of care or are medically unnecessary."[61]

HCFA is increasing the level of scrutiny around issues of potential fraud and abuse. Areas of special attention include billing for services not rendered; misrepresenting a diagnosis to justify payment; soliciting, offering, or receiving kickbacks; unbundling or exploding charges; falsifying certificates of medical necessity, plan of treatment, and medical records to justify payment; or billing for a service that was not furnished.[62] Case management staff are in a position to safeguard organizations against allegations of fraud or abuse by working closely with the health care team to ensure rigorous utilization and case management as well as complete and appropriate medical record documentation.

IMPLICATIONS OF THE BBA OF 1997[63]

The BBA was enacted with the intent of reducing Medicare spending, extending the life of the Medicare trust fund, increasing health care options for senior citizens and children, enhancing Medicare-covered wellness benefits, and increasing HCFA's attack on Medicare fraud and abuse. The creation of Medicare+Choice and the Program of All-inclusive Care for the Elderly (PACE) increased health care options for the elderly. The creation of the SCHIP increased access to health care services for low-income children. Under the BBA, Medicare Part B now covers additional preventive services including screening mammography, Pap smears, and pelvic exams; prostate and colorectal cancer screening; diabetes self-management programs; risked-base use of bone mass measurement; and the expansion of vaccination outreach programs.

A key strategic objective of BBA legislation was to shift a greater proportion of financial risk for the Medicare program to the private sector. That goal will be accomplished through the expansion of PPS programs for reimbursement of inpatient rehabilitation, SNF, hospital services provided in the outpatient setting, outpatient rehabilitation, and home health care services. Activating PPSs in these venues of care imposes the same incentive for ensuring clinical quality, rigorous utilization, and cost management as currently exists for acute inpatient care.

Hospital Transfer Rule[64]

The Hospital Transfer Rule is an example of a rule that was set up through the BBA to prevent hospitals and other health care organizations that also own home health agencies and other postacute care services from "double dipping." The Hospital Transfer Rule redefines the movement of patients from PPS facilities to postacute care providers (SNFs, PPS-exempt hospitals, and home health) as "transfers" as opposed to "discharges" for 10 designated DRGs (Exhibit 9–4).

As a result, the hospital DRG case-rate payment is essentially reduced to a per diem rate that usually results in lower total reimbursement to the hospital. Hospitals will get paid less than the full DRG payment when patients are transferred "early" to postacute venues. Payment for these postacute transfers cannot exceed the sum of 50 percent of the regular transfer payment and 50 percent of the regular DRG payment. The

Exhibit 9–4 10 DRGs Affected by the Hospital Transfer Rule

DRG 14	Cerebrovascular Disease except TIA
DRG 113	Amputation R/T Circulatory System Disorders
DRG 209	Major Joint Limb Reattachment of Lower Extremity
DRG 210 + 211	Hip and Femur Procedures w & w/o cc
DRG 236	Fracture of the Hip and Pelvis
DRG 263 + 264	Skin Graft &/or Debridement for Ulcer w&w/o cc
DRG 429	Organic Disturbances & Mental Retardation
DRG 483	Tracheotomy except face, neck, & mouth Dx

transfer rule can be applied to home health if the home health care service is for the same condition for which a person had an inpatient stay and is delivered within an appropriate time period.

OPPS[65–68]

The BBA created a prospective payment system for outpatient services that are performed in the hospital setting. The unit of payment used in outpatient prospective payment systems (OPPS) is the APC, which plays a role in outpatient hospital reimbursement similar to that of DRGs for inpatient. APCs group outpatient services that are alike from a clinical and resource utilization perspective. Like DRGs, APCs use a fixed or lump-sum payment mechanism. Unlike DRGs, multiple APCs can be assigned to a single claim. A complex set of rules (based on HCFA Common Procedure Coding System modifiers, revenue center, service unit, service date, condition codes, and type of bill) are required to determine the final APC payment rate. Beneficiary copayment amounts are "capped" under OPPS legislation, emulating the 80/20 Medicare/beneficiary payment responsibility mix.

APCs[69,70]

APCs are determined by a combination of CPT/HCPCS codes, involved body system, and the nature and relative cost of the procedure or service. Ambulatory surgeries and procedures, ancillary diagnostic services (other than clinical laboratory), medical visits, most drugs, and implantable items and supplies are "packaged" into their related APC and not paid separately. The "unit" for an APC is a visit, and a visit is defined as a single date of service. There is no "bundling" of services provided on other dates. Multiple APCs may be assigned for a given visit.

Unlike inpatient DRGs, some APCs are always paid at 100 percent of their schedule. Other APCs are subject to a 50 percent reduction when other procedures are performed on the same date. Each HCPCS code is assigned a "payment indicator status." This indicator determines how each HCPCS code will be paid within the context of other codes that may be reported (Table 9–4). Additional APC payments may be made for significant procedures performed in the emergency department or clinic that may increase total reimbursement for that visit.

Inpatient Only Procedures[71]

The OPPS Rule also provides a list of procedures that HCFA believes should not be performed on an outpatient basis. This list, which will be regularly updated, is available on-line via the HCFA Web site.

Observation Status under the BBA[72]

The OPPS Rule restated HCFA's earlier position that routine observation time preceding or

Table 9–4 Ambulatory Payment Category Indicators

Type of Service	*Indicator*	*Payment*
Significant procedures	S	All paid at 100%
Significant procedures	T	Subject to 50% multiple procedure reduction
Medical visits (emergency department, clinic)	V	All paid at 100%
Ancillary services	X	All paid at 100%
Partial hospitalization	P	Per diem payment
Inpatient only	C	Not paid as outpatient
Incidental/packaged	N	No separate payment

following a planned procedure cannot be reported separately. Specific HCPCS codes remain available for reporting legitimate observation services on a per hour basis and must be reported in multiple units of services for multiple hours of observation. Currently, there is no payment for observation services that are performed separately from emergency department services; however, HCFA may reconsider and provide payment for observation status by creating an APC during the next PPS year if justification can be adequately demonstrated.

REFERENCES

1. E.D. Hoffman Jr. et al. *Brief Summaries of Medicare & Medicaid Title XVIII and Title XIX of The Social Security Act as of July 1, 2000/National Health Care Expenditures.* Office of the Actuary, Health Care Financing Administration, U.S. Department of Health and Human Services. http://www.hcfa.gov/pubforms/actuary/ormedmed/default2. Accessed September 2000.
2. Hoffman et al., *Brief Summaries of Medicare & Medicaid.*
3. U.S. Department of Health and Human Services. "P.L. 105–33: Balanced Budget Act of 1997," *Legislative Summary.* http://www.hcfa.gov/regs/bbaupdat.htm. Accessed September 2000.
4. U.S. Department of Health and Human Services, "General Information about the Program/Administration of Medicare Program" in *Health Insurance for the Aged/Medicare Hospital Manual.* HCFA Pub. 10, PB 98–955100, sections 100–112.
5. Hoffman et al., *Brief Summaries of Medicare & Medicaid.*
6. U.S. Department of Health and Human Services, "General Information about the Program/Administration of Medicare Program," section 155.
7. Hoffman et al., *Brief Summaries of Medicare & Medicaid.*
8. U.S. Department of Health and Human Services, "Coverage of Hospital Services/Duration of Covered Inpatient Services" in *Health Insurance for the Aged/Medicare Hospital Manual.* HCFA Pub. 10, PB 98–955100, section 215.
9. Hoffman et al., *Brief Summaries of Medicare & Medicaid.*
10. U.S. Department of Health and Human Services, "Coverage of Hospital Services/Duration of Covered Inpatient Services," section 219.
11. Hoffman et al., *Brief Summaries of Medicare & Medicaid.*
12. U.S. Department of Health and Human Services, "General Information about the Program/Administration of Medicare Program," section 160.
13. Hoffman et al., *Brief Summaries of Medicare & Medicaid.*
14. *The Balanced Budget Act of 1997,* Public Law 105–33, "Subtitle A/Chapter 1 Medicare+Choice Program, Section 1851 Eligibility, Election, Enrollment." http://www.hcfa.gov/regs/subt_a.htm. Accessed September 2000.
15. Hoffman et al., *Brief Summaries of Medicare & Medicaid.*
16. U.S. Department of Health and Human Services, "Coverage of Hospital Services/Duration of Covered Inpatient Services," section 210.
17. *The Balanced Budget Act of 1997,* Public Law 105–33, "Subtitle F Provisions Related to Part B Only, Chapter 2 Payment for Hospital Outpatient Department Services, Section 4523 PPS for Hospital Outpatient Services." http://www.hcfa.gov/regs/subt_f.htm. Accessed September 2000.
18. Hoffman et al., *Brief Summaries of Medicare & Medicaid.*
19. U.S. Department of Health and Human Services, Health Care Financing Administration, "Overview of the Medicaid Program & Medicaid Eligibility." http://www.hcfa.gov/medicaid/mover.htm and http://www.hcfa.gov.medicaid/meligib.htm. Accessed September 2000.
20. U.S. Department of Health and Human Services, Health Care Financing Administration, "Medicaid Services." http://www.hcfa.gov/medicaid/mservice.htm. Accessed September 2000.
21. Hoffman et al., *Brief Summaries of Medicare & Medicaid.*
22. U.S. Department of Health and Human Services, "General Information about the Program/Administration of Medicare Program," sections 165–168.
23. U.S. Department of Health and Human Services, "General Information about the Program/Administration of Medicare Program," section 168.
24. U.S. Department of Health and Human Services, "General Information about the Program/Administration of Medicare Program," section 165–168.
25. U.S. Department of Health and Human Services, "General Information about the Program/Administration of Medicare Program," section 175.
26. Hoffman et al., *Brief Summaries of Medicare & Medicaid.*

27. *The Balanced Budget Act of 1997,* Public Law 105–33, "Subtitle F Provisions Related to Part B Only, Chapter 2 Payment for Hospital Outpatient Department Services, Section 4523 PPS for Hospital Outpatient Services." http://www.hcfa.gov/regs/subt_f.htm. Accessed September 2000.
28. Hoffman et al., *Brief Summaries of Medicare & Medicaid.*
29. U.S. Department of Health and Human Services, Health Care Financing Administration. "Medicaid Eligibility." http://www.hcfa.gov/medicaid/meligib.htm. Accessed September 2000.
30. Hoffman et al., *Brief Summaries of Medicare & Medicaid.*
31. U.S. Department of Health and Human Services, Health Care Financing Administration. "Medicaid Eligibility." http://www.hcfa.gov/medicaid/meligib.htm. Accessed September 2000.
32. Hoffman et al., *Brief Summaries of Medicare & Medicaid.*
33. U.S. Department of Health and Human Services, Health Care Financing Administration. "Medicaid Eligibility." http://www.hcfa.gov/medicaid/meligib.htm. Accessed September 2000.
34. U.S. Department of Health and Human Services, Health Care Financing Administration, "Section 3628 Deduction of Incurred Medical & Remedial Care Expenses (Spenddown), Section 3645 Pay-in Spenddown Option," *State Medicaid Manual—Part 03, Eligibility.*
35. U.S. Department of Health and Human Services, Health Care Financing Administration. "Medicaid Services." http://www.hcfa.gov/medicaid/service.htm. Accessed September 2000.
36. *The Balanced Budget Act of 1997,* Public Law 105–33, "Subtitle J, State Children's Health Insurance Program, Chapter 1, State Children's Health Insurance Program/ Chapter 2, Expanded Coverage of Children under Medicaid." http://www.hcfa.gov/init/kidssum.htm. Accessed September 2000.
37. U.S. Department of Health and Human Services, "General Information about the Program/Administration of Medicare Program," sections 165–168, 175.
38. U.S. Department of Health and Human Services, Health Care Financing Administration, "Section 3001 Hospital Insurance Entitlement/Section 3003 Supplementary Medical Insurance," in *Medicare Intermediary Manual Part 3.*
39. U.S. Department of Health and Human Services, Health Care Financing Administration. "Medicaid Eligibility." http://www.hcfa.gov/medicaid/meligib.htm. Accessed September 2000.
40. Social Security Administration/Social Security OnLine. "Supplemental Security Income (SSI)/Understanding SSI," *Supplemental Security Income (SSI) Overview.* http://www.ssa.gov.
41. U.S. Department of Health and Human Services/Health Care Financing Administration. *Medicare & You 2000,* Publication No. HCFA 10050. Revised January 2000, 11–16.
42. U.S. Department of Health and Human Services, Health Care Financing Administration, "Special Provisions Related to Payment, Section 3420," in *Medicare Intermediary Manual Part 3.*
43. U.S. Department of Health and Human Services, "General Information about the Program/Administration of Medicare Program," sections 134 and 290.
44. U.S. Department of Health and Human Services, Health Care Financing Administration, "Utilization Control, Section 9102/Scope of the UC Quality Review System" and "Exhibit 1, Sample Certification of Utilization Control For Inpatient Hospitals" in *State Medicaid Manual/ Part 09.*
45. U.S. Department of Health and Human Services, "General Information about the Program/Administration of Medicare Program," section 195.
46. U.S. Department of Health and Human Services, "General Information about the Program/Administration of Medicare Program," section 199.
47. U.S. Department of Health and Human Services, "General Information about the Program/Administration of Medicare Program," sections 195–196.
48. U.S. Department of Health and Human Services, "General Information about the Program/Administration of Medicare Program," section 196.
49. Health Care Financing Administration, "Review of Hospital Issued Notices of Non-coverage (HINN) and Notice of Discharge and Medicare Appeal Rights (NODMARs)," in *Peer Review Organization Manual, Part 7—Denials, Reconsiderations, and Appeals*, sections 7000–7055.
50. U.S. Department of Health and Human Services, "General Information about the Program/Administration of Medicare Program," sections 197 and 288.
51. Health Care Financing Administration, "Denial Determinations and Sections," "Reconsideration Determinations," and "Hearings and Further Appeals," in *Peer Review Organization Manual, Part 7—Denials, Reconsiderations, and Appeals*, sections 7100–7155, 7400–7440, and 7500–7580.
52. U.S. Department of Health and Human Services, "Coverage of Hospital Services/Duration of Covered Inpatient Services," section 230.6.
53. U.S. Department of Health and Human Services, Health Care Financing Administration, "Coverage of Services, Section 3112.8, Outpatient Observation Services," in *Medicare Intermediary Manual Part 3.*
54. U.S. Department of Health and Human Services, Health Care Financing Administration, Program Memorandum Carriers, "2001 Physician Fee Schedule for Payments." Transmittal B-00-65, Change Request 1438. http://

www.hcfa.gov/pubforms/transmit/b0065.pdf (21 November 2000). Accessed 27 March 2001.

55. Health Care Financing Administration. "Quality of Care Home Page." http://www.hcfa.gov/quality/defaults.htm. Accessed September 2000.
56. U.S. Department of Health and Human Services, Health Care Financing Administration, Quality of Care—Peer Review Organizations. "Medicare's Healthcare Quality Improvement Program," v5-2. Pub. no. 10156. http://www.hcfa.gov/quality/5b1.htm. Accessed 27 March 2001.
57. U.S. Department of Health and Human Services, Health Care Financing Administration, Quality of Care—National Projects. "National Projects Reports: PRO Results: Bridging the Past with the Future." http://www.hcfa.gov/quality/3k1.htm (September 1998). Accessed 27 March 2001.
58. U.S. Department of Health and Human Services, Health Care Financing Administration. "Part 11, Payment Error Prevention Program," *Medicare Peer Review Organization Manual.* Transmittal 83. http://www.hcfa.gov/pubforms/transmit/r83pro.pdf (5 October 2000). Accessed 27 March 2001.
59. U.S. Department of Health and Human Services, Health Care Financing Administration. "Part 4—Case Review, Section 4000-4080 Mandatory Case Review Requirements," *Peer Review Organization Manual (02-01),* Rev 86, p. 4-4 to 4-10. http://www.hcfa.gov/pubforms/19%5Fpro/pr04/.htm#_4000_0.
60. U.S. Department of Health and Human Services, Health Care Financing Administration. "Fighting Fraud and Abuse/What Is Medicare Fraud." http://www.hcfa.gov/medicare/fraud/DEFINI2.htm. Accessed September 2000.
61. U.S. Department of Health and Human Services, Health Care Financing Administration. "Fighting Fraud and Abuse/What Is Medicare Fraud." http://www.hcfa.gov/medicare/fraud/DEFINI2.htm. Accessed September 2000.
62. U.S. Department of Health and Human Services, Health Care Financing Administration. "Fighting Fraud and Abuse/What Is Medicare Fraud." http://www.hcfa.gov/medicare/fraud/DEFINI2.htm. Accessed September 2000.
63. U.S. Department of Health and Human Services, Health Care Financing Administration, Balanced Budget Act of 1997, Medicare & Medicaid Provisions.
64. U.S. Department of Health and Human Services, Balanced Budget Act of 1997, Medicare & Medicaid Provisions, Subtitle E – Provisions Related to Part A Only, Section 4407 Certain Hospital Discharges to Post Acute Care.
65. U.S. Department of Health and Human Services, Balanced Budget Act of 1997, Medicare & Medicaid Provisions, Subtitle F—Provisions Relating to Part B Only, Chapter 2, Payment for Hospital Outpatient Department Services.
66. U.S. Department of Health and Human Services, Health Care Financing Administration. "Hospital Outpatient Prospective Payment System." http://www.hcfa.gov/medicare/hopsmain.htm. Accessed September 2000.
67. Hale, G., "Outpatient Prospective Payment System/Overview and Operational Considerations." Cap Gemini Ernst & Young internal presentation, August 2000, 2–5.
68. U.S. Department of Health and Human Services, Health Care Financing Administration. "Outpatient Prospective Payment System—Quick Reference Guide." http://www.hcfa.gov/medlearn/refopps.htm.
69. QuadraMed, APC IQ, QuadraMed's Forum on Ambulatory Patient Classifications, *Summary* (www.apc-iq.com/summary.htm).
70. Hale, "Outpatient Prospective Payment System/Overview and Operational Considerations," 6–12.
71. Hale, "Outpatient Prospective Payment System/Overview and Operational Considerations," 14.
72. Hale, "Outpatient Prospective Payment System/Overview and Operational Considerations," 13.

SUGGESTED READINGS

U.S. Department of Health and Human Services, Health Care Financing Administration, *Medicare & You 2000*, Publication No. HCFA 10050. Revised January 2000.

U.S. Department of Health and Human Services, Health Care Financing Administration, *Medicare & You/Your Medicare Benefits 1999*, Publication No. HCFA 10116. Revised May 1999.

U.S. Department of Health and Human Services, Health Care Financing Administration, *Medicare & Home Health Care*, Publication No. HCFA 10969. September 1999.

U.S. Department of Health and Human Services, Health Care Financing Administration, *Medicare Hospice Benefits*, Publication No. HCFA 02154. Revised August 1999.

U.S. Department of Health and Human Services, Health Care Financing Administration, *Your Guide to the Outpatient Prospective Payment System*, Publication No. HCFA 02118. July 2000.

U.S. Department of Health and Human Services, Health Care Financing Administration, *Medicare Coverage of Kidney Dialysis and Kidney Transplant Services,* Publication No. HCFA 10128. August 2000.

SUGGESTED WEB SITES

U.S. Department of Health and Human Services, Health Care Financing Administration. "Health Care Financing Administration: The Medicare, Medicaid, and SCHIP Agency." http://www.hcfa.gov. Accessed 14 February 2001.

U.S. Department of Health and Human Services, Health Care Financing Administration. "The Official U.S. Government Site for Medicare Information." http://www.medicare.gov. Accessed 14 February 2001.

Part III

Documentation and Measurement

CHAPTER 10

The Role of the Case Manager in Hospital Preparation for Joint Commission Accreditation

Nancy H. Fullerton and Mary Ellen Kripp

TAKE THIS TO WORK

1. The best way to prepare for an accreditation survey by the Joint Commission on Accreditation of Healthcare Organizations (Joint Commission) is to incorporate Joint Commission performance standards into your day-to-day case management operations.
2. Interdisciplinary collaboration and preparation are key techniques for promoting positive survey outcomes.
3. By focusing on continuous performance improvement, your organization will be well prepared for your Joint Commission survey; moreover, your efforts will contribute to maintaining the highest quality of patient care and services (e.g., clinical practice guidelines for the management of patients with acute chest pain improve clinical outcomes by ensuring early intervention and treatment).

We have covered a great deal of material on care and utilization management (UM) and the many roles of the case manager in a broader context. Now we will discuss the role of the case manager in a specific set of circumstances—the preparation of a hospital for accreditation from the Joint Commission on Accreditation of Healthcare Organizations (Joint Commission).

The Joint Commission is a not-for-profit organization that evaluates and accredits health care organizations, including hospitals, health care networks, long-term ambulatory care facilities, home care organizations, clinical laboratories, and behavioral health care facilities, in the United States and other countries. Although accreditation by the Joint Commission is voluntary, many organizations pursue it because of the added value it can bring.

- Accreditation requires the organization to monitor and improve the quality of patient care through an ongoing and well-organized performance improvement effort.
- Accreditation provides an objective "report card" of an organization that can effectively enhance customer confidence and satisfaction.
- Accreditation maximizes the organization's ability to negotiate third-party reimbursement.

Acknowledgment: The authors wish to give special thanks to Brenda Carsten for her major role in preparation of this manuscript.

- Many Joint Commission standards meet or exceed federal and state licensure requirements.
- An accredited facility attracts top-notch leadership, medical, and clinical staff.

This chapter presents the steps case managers need to take to prepare a hospital for an accreditation survey. It also presents the key Joint Commission standards in which the case manager has a strong role.

GETTING STARTED

The volume of Joint Commission standards in the *Comprehensive Accreditation Manual for Hospitals (CAMH)* has grown steadily over the years, yet the accreditation decision remains focused on a single page of data, the accreditation grid (Exhibit 10–1).[1] A guiding principle in the efforts to prepare a facility for an accreditation survey is to focus on those elements that drive the accreditation decision and to incorporate the related tools and techniques for those standards into your daily routine. But where do you begin? The first step in preparing for a Joint Commission survey is to identify the "core" case manager team members. The identified case managers are responsible for ensuring compliance in case management-related areas as well as supporting the organization's overall survey preparation process.

Case managers should be assigned to their department's "patient-centered" and "organizational-centered" teams, as outlined in the accreditation grid. (Note: Although case managers will likely support activities in the structures with functions areas, those activities will not be covered here.) The role of the case manager includes the following:

- Review the assigned case management-related standards.
- Identify most problematic case management-related standards.
- Collaboratively develop process improvements with other key stakeholders.
- Implement process improvements in a timely fashion.
- Monitor process improvements on a regular basis.
- Meet regularly with "core" case management team members to discuss ongoing issues and develop additional improvement strategies (meeting more frequently as the actual Joint Commission survey approaches).
- Report case management progress back to the organization's Joint Commission team.

The Joint Commission accreditation survey lasts two to three days, depending on the organization's specific needs. A typical survey includes the following key case management-related elements:

- *Document review sessions*—These sessions include patients' medical records, policies, and procedures; reports to medical staff; committee minutes; and so forth. They survey how the hospital addresses important case management functions.
- *Interviews with hospital leaders*—These interviews address the collaboration of senior leadership and allow surveyors to address specific case management issues with hospital administration, medical staff and nursing leaders, and departmental directors.
- *Visits to patient care settings*—As much as half of the survey time can be spent in these visits. Surveyors assess how the hospital's case management functions come together in the places where patients receive care.
- *Function interviews*—Surveyors meet with interdisciplinary teams related to specific case management functions to follow up on issues raised in the earlier document review sessions and visits to patient care settings.
- *Feedback sessions*—Surveyors provide feedback at daily organizational briefings. At the exit conference, complete survey findings and a preliminary written report

Exhibit 10–1 Joint Commission Hospital Accreditation Services Accreditation Decision Grid

Organization:________________ Survey Date:________________

Location:________________ Survey Type:________________

PATIENT-FOCUSED FUNCTIONS

Patient Rights and Organizational Ethics

Patient Rights	
Organizational Ethics	

Assessment of Patients

Initial Assessment	
Pathology and Clinical Laboratory Services—Waived Testing	
Reassessment	
Care Decisions	
Structures Supporting for Specific Patient Populations	
Additional Requirements for Special Patient Populations	

Care of Patients

Planning and Providing Care	
Anesthesia Care	
Medication Use	
Nutrition Care	
Operative and Other Procedures	
Rehabilitation Care and Services	
Special Treatment Procedures	

Education

Patient and Family Education and Responsibilities	

Continuum of Care

Continuum of Care	

ORGANIZATIONAL FUNCTIONS

Improving Organizational Performance

Plan	
Design	
Measure	
Assess	
Improve	

Leadership

Planning	
Directing Departments	
Integrating and Coordinating Services	
Role in Improving Performance	

Management of the Environment of Care

Design	
Implementation	
Measure Outcomes of Implementation	
Social Environment	

Management of Human Resources

Human Resources Planning	
Orienting, Training, and Education of Staff	
Assessing Competence	
Managing Staff Requests	

1 = Substantial Compliance
2 = Significance Compliance
3 = Partial Compliance
4 = Minimal Compliance
5 = Noncompliance
N = Not Applicable
P = Defer to Primary Service

Summary Grid Score = ___%

ORGANIZATIONAL FUNCTIONS CONTINUED

Management of Information

Information Management Planning	
Patient-Specific Data and Information	
Aggregate Data and Information	
Knowledge-Based Information	
Comparative Data and Information	

Surveillance, Prevention, and Control of Infection

Surveillance, Prevention, and Control of Infection	

STRUCTURES WITH FUNCTIONS

Governance

Governance	

Management

Management	

Medical Staff

Organization, Bylaws, Rules, and Regulations	
Credentialing	

Nursing

Nursing	

Special Type I Recommendation(s)

1997 HAS Grid—Effective: January, 1995 © 1994

Source: © Joint Commission: *CAMH: Comprehensive Accreditation Manual for Hospitals.* Oakbrook Terrace, IL: Joint Commission on Accreditation of Healthcare Organizations, 1997, p. ADP-3. Reprinted with permission.

and accreditation decision are provided to the staff, at the discretion of the chief executive officer. A final report and rating are provided within an average of 45 days following completion of the survey.

THE MOCK SURVEY

The next step in the preparation process is to conduct a mock survey of your case management activities. The mock survey is a vital tool for measuring performance, providing feedback, and implementing improvements prior to undergoing the actual Joint Commission survey. The mock survey can be conducted by internal resources within the organization (e.g., performance improvement team members, nursing leadership) or with the assistance of outside consultants. Timing is crucial—the mock survey should be done at least 18 months prior to each scheduled Joint Commission survey. This allows 6 months for implementation of identified process improvements and 12 months for evidence of documented and sustained change. (Twelve months of compliance is required prior to a resurvey, which is performed every three years; four months of compliance is the minimum for an initial survey.)

When conducting the mock survey, you should ask questions of the staff as if you were the Joint Commission surveyor. You can prepare your staff for surveyor questions by observing case management activities and asking specific questions while pretending to be unfamiliar with the day-to-day case management operations. To reap the maximum benefits of your mock survey, it is imperative that you analyze the outcomes and incorporate recommended improvements in day-to-day case management processes. Depending on the outcomes, it may be necessary to complete additional mock surveys prior to the actual Joint Commission visit.

Appendix 10–A presents each standard in which the case manager plays a strong role. (This listing of case management-related standards in not intended to be all inclusive. Please refer to the *CAMH* for full details of all standards.) The appendix is a tool you can use to guide you through your mock survey. It is organized as follows:

- *Joint Commission standard number*—Key standards in which the case manager plays a strong role. A complete listing of standards can be found in the *CAMH.*
- *Definition of key Joint Commission case management-related standards*—Definition of key related standards.
- *Definition of key Joint Commission case management-related tools/techniques*—Tools and techniques you may or may not already have in place.
- *Definition of key Joint Commission case management-related mock survey questions*—Sample questions that might be posed to the staff during an actual Joint Commission survey. Practice answering these questions and try to probe beyond the "simple" answers into greater detail for maximum results.

Once case managers have been assigned their role (patient centered or organizational activities), your team can begin the preparation process.

CONCLUSION

It will be important to maintain ongoing communication to the organization prior to and throughout the preparation process. Useful tools for creating awareness and educating staff are "question of the week" messages, standing agenda items at case management staff meetings, and posters/fliers distributed in the departments. Be creative in your efforts to generate interest and encourage participation throughout your organization.

When you review the *CAMH,* it is important to recognize that the standards discussed above are not mutually exclusive; that is, leadership standards are measured not only within the framework of the leadership interviews, but may also be addressed in any of the other areas, such as the human resources, continuum-of-care, or medical staff interviews. Therefore, the information in this chapter should be used as a guide for survey preparation rather than as a solution.

REFERENCES

1. Joint Commission on Accreditation of Healthcare Organizations, *1999–2000 Comprehensive Accreditation Manual for Hospitals: The Official Handbook* (Oakbrook Terrace, IL: 2000).

SUGGESTED READINGS

M. Bell, "Hospital Uses Team Approach To Improve Processes, Reduce Costs," *AORN Journal 68,* no. 1 (July 1998): 68–72.

H. Boerstler et al., "Keys for Successful Implementation of Total Quality Management in Hospitals," *Health Care Management Review 41,* no. 2 (Winter 1996): 48–60.

C. Calomeni et al., "Nurses on Quality Improvement Teams: How Do They Benefit?" *Journal of Nursing Care Quality 13,* no. 5 (June 1999): 75–90.

T. Cesta, "The Link Between Continuous Quality Improvement and Case Management," *The Journal of Nursing Administration 23,* no. 6 (June 1993): 55–61.

J. Clark, *Ongoing Records Review: A Guide to Joint Commission Compliance and Best Practice* (Marblehead, MA: Opus Communications, Inc., 1998).

B. Dugar, "Implementing CQI on a Budget: A Small Hospital's Story," *The Joint Commission Journal on Quality Improvement 21,* no. 2 (February 1995): 57–69.

Joint Commission on Accreditation of Healthcare Organizations, *1999–2000 Comprehensive Accreditation Manual for Hospitals: The Official Handbook* (Oakbrook Terrace, IL: 2000).

D. Wakefield and B. Wakefield, "Overcoming the Barriers to Implementation of TQM/CQI in Hospitals: Myths and Realities," *QRB Quality Review Bulletin 19,* no. 3 (March 1993): 83–88.

APPENDIX 10–A

Joint Commission Standards Related to Case Management

Source: © Joint Commission: *Comprehensive Accreditation Manual for Hospitals: The Official Guidelines.* Oakbrook Terrace, IL: Joint Commission on Accreditation of Healthcare Organizations, 2000, Selected Standards. Reprinted with permission.

Standard Number	Description of Key Standards	Key Tools/Techniques	Key Mock Survey Questions
Patient-Focused Activities			
Patient Rights and Organizational Ethics			
RI.1.2	Patients are involved in all aspects of their care.	• Document initial and ongoing discharge planning activities in the patient's medical record • Document interdisciplinary care conferences in patient's medical record and/or care conference minutes • Hospital leaders, physicians, case managers (CMs), and clinical staff articulate how patients are involved in all aspects of their care, including the discharge planning process • Patients discuss how they are involved in all aspects of their care, including developing a realistic discharge plan • Related policies and procedures • Document managing pain effectively in the patient's medical record, especially as the patient transitions into the post-hospital setting* • Related policies and procedures	• How are patients included in developing their discharge plans? • If patients are unable to participate in developing their discharge plans, what is the mechanism for identifying discharge needs? Developing discharge plan? Implementing discharge plan? • Describe how patients are included in the development of their pain management plans for use in the post-hospital setting.*

continues

Standard Number	Description of Key Standards	Key Tools/Techniques	Key Mock Survey Questions
RI.1.2.2	The family participates in care decisions.	• Document CM/family discussions in the patient's medical record • Schedules of patient activities that include family involvement, e.g., interdisciplinary care conferences, support groups, and family education sessions • Hospital leaders, physicians, case managers, and clinical staff articulate how families are involved in all aspects of their relative's care, including the discharge planning process • Families discuss how they are involved in all aspects of their relative's care, including developing a realistic discharge plan • Related policies and procedures	• Describe how a patient's family participates in developing a realistic discharge plan. • If patients do not have family and/or primary care givers, what is the mechanism for ensuring a realistic and safe discharge plan?
RI.1.2.4	The hospital addresses advance directives.	• Document advance directives, resuscitation status, and using and removing life-sustaining treatment information in the patient's medical record • Related policies and procedures	• Describe the decision-making process for addressing advance directives, resuscitation status, and using and removing life-sustaining treatment. • How is advance directive, resuscitation, and using and removing life-sustaining treatment information communicated with the patient's post-hospital care providers? • Describe both inpatient and outpatient Hospice referral processes.
RI.1.2.5	The hospital addresses withholding resuscitation services.		
RI.1.2.6	The hospital addresses forgoing or withdrawing life-sustaining treatment.		

continues

Standard Number	Description of Key Standards	Key Tools/Techniques	Key Mock Survey Questions
RI.1.3.1	The hospital demonstrates respect for the patient's need for confidentiality.	• Policies related to Patient Confidentiality and Privacy • Policies related to Communicating with Third-Party Payers	• How does the CM demonstrate respect for the patient's confidentiality? • Describe the process for discussing confidential information with the patient/family.
RI.1.3.2	The hospital demonstrates respect for the patient's need for privacy.	• Policies related to Communicating with Post-Hospital Providers	• Describe how the CM communicates with the third-party payers. • Describe how the CM communicates patient's medical information with other providers, e.g., home care agencies, pharmaceutical and equipment companies. • How are medical records forwarded to the post-hospital provider, e.g., home care agencies, skilled nursing and rehabilitation facilities?
Assessment of Patients			
PE.1	Each patient's physical, psychological, and social statuses are assessed.	• Document physical, psychological, and social status in the patient's medical record • Discharge Planning Screening Criteria • Discharge Assessment Forms • Post-Hospital Provider Referral Forms • Related policies and procedures	• Does the discharge planning process apply to all patients? • How is each patient's physical, psychological, and social status assessed prior to discharge? • Are patients screened for potential discharge needs prior to or at the time of admission?
PE.1.1	The scope and intensity of any further assessment are based on the patient's diagnosis, the care setting, the patient's desire for care, and the patient's response to any previous care.	• Policies related to Utilization Management	• What determines the scope and intensity of additional patient assessments? • Describe how the CM uses established criteria for assessing intensity, severity, diagnostic screening, and appropriateness of service, e.g., InterQual, Milliman & Robertson.

continues

Standard Number	*Description of Key Standards*	*Key Tools/Techniques*	*Key Mock Survey Questions*
PE.1.4	Pain is assessed in all patients.	• Document initial and ongoing pain assessment in the patient's medical record • Physicians, case managers, and clinical staff articulate how patients participate in their pain assessment* • Patients articulate participation in their pain assessment* • Pain Assessment Evaluation Form • Related policies and procedures	• Describe the patient's initial pain evaluation process as completed by the CM. • Does the initial screening process include – history of pain – intensity and quality of pain – location of pain – duration of pain?
PE.1.6	The need for a discharge planning assessment is determined.	• Document discharge plan in the patient's medical record • Discharge Planning Screening Criteria • Discharge Assessment Form • Physician Order Form • Related policies and procedures	• Does the discharge planning process apply to all patients? • How are patients' discharge needs identified? • Can any member of the interdisciplinary team identify potential discharge needs? • Describe the physician's role in developing a discharge plan.
PE.2.1	Reassessment occurs at regular intervals in the course of care.	• Document any additional and/or revised discharge information in the patient's medical record • Related policies and procedures	• How often do CMs reassess their patients' discharge needs? Plans? • How often do CMs make "rounds"? • How often are interdisciplinary care conferences scheduled?
PE. 2.2	Reassessment determines a patient's response to care.		
PE.2.3	Significant change in a patient's condition results in reassessment.	• Document any significant patient changes (which may affect the patient's discharge status/plan) in the patient's medical record • Related policies and procedures	• What triggers the modification of the patient's discharge plan?
PE.2.4	Significant change in a patient's diagnosis results in reassessment.		

continues

Standard Number	Description of Key Standards	Key Tools/Techniques	Key Mock Survey Questions
PE.3	Staff members integrate the information from various assessments of the patient to identify and assign priorities to his or her care needs.	• Document the integration of various assessments in the patient's medical record, including the discharge assessment • Discharge Assessment Forms • Post-Hospital Provider Referral Forms • Related policies and procedures	• How does the CM staff integrate the information from various assessments of the patient in order to identify and assign priorities to the plan of care? Discharge plan?
PE.3.1	Staff members base care decisions on the identified patient needs and care opportunities.		
PE.4	The hospital has defined patient assessment activities in writing.	• Document initial discharge assessment and ongoing discharge plan in the patient's medical record • Discharge Assessment Forms • Post-Hospital Provider Referral Forms • Related policies and procedures	• How often do CMs document their case management activities, e.g., discharge planning? • Is the written discharge plan well-organized and legible?
Care of Patients			
TX1.1	Care, treatment, and rehabilitation are planned to ensure that they are appropriate to the patient's needs and severity of disease, condition, impairment, or disability.	• Document care, treatment, and rehabilitation plans in the patient's medical record, including any post-hospital plans • Policies and procedures related to patient assessment and care planning • Policies related to utilization management • Policies related to clinical practice guidelines/protocols/standing orders • Clinical practice guidelines • Clinical protocols/standing orders	• How are care, treatment, and rehabilitation planned to ensure that they are appropriate to the patient's needs and severity of disease, condition, impairment, or disability? • Describe how timely ordering, sequencing, and scheduling of tests and procedures ensure timely discharge of patients. • Describe how patients are assigned to appropriate clinical practice guidelines, protocols, and standing orders.
TX.1.1.1	Settings and services required to meet patient care goals are identified, planned, and provided if appropriate.		

continues

Standard Number	*Description of Key Standards*	*Key Tools/Techniques*	*Key Mock Survey Questions*
TX.1.2	Care is planned and provided in an interdisciplinary, collaborative manner by qualified individuals.	• Document interdisciplinary plan of care in the patient's medical record • Policies related to patient assessment and care planning • Policies related to interdisciplinary care conference • Policies related to clinical practice guidelines/protocols/standing orders • Interdisciplinary Team Conference Forms or Conference Minutes • Clinical practice guidelines • Clinical protocols/standing orders	• What mechanisms exist to ensure that care is planned and provided in an interdisciplinary, collaborative manner by qualified individuals? • Is there a clear focus on collaboratively working with physicians? • Describe how the CM communicates among the patient/family and members of the health care team. • How does the CM ensure communication among all members of the health care team? • How often are team conferences scheduled? • What if the patient requires more conferences? • Is the patient demographic and clinical information accessible to all members of the interdisciplinary team?
TX.1.3	Patients' progress is periodically evaluated against care goals and the plan of care and when indicated, the plan or goals are revised.	• Document patient progress in the patient's medical record, especially as it relates to his or her discharge plan • Related policies and procedures	• What is the process for evaluating patient's progress and how often is it done? • How does the CM ensure that all plans have compatible goals and objectives?

continues

Standard Number	Description of Key Standards	Key Tools/Techniques	Key Mock Survey Questions
Education (Patient/Family)			
PF.3	The patient receives education and training specific to the patient's assessed needs, abilities, learning preferences, and readiness to learn as appropriate to the care and services provided by the hospital.	• Document all patient/family educational needs, training activities, and response to training in the patient's medical record • Clinical practice guidelines/protocols and standing orders • Post-Hospital Referral Forms • Patient Education Evaluation Forms • Patient Education Progress Notes • Patient Education Materials • Discharge Instructions • Related policies and procedures	• How are the patient's/family's learning needs, abilities, preferences, and readiness to learn assessed? • Describe how the discharge needs for the child are assessed. • Describe how the patient's/family's response to learning is incorporated into the discharge plan. • Are discharge instructions given to the patient/family/organization responsible for continuing the patient's care?
PF.3.1	Based on assessed needs, the patient is educated about how to safely and effectively use medications, according to law and regulation, and the hospital's scope of services, as appropriate.	• Document any patient medication training in the patient's medical record, especially any medications ordered in the post-hospital setting • Related policies and procedures • Post-Hospital Referral Forms • Patient Education Evaluation Forms • Patient Education Progress Forms • Patient Education Materials (including those from outside vendor) • Discharge Instructions	• Describe how patients and their families are educated to safe and effective medication usage prior to discharge. • Describe the process for educating the patient and his or her family if home intravenous medications are required. • Describe process for outside vendor education prior to a patient's discharge. • For those patients receiving home intravenous medications, are they provided with any pharmaceutical vendor names and phone numbers?

continues

Standard Number	*Description of Key Standards*	*Key Tools/Techniques*	*Key Mock Survey Questions*
PF.3.3	The hospital assures that the patient is educated about how to safely and effectively use medical equipment or supplies, as appropriate.	• Document any medical equipment training in the patient's medical record • Post-Hospital Referral Forms • Patient Education Evaluation Forms • Patient Education Progress Forms • Patient Education Materials (including those from outside vendor) • Discharge Instructions • Related policies and procedures	• Describe how patients and their families are educated to safely and effectively using medical equipment or supplies. • Describe the process for educating the patient and his or her family if an outside vendor is required to provide necessary medical equipment. • How do you assess and provide for the education needs of children?
PF.3.6	The patient is educated about other available resources, and when necessary, how to obtain further care services or treatment to meet his or her identified needs.	• Document clear education plan in the patient's medical record, including patient's knowledge regarding availability of outside resources • Post-Hospital Referral Forms • Patient Education Evaluation Forms • Patient Education Materials • Discharge Instructions • Manual of community-based services • Brochures and/or community-based resource information • Related policies and procedures	• Describe how access to referral services is identified and addressed prior to discharge. • Describe the types of community resources utilized by your patients.
PF.3.7	The hospital makes clear to patients and families what their responsibilities are regarding the patient's ongoing health care needs, and gives them the knowledge and skills they need to carry out their responsibilities.	• Document clear discharge plan in the patient's medical record, including outlining patient and family responsibilities • Post-Hospital Referral Forms • Patient Education Evaluation Forms • Discharge Instructions • Related policies and procedures	• Describe how the organization identifies patient/family responsibilities.

continues

Standard Number	Description of Key Standards	Key Tools/Techniques	Key Mock Survey Questions
PF.3.9	Discharge instructions are given to the patient and those providing continuing care.	• Document discharge plan in the patient's medical record • Post-Hospital Referral Forms • Patient Education Evaluation Forms • Discharge Instructions • Related policies and procedures	• Are discharge instructions given to the patient/family/organization responsible for continuing the patient's care? • What information is included in the discharge instructions?
Continuum of Care			
CC.1	Patients have access to the appropriate type of care.	• Document patient's asessment in the patient's medical record • Document patient transfer and/or referral information in the patient's medical record • Related policies and procedures	• Describe how your patient assessment process ensures that the patients' needs are met.
CC.4	The hospital ensures continuity over time among the phases of service to a patient.	• Document in the patient's medical record • Criteria for selection and implementation of Clinical practice guidelines, protocols, and standing orders, if used	• Describe how your CM processes provide for continuity and coordination among interdisciplinary staff and settings. • Describe how the CM coordinates the patient's discharge plan and his or her transition to the post-hospital setting.
CC.5	The hospital ensures coordination among the health professionals within the services or setting involved in a patient's care.	• Copies of Clinical practice guidelines, protocols, and standing orders • Related policies and procedures	• Do your processes provide continuity across the continuum of care? • Has the hospital considered clinical practice guidelines in the design of improvement of clinical procedures? • If clinical guidelines are used, how do hospital leaders identify or set criteria for selection of the guideline?

continues

Standard Number	*Description of Key Standards*	*Key Tools/Techniques*	*Key Mock Survey Questions*
CC.6	The hospital provides for referral, transfer, or discharge of the patient to another level of care, health professional, or setting based on the patient's assessed needs and the hospital's capacity to provide the care.	• Document referral, transfer, or discharge information in the patient's medical record • Policies related to Referring Patients • Policies related to Transferring Patients • Policies related to Discharging Patients • Discharge criteria from key patient care areas, e.g., Emergency Department, Intensive Care, and other Specialty Units	• Describe the processes for referral, transfer, or discharge of a patient. • Does the CM identify ways to decrease LOS, place patient in alternate settings using alternative levels of care? • Describe how the CM communicates the patient's physical and emotional symptoms, e.g., pain, nausea, or shortness of breath, to alternate levels of care including the post-hospital providers.
CC.6.1	The discharge process provides for continuing care based upon the patient's assessed needs at the time of discharge.	• Document discharge plan in the patient's medical record • Related policies and procedures	• Describe the discharge planning process.
CC.7	The hospital ensures that appropriate patient care and clinical information is exchanged when patients are admitted, referred, transferred, or discharged.	• Document admission, referral, transfer, or discharge information in the patient's medical record • Related policies and procedures	• Describe your process for the exchange of patient information as patients are moved through the continuum of care, e.g., transferred to another department or discharged.

continues

Standard Number	Description of Key Standards	Key Tools/Techniques	Key Mock Survey Questions
CC.8	An established procedure(s) is used to resolve denial-of-care conflicts, services, or payment.	• Policies related to Denial Management, including addressing disagreements with third-party payers • Hospital leadership, physicians, and case managers articulate the process for resolving denial-of-care, services, and payments • Copy of Denial Letter • Copy of Appeal Letter	• What procedure is used to resolve denial-of-care conflicts over care, services, or payment? • Describe how insurance benefits are coordinated with the patient's plan of care. • How does the CM interact with the third-party payer? • How does the CM understand the patients' payment resources at or before the time of admission? • How do the physician and CM expedite the most effective plan of care within those parameters? • How does the CM provide timely assessment and communication for authorization of treatment? • Describe how the CM acts as a resource to staff regarding third-party payer issues. • Describe the role of the physician advisor in the denial management process.

continues

Standard Number	Description of Key Standards	Key Tools/Techniques	Key Mock Survey Questions
Organizational Activities			
Performance Improvement			
PI.1	The leaders establish a planned, systematic, organizationwide approach to process design and performance management, analysis, and improvement.	• Learn and facilitate understanding of performance improvement process within CM department and across interdisciplinary lines in assigned area of coverage (e.g., ICU, CCU, etc.) • Discuss PI issues as they are recognized both within CM department and across interdisciplinary lines • Provide specific feedback and recommendations for improvement based on collaborative efforts to Performance Improvement (PI) team; recommendations should include a course of corrective action and a measurement tool • Ensure accurate recording and sharing of case management information—data must be current and well organized; recommend action plans where performance goals are not met • Maintain an open line of communications within CM department and across interdisciplinary lines • Periodically review historic data for desirable and undesirable patterns or trends • Network with peers within and outside of the facility to identify PI initiatives that may provide benchmarks and strategic information	• How do you determine what and how will be measured for PI activities? • What is the feedback process for staff views regarding CM performance? • Are PI activities carried out in a collaborative fashion between CM and disciplines? • Do your design or improvement processes include planning, testing, assessing results (and redesigning if necessary), and implementing? • How were recommended actions to improve CM processes implemented?
PI.1.1	The activities are planned in a collaborative and interdisciplinary manner.		
PI.2	New or modified processes are designed well.		
PI.2.1	Performance expectations are established for new and modified processes.		
PI.2.2	The performance of new and modified processes is measured.		
PI.3	Data are collected to monitor the stability of existing processes, identify opportunities for improvement, identify changes that will lead to improvement, and sustain improvement.		

continues

Standard Number	Description of Key Standards	Key Tools/Techniques	Key Mock Survey Questions
PI.3.1	The organization collects data to monitor its performance.		
PI.3.1.1	The organization collects data to monitor the performance of processes that involve risks or may result in sentinel events.		
PI.4.2	The organization compares its performance over time and with other sources of information.		
PI.4.3	Undesirable patterns or trends in performance and sentinel events are intensively analyzed.		
Leadership			
LD.1.10	Clinical practice guidelines are considered for use in designing or improving processes.	• Documented clinical practice guidelines, protocols, and standing orders • Related policies and procedures	• Are clinical practice guidelines, protocols, and standing orders used as a resource for clinical PI activities? • If so, how do hospital leaders determine and measure criteria?
LD.1.10.1	When clinical practice guidelines are used, the hospital leaders identify criteria for their selection and implementation of clinical practice guidelines.		

continues

Standard Number	Description of Key Standards	Key Tools/Techniques	Key Mock Survey Questions
LD.1.3.3	Services are designed to respond to patient and family needs expectations.	• Proactively seek input of patient and family members in educational and care planning efforts • Provide patient and family feedback to CM staff	• How do you ensure the patients' needs and wishes are accounted for in the care planning process? • How do you involve family members in the decision process (when appropriate)?
LD.1.4	The planning process provides for setting performance-improvement priorities and identifies how the hospital adjusts priorities in response to unusual or urgent events.	• Develop strong understanding of CM performance improvement process and methodology of establishing priorities	• How have you established an environment that supports the hospital's services, policies, and mission? • How do you establish priorities in CM performance improvement?
LD.1.7	The scope of services provided by each department is defined in writing and is approved by the hospital's administration, medical staff, or both, as appropriate.	• Develop strong understanding of scope of services both within CM department, assigned department of coverage, and hospital-wide	• How was the scope of services of the CM department defined? • How do you ensure uniform performance of CM processes?
LD.1.9	The leaders develop programs for recruitment, retention, development, and continuing education of all staff members.	• Actively participate in CM educational and developmental programs • Encourage participation of coworkers	• Describe the CM education policy. • How does the hospital support the educational goals of the CM staff?
LD.1.9.1	The leaders implement programs to promote staff members' job-related advancement and educational goals.		

continues

Standard Number	Description of Key Standards	Key Tools/Techniques	Key Mock Survey Questions
LD.2.1	Directors integrate their department's services with the hospital's primary functions.	• Facilitate seamless delivery of service to patients by promoting cooperative efforts within and outside of CM department • Communicate related policies/procedures to CM staff in timely and regular manner • Perform regular reviews of historic and current data to promote continuous improvement by identifying areas for improvement and implementing action plans as needed • Provide CM staff ongoing education and developmental tools	• Are CMs qualified/educated to perform necessary function: UM, discharge planning, etc.? • Does director of CM department communicate on timely and regular basis with staff? • Describe the process for monitoring and improving CM performance.
LD.2.2	Directors coordinate and integrate services within their department and with other departments.		
LD.2.3	Directors develop and implement policies and procedures that guide and support the provision of services.		
LD.2.4	Directors recommend a sufficient number of qualified and competent persons to provide care.		
LD.2.6	Directors continuously assess and improve their department's performance.		
LD.2.8	Directors provide for orientation in-service training, and continuing education of all persons in the department.		

continues

Standard Number	Description of Key Standards	Key Tools/Techniques	Key Mock Survey Questions
LD.4.2	The leaders adopt an approach to performance improvement.	• Act as knowledgeable resource and role model in complying with performance improvement initiatives	• Do you actively participate in CM processes to improve and maintain performance? • What resources have you allocated for CM performance improvement?
LD.4.3.1	All leaders participate in interdisciplinary, interdepartmental performance-improvement activities.	• Collaborate at interdepartmental level at all stages of PI initiatives, not just when a problem has been identified • Forward relevant information to other leaders and coordinators of hospitalwide PI activities	• Do your leaders actively participate in CM processes to improve and maintain performance?
Environment of Care			
EC.1.8	A management plan addresses medical equipment.	• Knowledge and communication of biomedical department's policies and procedures regarding biomedical equipment, especially as it relates to using outside vendor medical equipment	• What is the procedure for training of staff on usage of outside vendor biomedical equipment, e.g., home infusion pumps, portable oxygen?
Human Resources			
HR.2	The hospital provides an adequate number of staff members whose qualifications are consistent with job responsibilities.	• CM department director retains sufficient number of qualified case managers • CM department director establishes policies/procedures to promote continual education/improvement of CMs	• How has the CM department director defined the appropriate level of qualification, responsibilities, and number of staff? • What is the system used to evaluate coverage of responsibilities?
HR.3	The leaders ensure that the competence of all staff members is assessed, maintained, demonstrated, and improved continually.		

continues

Standard Number	Description of Key Standards	Key Tools/Techniques	Key Mock Survey Questions
HR.4.2	Ongoing inservice and other education and training maintain and improve staff competence.	• Participate in available educational and development offerings • Encourage participation of co-workers in available educational and development offerings	• What education programs are offered to CMs?
HR.5	The hospital addresses each staff member's ability to meet the performance expectations stated in his or her job description.	• Provide thorough orientation to CMs	• How are CM staff oriented to their responsibilities, department and performance expectations?
Information Management			
IM.2	Confidentiality, security, and integrity of data and information are maintained.	• Ensure accurate recording and sharing of CM information • Recommend action plans where performance goals are not met	• Describe the training you have received in the principles of information management. • How do your CM processes ensure the confidentiality, security, and integrity of data? • How do your processes minimize bias in the data you record?
IM.3.2.1	Medical records are reviewed on an ongoing basis for completeness and timeliness of information, and action is taken to improve the quality and timeliness of documentation that impacts patient care.	• Ensure accurate recording and sharing of CM information • Recommend action plans where performance goals are not met	• Describe your medical record review process. • How are recommendations for improvement answered?

continues

Standard Number	*Description of Key Standards*	*Key Tools/Techniques*	*Key Mock Survey Questions*
IM.7	The hospital defines, captures, analyzes, transforms, transmits, and reports patient-specific data and information related to care processes and outcomes.	• Document in patient's medical record • Document in Case Manager's Worksheet • Work collaboratively with interdisciplinary team to ensure complete and accurate recording of information	• How do your processes ensure the standardization of data formatting and dissemination? • How do your processes ensure timely, accurate delivery of information?
IM.7.2	The medical record contains sufficient information to identify the patient, support the diagnosis, justify the treatment, document the course and results, and promote continuity of care among health care providers.		
IM.7.3.4.1	Compliance with discharge criteria is fully documented in the patient's medical record.	• Document in patient's medical record • Document in Case Manager's Worksheet	• How do your processes ensure compliance with discharge criteria?

*Indicates that standard will not be scored for completion in the year 2000, but at a later date to be determined.

Chapter 11

The Case Manager as a Facilitator of Accurate Medical Record Documentation

June M. Laing

TAKE THIS TO WORK

1. If it isn't documented, it wasn't done.
2. Everything of importance must be charted and the documentation must be specific.
3. An omission or obscurity in documentation can be the precursor to a subsequent denial or decreased payment.
4. The hospital is paid a fixed amount for treating patients in the same diagnosis-related group regardless of the services actually provided or the severity of their condition.
5. The incentive for effective management of medical care is that cost-efficient hospitals can keep any surplus in the DRG payment over costs while inefficient hospitals must absorb any loss.
6. The importance of consistent, complete documentation in the medical record cannot be overemphasized. Without such documentation, the application of all coding guidelines is a difficult, if not impossible, task.
7. The principal diagnosis is the starting point for the DRG assignment process: What condition ultimately had to be treated in order to make the patient well?
8. "Whose documentation is needed for coding purposes?" The rule-of-thumb answer is the physicians who actually see the patient, take a history, and perform a physical examination.
9. There are few people who work with records who would not rank improved documentation among the first three items that would improve the quality of their work life.
10. Improved payment accuracy is an important result of documentation accuracy.

The oft-quoted axiom, "If it isn't documented, it wasn't done" is never more applicable than in the health care sector, and this chapter could not be written without its repetition here. Although documentation specificity has always been encouraged, under Medicare's prospective payment system (PPS), it has become mandatory. Indeed, since the inception of PPS, many facilities have experienced costly payment denials because supportive documentation for diagnoses and procedures was not in evidence.

THE MEDICAL RECORD AS A MEDICAL DOCUMENT

From the time of a patient's admission to discharge, the medical record is the document that charts the progress of the patient's condition and treatment as recorded by all members of the patient's health care team. This documentation establishes both a continuity in the present treatment regimen, through the interaction of the caregiver disciplines, and a historical record for the future care of the patient. This emphasizes two important points.

1. Everything of significance must be charted.
2. The documentation must be specific.

THE MEDICAL RECORD AS A CONFIDENTIAL LEGAL DOCUMENT

The medical record is also a legal document because it contains privileged information about the patient. The information is protected by law from any reviewer not designated by the patient on a release of information form. Certain records—those of drug and alcohol abuse and psychiatric patients—are protected by federal law against disclosure to anyone other than those persons designated by the patient on a special release form. Some state laws go even further to govern the confidentiality of additional diagnoses, such as human immunodeficiency virus (HIV) and epilepsy. These federal and state statutes are the ultimate in protection that can be afforded any patient's record.

MEDICAL RECORD OWNERSHIP AND RESPONSIBILITY

A patient has the right to decide who may see his or her medical record, but the record itself is the physical property of the facility. As such, it is the facility's responsibility to preserve and protect the document from being altered or destroyed. It is not uncommon for a health information management (HIM) director to be served with a subpoena to produce a patient's record for a court case that may be against another person, the facility, or a member of the medical or nursing staff. It is the HIM director's responsibility, as custodian of the records, to keep the records secure so they cannot be altered in any way.

STATISTICS

Narratives of patients' diagnoses and procedures are recorded in coded form on their charts using the *International Classification of Diseases, 9th Revision, Clinical Modification (ICD-9-CM)* and the *Current Procedural Terminology (CPT)*. The *ICD-9-CM* is a U.S. expansion of the World Health Organization's 9th Revision, *International Classification of Diseases (ICD-9),* which is used to (1) classify international morbidity and mortality information for statistical reasons and (2) index medical records by disease and procedure for storage and retrieval purposes. The *ICD-9-CM* provides about 17,000 diagnosis codes and procedure codes for inpatients. The *CPT,* produced by the American Medical Association, is used to code outpatient and emergency room procedures. The clinical statistics derived from coded data are used internally by the facility for marketing, forecasting, and planning purposes. External users of the statistical data range from the local community (e.g., insurance companies, health departments, etc.) to the international community (i.e., the World Health Organization).

This introduction to medical record documentation is meant to convey the seriousness with which it should be viewed. An omission or obscurity in the documentation can be the precursor to a subsequent denial or decreased payment because the equity between the patient's medical condition and the treatment it required—the resource utilization—was not supported through documentation in the record.

THE PPS

The following is a brief, elementary explanation of the PPS. Though simple in concept, this system has a highly complex, technical infrastructure. A glossary containing terms commonly associated with the PPS can be found at the end of this book. This history will be more meaningful if the terms are reviewed first.

When Medicare was implemented in 1965, federal expenditures for health care spiraled in an upward direction for several reasons. For some beneficiaries, it was first-time insurance coverage, and they used services that had not been available to them before. Some beneficiaries dropped other policies and made Medicare their primary and *only* health care insurance—which had not been the program's intent. The Medicare program at that time did not contain incentives for providers to control costs. In October 1983, the PPS was legislated by the federal government as a way to change hospital behavior through financial incentives that would encourage more cost-efficient management of medical care.

How the PPS Works

Under the PPS, Medicare discharges that are similar both clinically and in hospital resource consumption are classified into *one* of several hundred diagnosis-related groups (DRGs) based on information abstracted from their medical record and reported on the inpatient bill. The hospital is paid a fixed amount for treating patients in the same DRG regardless of the services actually provided or the severity level of the patients' condition. The incentive for effective management of medical care is that cost-efficient hospitals can keep any surplus in the DRG payment over costs, whereas inefficient hospitals must absorb any loss.

The DRG assignment is calculated by the DRG grouper, a specialized computer software program that incorporates patient attributes (e.g., principal diagnosis [PDX], secondary diagnoses [SDXs], procedures, age, gender, and discharge status) and DRG hierarchy in determining a DRG assignment. This program is updated annually by the Health Care Financing Administration (HCFA).

A *relative weight* (r.w.) is assigned to each DRG to indicate the average cost of resources used to treat Medicare patients in each DRG relative to the national average cost of resources used to treat *all* Medicare patients. For example, a patient in a DRG with a relative weight of 3.000 would mean that, on an average, it would take *three* times the amount of resources to care for the patient in that DRG as it would to care for the average Medicare patient, or a patient in a DRG with a relative weight of 1.000. The DRG relative weights are recalculated on an annual basis by HCFA to make adjustments for fluctuations reported in the previous year's statistics.

Additionally, each hospital is assigned a hospital-blended rate (a dollar amount), adjusted annually by HCFA to reflect inflation, technical adjustments, and budgetary constraints. Each facility's blended rate also reflects geographic location, with special rates for urban and rural hospitals. Technical adjustments include those made for local wage variations, teaching hospitals, and hospitals with a disproportionate share of indigent patients.

The DRG payment for a Medicare inpatient is determined by multiplying the relative weight of the patient's DRG by the hospital's blended rate:

DRG relative weight x hospital's blended rate =
DRG payment

(DRG 127 w/ a r.w. of 1.0144 ×
hospital's blended rate of $4,000 =
a payment of $4,058)

The *average* DRG weight for all of a hospital's Medicare business is called the *case mix index* (CMI). The CMI indicates the relative severity of the hospital's patient mix and is directly proportional to the basic DRG payment. It is calculated by multiplying the number of discharged patients assigned to each DRG by the relative weight for that DRG, adding all the patients and the total DRG weights, and dividing the total of the DRG weights by the total patients in the calculation.

DRG 079 FY 2000 r.w. 1.6439 × 128 patients =
210.4192 total r.w.

DRG 089 FY 2000 r.w. 1.0855 × 361 patients =
391.8655 total r.w.

DRG 127 FY 2000 r.w. 1.0149 × 413 patients = 419.1537 total r.w.

DRG 184 FY 2000 r.w. 0.5286 × 145 patients = 76.6470 total r.w.

DRG 209 FY 2000 r.w. 2.1175 × 347 patients = 734.7725 total r.w.

DRG 210 FY 2000 r.w. 1.8028 × 102 patients = 183.8856 total r.w.

1,496 patients 2016.7435 total all DRG r.w.

2016.7435 ÷ 1,496 = 1.3480 Case Mix Index

The total annual Medicare payment to a hospital is calculated by multiplying the CMI by the hospital's blended rate and then by the total number of Medicare patients discharged from the hospital during the year.

The underlying concept of Medicare's PPS is simple: Medicare will pay for care for patients on the understanding that (1) the patient had the diagnoses that are submitted on the inpatient bill, and (2) they were treated. In essence, Medicare will pay for resource consumption.

Official Coding Guidelines

The *Official Coding Guidelines* are authored by the four cooperating parties: the American Health Information Management Association (AHIMA), the American Hospital Association (AHA), the National Center for Health Statistics (NCHS), and HCFA. Official coding guidelines and advice are published quarterly in the *Coding Clinic for ICD-9-CM* by the AHA's Central Office on ICD-9-CM. The introduction to the "Guidelines for Selection of Principal Diagnosis" states that "the importance of consistent, complete documentation in the medical record cannot be overemphasized. Without such documentation, the application of all coding guidelines is a difficult, if not impossible, task."

The DRG Hierarchy

Major Diagnostic Categories (MDCs)

At the top of the hierarchy are the 25 mutually exclusive major diagnostic categories (MDCs), most of which are based on an organ system instead of an etiology. Discharges with diseases involving both an organ system (digestive) and an etiology (adenocarcinoma of the stomach) are grouped to the MDC to which the *organ* system is assigned. There are conditions that could not be assigned to an organ-system-derived MDC, so several etiological MDCs were created for them (e.g., MDC 22 Burns). Each of the several hundred DRGs is assigned to *one* MDC.

DRG Partitioning Factors

The major factors in determining the DRG assignment include the patient's

- PDX
- principal procedure
- complications/comorbidities (CCs)
- gender
- age
- discharge status

PDX. The PDX is defined in the Uniform Hospital Discharge Data Set (UHDDS) as "that condition established *after study* to be *chiefly* responsible for occasioning the admission of the patient to the hospital for care." As its name indicates, this diagnosis is *sequenced* first. *Sequencing* refers to the order in which diagnoses and procedures are listed on the Uniform Bill-92 (UB-92), the billing form for a patient's care that is submitted to Medicare and other third-party payers for payment.

The PDX is the *starting point* for the DRG assignment process. Usually, the selection of the PDX is straightforward. At other times, obscurity or the presence of several conditions on admission may cloud the issue. Establishing this diagnosis is often a more difficult task than listing the SDXs and the procedures. The patient either had the SDX or he did not. Likewise with procedures—a procedure was either performed or it was not. However, detection of the PDX depends on differentiating an etiology from its associated manifestations, signs, or symptoms; therefore, the documentation to substantiate this diagnosis is essential.

When selecting the PDX, it may be helpful to ask the following questions:

- *Was there a stated reason for the admission?* (e.g., "The patient is being admitted for further evaluation and treatment of her peripheral vascular disease. It is noted that she also has a urinary tract infection for which she has been receiving treatment." In this case, the urinary tract infection, though present on admission and subsequently treated, would be considered a comorbidity in the face of the physician's *stated* reason for the admission, and it would be recorded as an SDX.)
- *Did the circumstances of the admission suggest the PDX?* (e.g., "The patient has developed an acute myocardial infarction and needs a cardiac cath. He is being transferred to Best Hospital for this procedure." The transferring hospital's PDX is that condition for which the patient was admitted there, but the receiving hospital's PDX is the acute myocardial infarction [AMI]—the diagnosis for which he was being transferred to receive treatment.)
- *What condition ultimately had to be treated in order to make the patient well?* (e.g., "The patient was admitted after being found to be anemic in our office. Her hemoglobin dropped 2 grams in the first hospital day and she was found to have a bleeding lesion in her colon. This was resected and the Path Report indicates a malignancy in the colon specimen." Although the patient was admitted because she was found to be anemic from a gastrointestinal bleed, what had to ultimately be treated in order to make the patient well was to resect the colon cancer. When this was done, it took care of the anemia and the bleed, which were manifestations of the cancer.)

An appendix is provided at the end of the chapter with additional detail on coding in the form of guidelines for selection of a principal diagnosis. These guidelines have to be strictly followed by the medical record coders. The assistance of the case managers in helping to clarify the documentation that determines the PDX will help the coders. The clarification will also assist the case manager and the case management process in general by helping to (1) put the patient on the correct pathway, (2) clarify information needed to obtain the appropriate certifications and recertifications, (3) manage variances from plan, and (4) improve the overall quality of care delivered.

Finally, a PDX may be assigned to only *one* DRG out of the hundreds in the PPS and *one* MDC of the 25. This underscores the importance of having the correct "starting point."

Principal Procedure. Procedures are considered either *therapeutic* or *diagnostic* in nature. A procedure performed for therapeutic purposes should be sequenced before one done for diagnostic reasons. Many diagnostic procedures, and some therapeutic ones, are not designated as "valid operating room (OR) procedures" by HCFA. Some procedures can be performed in an OR and do not qualify for consideration in a surgical DRG (e.g., chest tube insertion); others can be done at the patient's bedside and be included in the operative category (e.g., excisional debridement). Valid OR procedures are defined as ones that carry an operative or anesthetic risk, require highly trained personnel, or require special facilities or equipment.

CCs. Some DRG assignments are also determined by the presence of SDXs that affect the consumption of hospital resources. SDXs are those conditions, in addition to the PDX, that are associated with the *current* hospital episode. Certain significant SDXs, when present with a particular PDX, will usually affect the treatment received, length of stay (LOS), and cost of medical care. This subsequently affects the DRG assignment and results in an increased Medicare payment. These significant SDXs that cause DRG partitioning are called CCs.

- *comorbidity*—a condition, such as diabetes mellitus or chronic obstructive pulmonary disease (COPD), that coexists at the time of admission
- *complication*—a condition that develops after admission, such as a fracture caused by a fall from the hospital bed

The same basic list of CCs is used for most DRGs. However, some diagnoses on the CC list may be "excluded" from influencing DRG assignment if they are closely related to a particular PDX—that is, if they could be expected to occur with that PDX. For example, urinary retention is a CC for a patient admitted with congestive heart failure (CHF) because urinary retention is not "expected" to occur in CHF. However, urinary retention often accompanies a PDX of benign prostatic hypertrophy (BPH) and is, therefore, "excluded" as a CC when it occurrs with BPH.

Gender. There are certain diagnoses and procedures that are specific to only one gender (e.g., cervical cancer, prostatectomy), and certain DRGs were created to achieve clinical coherence for these patients.

Age. Some DRGs are partitioned by patient age. For the most part, DRGs are structured for patients of any age, except for certain categories. For example, neonates/newborns have seven exclusive DRGs, pediatric patients are assigned to DRGs for ages 17 years and younger, and one DRG is for *childhood* mental disorders.

Discharge Status. The discharge status of a patient is another decision factor in DRG assignment. Alcohol and drug abuse patients who leave the facility against medical advice are classified to a specific DRG. Burn patients and neonates who are transferred to another acute care facility are assigned to DRGs 456 and 385, respectively. AMI patients who expire before discharge also have an exclusive DRG assignment.

The DRG Grouping Process

After all the diagnoses and procedures on a case are established, the grouping process that will lead to the DRG assignment begins. The first partition occurs if there was a valid OR procedure performed during the hospital stay. Medical and surgical cases differ in resource consumption, and provision for this difference was made by creating medical and surgical DRGs. As might be expected, the surgical DRGs, as a rule, have higher relative weights. If a code for a valid OR procedure is listed, the case groups to a surgical DRG. If there is no valid OR procedure, the case remains in the medical DRG assigned to the PDX.

It is not unusual for two or more surgeries related to the same PDX to occur during a hospital episode, especially on a complicated case. In this instance, the question arises as to which procedure is considered the *principal* procedure. Recognizing the potential for this situation to occur, a surgical DRG hierarchy was structured for each MDC and its DRGs. Surgical DRGs are assigned to "classes" within the MDC (e.g., craniotomy, spinal procedures, extracranial vascular procedures, carpal tunnel release, and peripheral and cranial nerve and other OR nervous system procedures are classes within MDC 01, Diseases & Disorders of the Nervous System). Therefore, if two procedures *within the same MDC* are performed, the assigning DRG will depend on which *class* is sequenced highest on the surgical hierarchy. Of note is the fact that the surgical hierarchy assignment will place the case in the most resource-intensive *surgical class*, whether or not that particular case is in the most resource-intensive *DRG*.

If the scenario above were revised and one procedure is in the same MDC as the PDX and another is not, the procedure whose MDC matches that of the PDX will be designated as the principal procedure in order to keep the surgical DRG assignment in the same body system. The grouper program will *always* match procedure MDC to PDX MDC first.

Provision is also made for cases in which the procedure performed during an admission is *not* in the same MDC as the PDX. There are three specific DRGs for procedures that are *unrelated* to the PDX. The first partition considers whether the procedure is a prostatic procedure. If so, then DRG 476, "Prostatic O.R. Procedure Unrelated to Principal Diagnosis," is assigned. If there is no prostatic procedure, the grouper compares the procedure code with those assigned to DRG 477, "Non-extensive O.R. Procedure Unrelated to Principal Diagnosis." If a match is found, the case groups to DRG 477. If no match is found in the nonextensive procedures, the case is finally grouped to DRG 468, "Extensive O.R. Procedure Unrelated to Principal Diagnosis."

In the grouping process, CCs and the patient's gender, age, and discharge status are also evaluated for particular DRGs. This is the *basic* partitioning process, which is depicted in Figure 11–1. However, not *every* DRG requires a CC, is gender or age specific, or is affected by the discharge status. There are some DRGs that need a combination of particular diagnoses or procedures, others need specific complications, and one DRG requires a certain number of specific traumatic injuries. There are several handbooks published that list the MDCs, their DRGs, and the diagnoses and procedures assigned to each DRG. It is recommended that the case manager use one of these to assist in projecting a DRG for a case.

Other Factors Influencing the Inclusion and Sequencing of Diagnoses

The official "Guidelines for Selection of a Principal Diagnosis," published in *Coding Clinic*, Second Quarter 1990, are listed in an appendix at the end of the chapter. There are other factors that also influence the inclusion and sequencing of diagnoses. For instance, information found on laboratory test results, radiology reports, EKGs, and so forth may not be used by coders to list diagnoses. Radiology reports can be referenced to identify the specific location of a fracture, but the fracture itself must be acknowledged by the physician in the progress

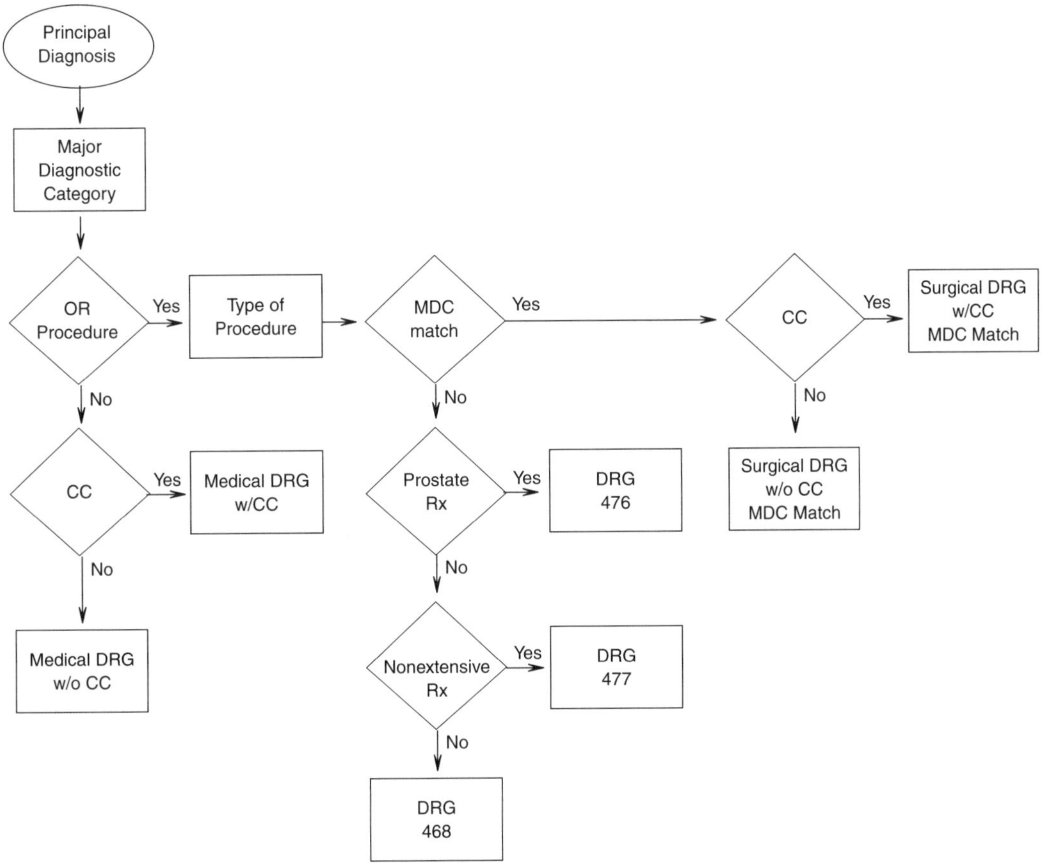

Notes: OR, operating room; MDC, major diagnostic category; CC, complication/comorbidity; DRG, diagnosis-related group.

Figure 11–1 Basic DRG Assignment Structure

notes, consultation report, or discharge summary. If a physician only states in the progress notes that the patient's sodium has decreased and he or she will order intravenous (IV) normal saline to correct the imbalance, what the physician has documented is a lab result and a treatment modality. What the physician has *not* indicated is a diagnosis. If the physician does not document a diagnosis, the discrepancy must be brought to his or her attention and the information recorded on the chart.

A question that often arises is, "Whose documentation is needed for coding purposes?" The rule-of-thumb answer is the physicians who actually see the patient, take a history, and perform a physical examination. This usually includes the emergency room physician, the attending physician, any consulting physician, and the anesthesiologist. Mention of the anesthesiologist sometimes surprises reviewers, but there is often valuable information on the preanesthesia evaluation concerning diagnoses not previously documented by the attending or consulting physicians, or it may clarify diagnoses they have mentioned. Interventional radiologists who do a history and physical examination on the patient are another source, and the documentation of resident physicians may be included *if the attending physician has countersigned the entry.*

This is not to say that documentation by other members of the provider team is not significant. To the contrary, it offers important "clues" that can be used to query the physician further. For instance, if a nursing home patient with a history of a previous cerebral infarction is admitted with a fever and the nursing staff describe his dysphagia, radiology reports patchy infiltrates in his right middle and lower lobes, and speech therapy performs a swallowing study that reveals aspiration and recommends a pureed diet, the physician may document the diagnosis as "pneumonia." However, this is an opportunity for the case manager to query the physician as to whether the patient has *aspiration* pneumonia, seeking the adjective that describes the specific *type* of pneumonia. This specificity provides a more accurate clinical profile of the patient as his care addresses the aspiration component, as opposed to a community-acquired pneumonia. In other words, aspiration pneumonia more appropriately reflects the clinical severity, resources utilized, and LOS.

In the case of nonspecific information, if an attending physician states that the patient has diabetes mellitus and the consulting endocrinologist states that it is insulin-dependent diabetes, it is appropriate to use the endocrinologist's specific, expanded diagnosis because this is in his or her field of expertise and there is no contradiction of the attending physician's diagnosis. However, if two or more physicians document conflicting information, the attending physician must be queried for the definitive diagnosis. For example, if the attending physician states that the above patient has non-insulin dependent diabetes, in conflict with the endocrinologist's diagnosis, the attending physician must be questioned to arrive at the correct answer.

What if, instead of omissions, the physician documents diagnoses that are *not* clinically supported—no workup or treatment was initiated? Remembering the simple concept of Medicare payment being based on resource consumption, the case manager must also bring this discrepancy to the physician's attention for correction—either to provide documentation of treatment or to delete the diagnosis.

Occasionally, physicians will list in the discharge summary or on the face sheet diagnoses that occurred previously but have no bearing on the current hospital admission. It was stated earlier that these conditions are *not* to be reported. However, there are certain systemic diagnoses (e.g., hypertension, diabetes mellitus, Parkinson's disease, COPD) that should be listed, along with other conditions (e.g., blindness, status following cardiac valve replacement, status post leg amputation) because, once there, they never leave, and they affect the management of the patient.

Everything up to this point has been to lay a foundation for understanding the official coding guidelines, the PPS, and the importance of medical record documentation. Medicare has set the expectation, as a requisite for payment, that *all diagnoses and procedures will be substantiated by physician documentation within the medical record.* Those persons who have been imprisoned and facilities that have been fined hundreds of thousands of dollars know too sadly the price for conducting business in a fraudulent manner.

THE BUSINESS OF ACHIEVING ACCURATE, THOROUGH, CONSISTENT DOCUMENTATION

There is a new, challenging career opportunity for case managers in a cutting-edge movement to realize improved hospital and physician profiles, improved data quality and compliance, improved medical record efficiency, and improved payment accuracy. It is the role of facilitator for accurate medical record documentation. There are few individuals who work with records who would not rank improved documentation among the first three items that would improve the quality of their work life. So, as a facilitator of accurate medical record documentation, what does one have to do?

Why Case Managers?

Case managers are the natural selection for this role for the following reasons:

- *They already review the record* from a clinical and resource utilization perspective. The information used to determine medical necessity of admission is the same as that used to determine the PDX. Accurate documentation of all conditions present and treated during the patient's hospital stay will provide a more specific picture of the severity of illness to the entire health care team and reviewing agencies.
- *They have established relationships with physicians* as they have discussed the management of patients. Clinical specificity derived from these encounters provides the case manager with information for medical necessity and continued stay rationale. It also gives the physician an opportunity to discuss the patients with another clinician.
- *They possess the clinical knowledge* to know when there is an obscurity or absence of information that would more accurately reflect the patient's medical profile.

Timeliness

A case manager's association with a patient usually starts with the patient's arrival on the floor, so case managers can influence thorough documentation from the beginning. Documentation about all of the diagnoses that are being treated or regarded on the present admission should be found *throughout* the medical record. Difficulties often arise for facilities when there are single-entry "surprises" in the discharge summary that document the only CC on the case or a more specific type of pneumonia, causing the case to group to a higher-weighted DRG.

Facilitating Physician Education—or Improved Profiles

The Office of the Inspector General's (OIG's) *Compliance Program Guidance for Hospitals* states:

> Accurate coding depends upon the quality and completeness of the physician's documentation. Therefore, the OIG believes that active staff physician participation in educational programs focusing on coding and documentation should be emphasized by the hospital.

In just the past 20 years, we have seen a movement from the *art* of medicine to the *science* of medicine to the *business* of medicine. Although younger physicians are knowledgeable about the PPS and DRGs, understanding the coding classification and guidelines and the importance of thorough, specific documentation are still underdeveloped areas.

Perhaps the easiest explanation one can use to illustrate specificity is to note that if there is more than one adjective that can be applied to a condition or procedure, the modifier applicable to the present situation must be stated in order to capture certain information—to establish both a continuity in the present treatment regimen and a historical record for the future care of the patient. Some physicians ask why they should make this effort. The answer is that it not only benefits the patient and the facility, but it more accurately represents a physician's medical practice. This is especially important because data from physician practice profiles have started to become available to the public.

A common scenario is that of a patient evaluation in the physician's office on Wednesday for symptoms and signs suggesting a urinary tract infection. She is given an antibiotic and sent home. However, she comes in Friday to the emergency room with a 103° temperature, shaking chills, and malaise. Her admitting blood cultures are positive for a pathogen. She is put on IV gentamicin and admitted to the intensive care unit (ICU), and has a 7-day LOS. Invariably, when the patient is discharged, the PDX will be "urinary tract infection." Sometimes, the diagnosis is "urosepsis." The problems are these:

- The patient was not admitted on Wednesday for a urinary tract infection and it does not argue well that she was admitted on Friday for that same diagnosis.
- Urinary tract infections often will not meet the criteria for *inpatient* admission and treatment.
- Urinary tract infections, as a rule, do not necessitate the intense resource consumption seen on this case.

The positive blood cultures and subsequent treatment would actually substantiate a diagnosis of septicemia. Septicemia would justify the intense resource consumption and would meet the criteria for admission to the ICU. In other words, septicemia would bring equity to the diagnosis–treatment relationship.

Usually, when physicians document the diagnosis as "urosepsis," they believe they are indicating sepsis that started with a urinary tract infection—that is why they record "urosepsis" instead of urinary tract infection. Ironically, in the *ICD-9-CM,* the diagnosis of urosepsis is assigned to the same code as a *urinary tract infection.* The case manager should query physicians about whether they were treating a localized urinary tract infection or a more systemic infection (septicemia).

Another indication for documentation improvement is the circumstance in which a medication is listed on the medication administration record, but there is no corresponding diagnosis to explain the resource consumption.

Say, for example, that a patient presents to the hospital with lower extremity edema and the chest X-ray shows an enlarged cardiac profile and bilateral pleural effusions. The home medications include Lasix, which is also administered during the hospital episode.

In this instance, the case manager should ask the physician if the patient is being treated for CHF, as the term was not found in his or her progress notes. CHF, a CC, will affect the DRG assignment and increase the payment for the patient's care.

Similarly, it is often noted that a patient is treated at home and in the hospital with coumadin, but no diagnosis is found in the documentation to warrant the medication. Inquiry about a diagnosis of atrial fibrillation would be justified in this case.

Another reason for physician query is for the patient who has a long history of excessive tobacco use and a chest X-ray finding of "decreased pulmonary perfusion in the upper lung zone along with larger than normal lung volume, consistent with chronic obstructive pulmonary disease." COPD is also considered a CC. However, unlike most other CCs, COPD does not have to be actively treated during the hospitalization in order for it to appear on the diagnosis list. Its very presence is justification enough for inclusion.

Frequently, a patient is admitted with acute exacerbation of chronic asthma or CHF, but has a white blood count of 23,000, with 15 bands—probably indicating the presence of a bacterial infection. The physician's admitting orders include IV Ceftriaxone and Gentamycin and serial chest X-rays. It is important for the case manager to follow the progress of the clinical picture and to inquire about the possibility that the exacerbation is in the form of a bacterial pneumonia.

For a final example, one of the highly underdocumented diagnoses is dehydration. Patients will be given IV fluids at 125 cc per hour—sometimes after a bolus—but the physician will not have recorded that he or she is treating dehydration. This diagnosis is important for the patient's medical profile and resource consumption, and physicians should adopt the habit of recording the diagnosis consistently.

Sometimes, when the case manager reviews the medical record, medications will have been ordered, but there will be no corresponding diagnosis documented for which the medication would be used. The case manager would have to query the physician for a diagnosis to qualify the resource consumption.

As was discussed in the section on how the PPS works, the facility's CMI indicates the relative severity of its patient mix and is directly proportional to the basic DRG payment. If the severity of less than 100 percent of a facility's patients is accurately reflected in their diagnoses, *the basic DRG payment will be less than 100 percent correct.*

Improved Compliance

To help facilities use the rules and regulations of the PPS, Medicare grants contracts to peer review organizations (PROs) in each state to evaluate the accuracy of the diagnoses and procedures reported to Medicare for payment. Detected errors can cause the facility to be placed on intensified review, featuring review of *all* Medicare cases (rather than a sample) and loss of payment.

PROs focus on hospital compliance with federal rules and regulations, looking at necessity of admission, quality of care, premature discharge, accuracy of coding and DRG assignment, and insufficient physician documentation. Under their sixth scope of work, PROs entered the fraud and abuse arena by participating in the Payment Error Prevention Program (PEPP). The OIG of the Department of Health and Human Services, the Department of Justice, the Treasury Department, the Federal Bureau of Investigation, the U.S. Postal Service, and numerous other state and federal law enforcement agencies participated in Operation Restore Trust to fight health care fraud. Millions of dollars have been paid in retribution and fines by facilities that were found to misrepresent claims that were paid by Medicare. The Health Insurance Portability and Accountability Act (HIPAA) of 1996 has incorporated many of the concepts used in Operation Restore Trust in a mandate to the U.S. Attorney General and the OIG to implement a comprehensive national Health Care Fraud and Abuse Control Program.

Additionally, to close a loophole, the old saying of "ignorance of the law is no excuse" is reinforced by these investigating agencies. The federal law

> prohibits presenting or causing to be presented to the United States government, any State agency or any agent thereof a claim: for a medical or other item or service that the person *knows or should know* was not provided as claimed, including a pattern or practice of presenting or causing to be presented a claim for an item or service that is based on a code that such person *knows or should know* will result in a *greater payment* to the claimant than the code such person *knows or should know* is applicable to the item or service actually provided.

A program for volunteer disclosure is in effect for those facilities that have audited themselves and found errors. They still have to return overpayments, but their fine is substantially less than those facilities that do not self-report but are found delinquent.

Improved Medical Record Efficiency

Traditionally, when the medical record comes to the HIM department, the coder may find "holes" in the documentation that present a barrier to obtaining a specific diagnosis, and a query is made retrospectively to the physician for clarification. This wait for an answer holds up the coding and billing processes. Sometimes, the wait is in vain. If the case manager can intervene while the patient is still in the hospital and obtain specific information from the physician, this delay is avoided. The bill can be dropped in a timely fashion, the hospital will receive its correct payment, and there is a greater possibility for realizing the deserved CMI.

Improved Payment Accuracy

Improved *payment* accuracy is an important result of *documentation* accuracy. When the information on the bill sent to Medicare is accurate, the facility has the opportunity to realize its full payment and, at the same time, reduce the risk of noncompliance. Failure to achieve correct payment can impede future plans because the resources might not be available, or, more immediately, compromise the solvency of the hospital.

REFERENCES

Coding Clinic for ICD-9-CM, Second Quarter 1990: 3–12. (Chicago: American Hospital Association, 1990).

Diagnosis Related Groups Definitions Manual, Version 15.0. (Salt Lake City, UT: 3M).

For the Record (June 1, 1999): 38–41. (Valley Forge, PA: Great Valley Publishing Company, Inc.)

SUGGESTED READINGS

ADVANCE for Health Information Professionals (King of Prussia, PA: Merion Publications, Inc.).

Federal Register, DHHS: Final Rules for Medicare Inpatient Prospective Payment System (Washington, DC: U.S. Government Printing Office).

Journal of AHIMA, American Health Information Management Association, Chicago.

APPENDIX 11–A

Guidelines for the Selection of a Principal Diagnosis

The following are the official guidelines for selection of a principal diagnosis. Review of them will help the case manager recognize that condition. The diagnosis listed *first* in the sequencing section is the principal diagnosis, followed by secondary diagnoses that occurred during the current hospital admission. *Sequencing* refers to the order in which diagnoses and procedures are listed on the Uniform Bill-92 (UB-92), the billing form for a patient's care that is submitted to Medicare and other third-party payers for payment.

PDX 1: Codes for symptoms, signs, and ill-defined conditions ***from Chapter 16 in the ICD-9-CM are not to be used as the PDX when a related definitive etiology is present.***

Example: Syncope secondary to bradycardia

Sequencing: bradycardia

Syncope is a symptom/sign (located in Chapter 16) of the cardiac dysrhythmia; therefore, the latter is the PDX. (Syncope does not actually need to be listed in this case, since it does not influence the type of treatment given, the length of stay, nor is it important for statistical or retrieval needs.)

PDX 2: Italicized codes or codes in slanted brackets ***can never be sequenced as the PDX. There are certain diseases (e.g., diabetes mellitus, tuberculosis) that have their manifestations noted by italicized codes or codes in slanted brackets. Manifestations thus denoted must always be sequenced following the underlying disease. The case manager may have to work in conjunction with the coding staff to gain recognition of these particular etiologies.***

Example: Foot ulcer *[ICD-9-CM code 707.1]* due to insulin dependent diabetes mellitus (code 250.81)

Sequencing: Insulin dependent diabetes mellitus with other specified manifestation, foot ulcer

PDX 3: Acute (subacute) and chronic descriptions for the same condition ***are sequenced with the acute condition first.***

Example: Acute and chronic cholecystitis

Sequencing: Acute cholecystitis, chronic cholecystitis

PDX 4: When two or more interrelated conditions (such as diseases in the same ICD-9-CM chapter or manifestations characteristically associated with a certain disease) are present on admission, each potentially meeting the definition for PDX, ***either condition may be sequenced first, unless the circumstances of the admission, the therapy provided, the Tabular List, or the Alphabetic Index indicate otherwise.***

Example: A patient was admitted in atrial fibrillation and acute congestive heart failure (CHF). The dysrhythmia was treated with digoxin and the heart failure with IV Lasix. Both conditions potentially meet the definition of PDX and either may be sequenced as such. When the diagnoses are grouped, the DRG for CHF has the higher relative weight and it is selected as the PDX.

Sequencing: Congestive heart failure, atrial fibrillation

PDX 5: In the unusual instance when two or more diagnoses equally meet the criteria for PDX ***as determined by the circumstances of admission, diagnostic workup and/or therapy provided, and the Alphabetic Index, Tabular List, or another coding guideline does not provide sequencing direction, any one of the diagnoses may be sequenced first.***

Example: The patient in the case above also has an acute overlying pneumonia on admission, and sputum cultures done in the ER are positive for *Klebsiella.* Intravenous antibiotics and aggressive respiratory therapy are begun immediately, as well as therapy for the CHF and atrial fibrillation. The *Klebsiella* pneumonia meets the criteria for PDX and grouping shows it is in a higher-weighted DRG than the heart failure.

Sequencing: *Klebsiella* pneumonia, congestive heart failure, atrial fibrillation

PDX 6: In those rare instances when two or more comparative or contrasting conditions ***are documented as either/or, they are listed as if the conditions were confirmed and the diagnoses are sequenced according to the circumstances of the admission. If no further determination can be made as to which diagnosis should be the PDX, either diagnosis may be sequenced first.***

Example: A patient is diagnosed with acute pancreatitis and malignant neoplasm of the pancreas head, but neither can be singularly confirmed as the cause of the patient's jaundice. Grouping the two diagnoses reveals the malignancy is in a higher-weighted DRG.

Sequencing: Malignant neoplasm of the pancreas head, acute pancreatitis

PDX 7: When a symptom is followed by contrasting/comparative diagnoses, ***the symptom is sequenced as the PDX. The potential etiologies should be listed as confirmed conditions and sequenced as secondary diagnoses (SDXs).***

Example: Abdominal pain due either to possible acute pancreatitis or possible acute cholecystitis.

Sequencing: Abdominal pain, acute pancreatitis, acute cholecystitis

(A good way to remember this rule is to code what seems known first [pain] and then what might have caused it [pancreatitis vs. cholecystitis].)

PDX 8: When a patient is admitted for observation and evaluation of a suspected condition, ***but no subsequent confirming evidence is found and no treatment is rendered, a choice is made from the Observation and Evaluation for Suspected Conditions series (V71.0-V71.9).***

Example: A patient is admitted after a motor vehicle accident for a possible concussion. After evaluation, it is determined the patient only suffered minor cuts and bruises of the head.

Sequencing: Observation following other accident (V71.4), minor cuts and bruises of head

PDX 9: When the original plan of treatment is not carried out ***due to unforeseen circumstances, the condition after study which occasioned the patient's admission to the hospital should still be sequenced as the PDX.***

Example: A patient with degenerative arthritis is admitted for a total knee replacement but develops severe chest pain the morning of surgery. Evaluation reveals this to be unstable angina. The knee surgery is delayed and the patient is scheduled for a heart cath.

Sequencing: Degenerative arthritis, unstable angina; heart cath

PDX 10: The residual condition or nature of a late effect ***is sequenced first, followed by the*** **cause** ***of the residual condition (Example 1 below), except in a few instances where the Alphabetic Index directs otherwise (Example 2 below).***

Example 1: Patient with arthritis of the elbow due to an old fracture of the humerus suffered five years ago.

Sequencing: Traumatic arthritis, late effect of fracture of upper extremity

Example 2: Patient with curvature of the spine [737.40] due to previous tuberculosis (015.0)

Sequencing: Late effect of tuberculosis, curvature of the spine

PDX 11: When multiple burn sites exist, ***sequence the most serious (the highest degree) as the PDX.***

Example: A patient is admitted with second-degree burns to both arms and third degree burns to the chest wall.

Sequencing: Third degree burns on chest wall, second degree burns on arms

PDX 12: When multiple injuries exist, ***sequence the most severe injury as determined by the attending physician as the PDX.***

Example: A patient is admitted with fractures of three ribs, a mid-shaft fracture of the left ulna, and an open fracture of the left humeral head. The attending physician determines the open fracture to be the most severe injury because it requires the most extensive treatment.

Sequencing: Open fracture of humeral head, closed fracture of three ribs, closed fracture mid-shaft of ulna

PDX 13: When an ambulatory surgery outpatient is admitted to inpatient status—***directly or after a period of observation—due to a complication following the day surgery, the*** **condition causing the inpatient admission** ***is the PDX, followed by the diagnosis that necessitated the surgery. The procedure is also included on the inpatient chart. NOTE: This may cause the case to group to DRG 468, Extensive O.R. Procedure Unrelated to Principal Diagnosis, but this is the correct sequencing. (See more about procedures unrelated to principal diagnoses under*** **B. Procedures.*)***

Example: The patient has a needle biopsy of the lung performed in day surgery to determine the presence of a malignancy. In the PACU, she goes into acute respiratory failure secondary to a collapsed lung, is intubated and put on a ventilator, and admitted to the hospital.

Sequencing: Acute respiratory failure, post-op atelectasis, CA of the lung; lung biopsy, intubation, mechanical ventilation

PDX 14: Neoplasms. ***When selecting the PDX on a cancer case, it may be helpful to consider the following questions:***

- Was the *focus* during the admission on the primary neoplasm or a metastasis?
- Was the *treatment* during this admission directed toward the neoplasm or toward a complication of the neoplasm or its therapy?
- Was *radiotherapy or chemotherapy* the reason the patient was admitted?

A. If the treatment is directed at the malignancy, **designate the malignancy as the PDX, except when the purpose of the admission is for radiotherapy or chemotherapy, in which instance the malignancy is sequenced as a SDX.**

B. When a patient is admitted for the purpose of radiotherapy or chemotherapy and develops complications, **such as uncon-**

trolled nausea and vomiting or dehydration, the PDX is Admission for radiotherapy or Admission for chemotherapy.

C. When an episode of inpatient care involves surgical removal of a primary or secondary site malignancy followed by adjunctive chemotherapy or radiotherapy, **sequence the malignancy as the PDX.**

D. When the reason for admission is to determine the extent of the malignancy, or for a procedure such as a paracentesis or thoracentesis, **the malignancy is designated as the PDX, even though chemotherapy or radiotherapy is administered.**

E. When the primary malignancy has been previously excised or eradicated from its site and there is no adjunctive treatment directed to that site and no evidence of any remaining malignancy at the primary site, **a History of primary malignancy diagnosis applies. However, it can never be a PDX—it is always a SDX. (However, if the patient is still receiving any treatment for the malignancy, the *active* malignancy diagnosis is sequenced as a SDX if the admission is for chemotherapy or radiotherapy.) Any mention of extension, invasion, or metastasis to a nearby structure or organ or to a distant site is listed as a secondary malignancy and may be the PDX.**

F. When a patient is admitted for surgical intervention of a known malignancy and a secondary site is discovered at the time of surgery **and a biopsy of the metastasis is also performed, the PDX is the known-at-admission malignancy for which the patient was admitted. The metastasis is also listed and is sequenced as a SDX.**

G. When a patient is admitted for pain and primary and secondary malignancy sites are both discovered at the time of surgery **and surgery is performed on both, either may be sequenced as the PDX, since their discovery was simultaneous and not known at admission.**

H. When a patient is admitted because of a primary neoplasm with metastasis and treatment directed toward the secondary site only, **the secondary neoplasm is designated as the PDX, even though the primary malignancy is still present.**

I. Symptoms, signs, and ill-defined conditions listed in Chapter 16 (code range 780–789) characteristic of, or associated with, an existing primary or secondary malignancy **cannot be used to replace the malignancy as the PDX, regardless of the number of admissions for treatment and care of the neoplasm. Examples of these conditions would include pain, syncope, nausea, and vomiting.**

J. Listing and sequencing complications associated with the malignant neoplasm or with the therapy thereof are subject to the following guidelines:

- When admission is for management of an anemia associated with the malignancy, and the treatment is only for anemia, the anemia is designated as the PDX and is followed by the malignancy diagnosis.
- When the admission is for management of an anemia associated with chemotherapy or radiotherapy and the only treatment is for the anemia, the anemia is designated as the PDX and is followed by the malignancy diagnosis.
- When the admission is for management of dehydration due to the malignancy or the therapy, or a combination of both, and only the dehydration is being treated (IV rehydration), the dehydration is the PDX, followed by the malignancy diagnosis.
- When the admission is for treatment of a complication resulting from a surgical procedure, such as a colon resection performed for the treatment of an intestinal malignancy, the complication is designated as the PDX if treatment is directed at resolving the complication. Examples

of conditions that would be designated as the PDX in this case would be postsurgical nonabsorption syndrome, malfunction of a colostomy, and complications of implants.

- When the admission is for control of intractable pain due to the malignancy, the malignancy is the PDX. There is no code in the ICD-9-CM for intractable pain; therefore, intractable pain is classified to its cause.
- When admission is for treatment of toxic effects of a chemotherapeutic drug, the toxic effect (e.g., uncontrolled vomiting) is the PDX.

PDX 15: When sequencing a poisoning or reaction to the improper use of a medication ***(e.g., wrong dose, wrong substance, wrong route of administration), the poisoning is sequenced as the PDX. This includes the use of unprescribed medications, medications taken in combination with other drugs without a physician's knowledge, or medications taken with alcohol.***

Example: Coma due to digoxin overdose

Sequencing: Digoxin poisoning, coma

PDX 16: When sequencing an adverse effect to the proper use of a medication, ***the manifestation (e.g., palpitations, coma) is sequenced as the PDX.***

Example: Coma despite proper use of digoxin

Sequencing: Coma, adverse effect of digoxin

PDX 17: When the admission is for treatment of a complication of surgery or other medical care, ***the complication (from the 996–999 series) is sequenced as the PDX. Accuracy must be exercised in using this series since the complication*** **must be due to a procedure** ***or other medical care and not one that just happened to have occurred in the postoperative period (e.g., a postoperative infection versus a fracture from a fall out of the hospital bed following surgery).***

A. When the complication is due to the presence of an internal device, implant, or graft, a code from the 996 series, Complications Peculiar to Certain Specified Procedures, must be used.

- If there is a *mechanical* malfunction of the device, implant, or graft (e.g., breakdown, displacement, leakage, mechanical obstruction, perforation, or protrusion), the PDX must come from the 996.0–996.59 series.
- If there is an *infection or inflammatory reaction* due to an internal prosthetic device, implant, or graft, the PDX must come from the 996.6 series.
- If there are *other complications* of an internal (biological) (synthetic) prosthetic device, implant, or graft (e.g., occlusion, embolism, fibrosis, hemorrhage, pain, stenosis, thrombus, or unspecified complication), the PDX must come from the 996.7 series.
- If there are complications of a *transplanted organ*, the PDX must come from the 996.8 series.
- If there are complications of a *reattached extremity or body part*, the PDX must come from the 996.9 series.

B. If the complications affect specified body systems and are not elsewhere classified, the PDX will come from the 997 series, Complications Affecting Specified Body Systems, Not Elsewhere Classified.

C. If the complications of procedures are not elsewhere classified, the PDX will come from the 998 series, Other Complications of Procedures, Not Elsewhere Classified.

D. If the complications of medical care are not elsewhere classified, the PDX will come from the 999 series, Complications of Medical Care, Not Elsewhere Classified.

E. If the complication is classified to the 996–999 series, an additional diagnosis for the specific complication may be added.

Example 1: A patient returns three weeks post hip replacement with pain due to a protruding screw.

Sequencing: Mechanical complication of an internal orthopedic device, implant, graft (996.4)

Example 2: The patient with an indwelling Foley catheter is admitted with a diagnosis of septicemia due to the catheter.

Sequencing: Infection/inflammation due to indwelling urinary catheter (996.64), sepsis (038.9)

Example 3: Four days after discharge for a laparoscopic cholecystectomy, the surgical wound becomes infected, the patient becomes very ill, and is readmitted with a diagnosis of postop septicemia.

Sequencing: Postoperative septicemia (code 998.59)

PDX 18: Conditions in the final diagnosis stated as suspected, questionable, possible, probable, etc., are listed as confirmed diagnoses. ***Diagnoses that have* not *been ruled out by the time of discharge are also listed as confirmed diagnoses. A diagnosis with the phrase "ruled out" at the end is treated as no evidence was found to substantiate the diagnosis and it, consequently, is not listed.***

Part IV

Transition from Discharge Planning to Community-Based Case Management

CHAPTER 12

Transition Planning (Discharge Planning)

Sara Atwell

TAKE THIS TO WORK

1. Case managers need to act proactively in identifying and planning the patient's transition from one level of care to the next.
2. The case manager needs to plan using the entire care team to facilitate the transition planning process.
3. There are four major stages in transition planning: assessment, planning, implementation, and evaluation.
4. The key driver for transitional activity is a set of level-of-care criteria.

Transition planning (known to most as discharge planning) has been in existence in some form for more than a century. In 1886, the Boston Visiting Nurses Association and Massachusetts General Hospital created the first continuing care agreement in the United States. This agreement was instrumental in linking the acute care hospital with nonacute community-based services. Since then, a series of events have helped shape how case managers prepare and plan transition/discharge for patients. In 1909, Metropolitan Life Insurance Company extended its insurance coverage to include home health care. In 1965, Medicare was enacted, fundamentally changing the way in which the elderly population can be cared for and the services that can be provided under Medicare coverage. Stanford Medical Center was one of the first hospitals to create a role for care coordination posthospitalization. This nurse was called the posthospital nurse care coordinator.

Understanding the provision of postacute services and the benefits offered to patients requiring postacute care is an essential component of the transition planning process. It was not until 1976 that the National League of Nurses published discharge planning guidelines. These guidelines provided the first written guide offering ways to assist in planning for discharge. From 1983 to the present, the Health Care Financing Administration's (HCFA's) regulatory requirements have made the most significant changes in health care delivery.

- 1983—Diagnosis-related groups (DRGs) are introduced.
- 1987—Nationwide, length of stay (LOS) is shortened by three days.
- 1997—Integrated delivery systems (IDSs) focus on transition management and full utilization of the IDS continuum of services.

- 1997—The Balanced Budget Act (BBA) begins a phased-in approach to reimbursement changes across the continuum (prospective payment having the greatest impact).
- 1999—Blending of acute care and post-acute services occurs.
- 2000—Prospective payment continues to spread across the nonacute care environments.

All of these changes have significantly impacted the way in which case managers help patients and families maneuver through the health care maze.

DRIVING FORCES THAT HAVE INFLUENCED TRANSITION PLANNING

There are five driving forces that have contributed to and influenced the process of transition planning.

1. managed care
2. competition
3. health care budgets
4. cost management
5. accountability for health status

Managed Care

Managed care is a system of health care delivery that tries to manage cost, quality, and access to health care. As health care costs continue to rise, managed care organizations (MCOs) are looking at the lowest cost care settings that can appropriately deliver the care needs to the patient. The focus continues to be on a decrease in the LOS within the most expensive care setting, the hospital.

Competition

Market competition is what drives hospitals to perform at the most efficient and effective level, with the ultimate focus on quality patient outcomes. Consumers are becoming wise to health care, and thus, more influential with payers and providers regarding their care choices.

Budgets and Cost Management

Budgets and cost management of both the payer and provider organizations are driving efficient and effective transition planning processes. Proactive transition planning can have a direct effect on the volume, cost, and quality of care.

Accountability

More so than ever before, providers and payers are being held accountable for meeting the moral and ethical standards of health care delivery. The continuing changes in regulatory requirements have forced accountability back onto the delivery system as well as the payer and the consumers themselves.

WHAT IS TRANSITION PLANNING?

Transition planning is a process of always looking forward. In transition planning, the attention of the case manager and caregivers is directed to the next stage of care, and timely communication and a systematic handoff of the patient's needs and services to the subsequent caregivers is provided. Case managers have become coordinators of patient care, with an unprecedented role in planning for discharge and transition.

The American Nurses Association defines discharge planning as the part of the continuity-of-care process that is designed to prepare the patient and his or her family for the next phase of care and to assist in making any necessary arrangements for that phase of care, whether it be self-care, care by family members, or care by an organized health care provider.

As case managers, transition planning means to facilitate and coordinate a plan of care that will assist and prepare the patient and family for transition from one level of care to another.

The emphasis in discharge/transition planning when done correctly is to ensure that at each point in the patient's course of treatment, care is delivered in the optimum setting. The optimum setting is determined by clinical appropriateness and appropriate utilization of resources. When determining the optimum level of care, the case manager should always ask if the patient is clinically appropriate for that particular level of care. Does the patient meet the criteria for service? Are the resources utilized appropriate for the services rendered and the outcome desired?

Transition/discharge planning involves

- early assessment of anticipated patient care needs
- concern for the patient's total well-being
- open communication with the patient, family, and caregivers to effectively transition the patient to venues of care across the continuum
- collaboration and coordination among the patient and family, the entire care team, physicians, and the payer
- knowledge of all levels of care and continuity-of-care resources to effectively transition patients to the most appropriate service

Transition/discharge planning is not

- limited to the concern about the physical transfer of the patient
- focused only on the physical needs of the patient
- done to or for the patient without his or her active involvement

PURPOSE, GOALS, AND OBJECTIVES OF THE TRANSITION PLAN

Purpose

The purpose of the transition plan is to meet the patient's needs while promoting efficient and effective communication among the patient, the patient's family, physicians, the case manager, payers and other postacute and community providers, and the hospital health care team in the discharge and transition process.

Goals and Objectives

Goals

- The transition plan must be focused on the patient.
- The transition plan must be clinically and fiscally appropriate.
- The transition plan must be cost effective to the patient, the provider, and the payer.

Objectives

- A successful transition plan encompasses timely communication throughout the transition process, continuing to manage the plan through all stages: assessment, planning, implementation, and evaluation.
- The transition plan, if managed appropriately, should contribute to a decrease in acute readmissions through ongoing education and post-transition follow-up.
- The transition plan will help to optimize the use of appropriate resources to avoid over- or underutilization.
- The transition plan will promote optimal clinical, financial, and satisfaction outcomes.

THE TRANSITION PLANNING PROCESS

Transition planning is an iterative process based on ongoing assessment, planning, implementation, and regular plan validation. The process itself is fluid and requires the case manager to be proactive and flexible during all of the transition planning stages.

Transition Planning Stages

Assessment

Planning for transition begins the minute the patient comes in contact with the organization. This could be in the physician's office, the clinic, the postprocedure area, admitting, or the emergency department. Once the patient has access to the system, the system has access to the patient. This is the time to gather clinical, social, and benefits information. If appropriate, start to discuss with the patient and/or family the plan of care, expected outcomes, and support mechanism in place to facilitate identifying the next level of care.

Planning

The transition plan coordinates with the clinical plan of care and should always "begin with the end in mind" (a Stephen Covey quote). When looking at the next venue of care, the case manager should always work up two potential transition plans. For example, the patient with a right hemipariegic stroke may be worked up for an acute rehabilitation stay postacute hospitalization and a skilled nursing rehabilitation stay. The patient's progress in the acute environment and his or her ability to tolerate therapy will determine the most appropriate postacute setting once he or she is discharged from the acute hospital.

Case managers must remain flexible in their plan and have the ability to adapt to changes in their patient's condition at any given notice. The transition plan may be coordinated by the case manager, but it takes a team approach to make it happen. The plan is forever evolving with the patient. The entire patient's care team should have input into the transition plan. The transition plan is best executed when the patient's care team, the physician, and the patient and family are involved from the start.

Implementation

Smooth implementation requires timely execution and coordination among all parties involved in the plan. It is essential that the team on the receiving end be synchronized with the case manager and the originating care team. It is at this time that if the plan has not been carefully thought through and planned appropriately, the transition becomes rocky and uncomfortable for the patient, family, and all involved.

Evaluation

Evaluation should occur throughout the process of assessment, planning, and implementation. If the case manager is evaluating while conducting the assessment, the evaluation becomes part of the assessment and the process of designing an appropriate transition plan. Evaluation during the planning stages requires input from the care team and could necessitate change due to recommendations made by other caregivers, the patient, and the patient's family. Evaluation of the plan also occurs as the patient's episode of care changes and his or her clinical picture improves or deteriorates. Evaluation during implementation includes evaluation of the implementation process, the associated outcomes achieved due to the plan's implementation, and satisfaction of the patient, family, and care team.

FORMULATING THE TRANSITION PLAN

There are four essential steps in formulating the transition plan.

1. Conduct the assessment.
2. Identify the target LOS.
3. Develop and communicate a systematic approach to the transition plan.
4. Identify the most appropriate settings, based on the patient's profile.

Conduct the Assessment

During the assessment stage of the transition planning process, the necessary clinical, psychosocial, and financial data are gathered. It is never too early to start planning. Case managers must have access to all aspects of data in order to adequately assess the needs of the patient and family as well as to coordinate the transition plan with the clinical plan of care. Remember, case managers will most often want to develop two plans simultaneously in order to be prepared for deviations from the original clinical course.

There are six basic steps that are conducted during an assessment.

1. Complete the care management intake assessment form.
2. Carefully review the medical record.
3. Conduct interviews with the patient and the patient's family.
4. Evaluate the patient's financial and benefits status.

5. Communicate with the payer (if the payer is involved in the patient's care).
6. Attend rounds and interdisciplinary planning meetings (often, it is the case manager who leads the interdisciplinary team planning meetings).

Complete the Intake Assessment Form

This form is one of the most valuable tools that case managers have at their disposal. The form can be a manual tool that is used throughout the episode of care to document clinical, social, and financial data. Many organizations have integrated this tool with their information systems utilization management (UM) software. This tool then becomes the information warehouse for the case manager as well as the communication tool among the rest of the care team.

Review the Medical Record

The medical record is the one comprehensive source for collecting and monitoring the patient's clinical progress during the episode of care. It provides the patient's past and current clinical picture, pertinent day-to-day updates to the medical plan, and a reference to monitor resource utilization and care team interactions.

Interview the Patient and Family

An interview with the patient and/or the patient's family provides the case manager with insight that is not necessarily obtained in any record. Good interviewing skills will allow the case manager to gather information that is not documented anywhere. It also helps to lay the foundation for establishing a relationship with the patient and family built on mutual trust. It is at this time that transition planning should be thoroughly explored and options laid out for the patient and family. During this process and throughout the episode of care, patients and their families will rely on you to educate them regarding postacute care venues, insurance coverage, and community support.

Evaluate Patient's Financial and Benefits Status

It is important to understand the patient's benefit package and the inclusion and exclusion of posthospital benefit coverage. The best transition plan for the patient can be sabotaged by the lack of benefits or funds under the benefit package to cover the postacute resources or placement necessary for posthospital care. Prior to discussing the optimal plan with the patient, the case manager must investigate thoroughly the necessary benefits and funds for carrying out the plan. Often alternative benefit coverage such as Medicaid (if qualified) can be initiated during the patient's hospitalization. Understanding the benefits is only half the battle. It is essential for the case manager to know the availability of those benefits and to what extent the patient has already used parts of his or her coverage. For example, a patient is covered for 80 skilled days under a commercial insurance plan and used 40 of those skilled days in a previous postacute skilled stay, ending just 3 weeks prior to the current hospitalization. This may impact the case manager's transition plan and the options available to the patient. It is the case manager's responsibility to work with the patient's insurance plan and the hospital's business office to gather the correct benefit data to support a smooth transition plan.

Communicate with the Payer

Timely communication is key to successful payer and provider relationships. Understanding the payer expectations of the provider will help in early transition planning. Answer the following questions: Is there a long-standing history with the payer and the patient? What is the best mode of communication regarding concurrent review of clinical data? How often are clinical reviews communicated? What is the contractual relationship that the payer and the provider share? What are the expected LOS and the conditions for postacute provisions? Knowing and understanding the answers to these questions will set the stage for a mutually beneficial relationship between the payer, the provider, and the patient. Planning smooth transitions requires input and participation from all members of the team.

Attend Rounds and Planning Meetings

Transition planning is integrated with daily care facilitation. Facilitating care and planning for discharge are interdependent processes. Rounding with physicians and the care team will help to expedite the planning, allow for input from clinical experts, and establish a forum for ongoing communication. It may not be possible for case managers to attend daily physician patient rounds, especially in an academic medical center environment. These rounds are time consuming and not necessarily compatible with the case manager's schedule. If case managers are unable to attend walking rounds with physicians, they need to set up alternative arrangements for reviewing daily patient's progress and discussing transition planning with the physician. This may take the form of telephone patient updates or worksheet updates on the unit with the physician (similar to nursing Kardex rounds) to review daily plans of care and discharge/transition planning progress. Establishing a strong relationship with attending physicians and specialists—one that demonstrates the case manager's ability to effectively, proactively coordinate and communicate the transition/discharge plan of care to the physician—will promote the value of the case manager's role in meeting the patient's needs and assisting the physician in care coordination.

Unit-based interdisciplinary planning meetings provide for information exchange and offer the case manager an opportunity to elicit input from other care team members collectively. These should occur twice a week to allow for timely clinical and transition planning updates. Patients and family members are often invited to these meeting to educate and actively involve them in the plan of care and discharge. Guidelines for rounding include the following:

- Review all medical needs.
- Discuss and gather new information from the team.
- Resurface previously identified issues that need clarification or ongoing resolution.
- Promote discussion to expedite care.
- Ensure ongoing communication of the transition plan with expected LOS.
- Request necessary orders to expedite the transition planning process.
- Integrate and communicate with the next level of care and community providers involved in the continuum-of-care process.

Identify the Target LOS

The target LOS has been established to guide the physicians, case managers, clinical care team, providers, and payers in providing efficient, cost-effective, quality care within a given reasonable time frame associated with the diagnoses and treatment interventions. It is meant to be used as a guide to aid in delivering focused care to patients within a given diagnosis that is typical and noncomplicated. The industry looks toward standards that have been set by HCFA (Medicare DRG mean LOS) and Milliman & Robertson, to name a few.

Part of the case manager's role is to identify the appropriate target LOS and communicate this target LOS to the physician and other care team members. Once established, this LOS will help guide the plan of care and establish an anticipated transition date. In communicating the target LOS to the physician, the case manager should remind the physician that this is a tool to help focus the plan and will vary with changes in patient clinical condition and anticipated next level of care.

Develop and Communicate a Systematic Approach to the Plan

Once the initial assessment is complete, the target LOS is assigned, and team meetings have taken place, the formation of a realistic transition plan is well under way. The plan or plans of care must be communicated with and collaborated by the physician, patient, and family. Alternative setting options must be reviewed by the patient and family so they can make an informed choice regarding the next steps in the episode of treatment. Communication with the payer to verify options and coverage should occur at the time of admission. This will enable the case manager to appropriately match the benefits with the next level or venue of care proactively.

Modify the Plan

As the patient progresses with the course of treatment, the transition plan may require alteration secondary to a change in the patient's need or clinical status. The transition plan acts as a guide to action. The plan performs this function only if it is current, complete, and ready to initiate. Case managers should ask themselves daily if this is still an appropriate transition plan.

Triggers that suggest that the plan may need alteration include the following:

- improvement or deterioration of the patient's condition
- change in lab values, diagnoses, and/or vital signs
- patient and/or family conflict
- issues regarding transfer and/or transition to a new level or setting

Any one of the above triggers can necessitate a change in the transition plan. When modifying the plan of care, consider the following steps:

- Evaluate the current plan to determine the magnitude of change.
- Identify the barriers, constraints, and necessary changes.
- Notify immediately the facilities, agencies, and/or services that have required modification.
- Notify the payer of a change in the plan and the supporting clinical and social data to support the change.
- Outline the next steps with the patient, family, physician, internal and external care team, and payer.
- Document thoroughly events leading up to the change in plan, and the new plan in progress.

As much as possible, case managers need to anticipate change, evaluate a new plan, and be responsive to the needs of the patient while effectively and efficiently coordinating with all members of the care team.

Identify the Most Appropriate Settings

An understanding of the levels of care, criteria for admission, and postacute options is essential in developing a proactive plan of care. Case managers have access to specific level-of-care criteria that help appropriately move the patient, when ready, to the next level of care. Most hospitals use InterQual criteria or similar criteria to set level-of-care admission and discharge criteria. This criterion is one of the many tools used by case managers to establish the transition plan and execute it appropriately. Outlined below are acute level-of-care criteria. (Postacute criteria are reviewed in detail in Chapter 13.)

Level-of-Care Criteria

Critical Care. To meet general critical care criteria, the patient must be hemodynamically unstable or require frequent monitoring.

The patient meets medical cardiac criteria under any one of the following circumstances:

- The patient needs continuous cardiac monitoring.
- The patient requires monitoring with intervention at least every two hours.
- The patient requires invasive hemodynamic monitoring.
- The patient requires titration of intravenous (IV) vasoactive agents every two hours.
- The patient has temporary pacemaker placement.
- The patient is on mechanical ventilation.

The patient meets trauma surgical criteria under the following circumstances:

- The patient has undergone a major surgical procedure.
- The patient experiences surgical complications (e.g., disseminated IV coagulation).
- The patient has an acute traumatic event (e.g., severe head injury).
- The patient requires invasive hemodynamic monitoring.
- The patient requires titration of IV vasoactive agents every two hours.
- The patient is on mechanical ventilation.

Intermediate Level of Care. Intermediate level of care in the acute care setting is defined by the delivery of required care elements and not by hospital unit or area. Intermediate care can be provided in a defined intermediate care unit or, if not available, in a critical care unit. There are two required elements for intermediate level of care: patient is hemodynamically stable and requires frequent monitoring.

The intermediate treatment area must be able to provide the following:

- continuous cardiac monitoring
- monitoring and intervention at least every four hours
- titration of IV vasoactive agents at least every four hours
- pacemaker monitoring

Medical–Surgical Units. Criteria for medical–surgical units are based on severity of illness (SI) and intensity of service (IS) criteria specific for each clinical service line/major diagnostic category. SI criteria answer the question of how sick the patient is. To meet SI criteria, the patient must have documented clinical findings that support hospitalization. IS criteria validate the severity of the patient's illness based on the treatments and interventions ordered by the physician. A patient must be evaluated daily to determine SI/IS criteria. Examples of the major diagnostic categories are as follows:

- hematology/oncology
- infectious disease
- obstetrics preterm < 37 weeks
- obstetrics term > 37 weeks
- respiratory/chest
- skin connective tissue
- surgery/trauma
- cadiovascular/peripheral vascular
- chemical dependence
- central nervous system/muscular skeletal
- endocrine/metabolic
- eyes, ears, nose, and throat
- gastrointestinal, biliary, and pancreatic

Observation Status. Observation status is considered outpatient status and is used when patients do not meet acute SIIS criteria but need continued monitoring to determine level of care or appropriate setting. Guidelines for using observation status include the following:

- Patient must have an unstable medical condition requiring evaluation, assessment, and/or frequent monitoring to determine the need for inpatient admission (e.g., uncertain diagnosis of myocardial infarction).
- Determination of observation status must be patient specific.
- If used following an outpatient procedure, observation status must include documentation of an adverse reaction or a complication triggering observation monitoring.
- Observation status must be documented. Documentation must support active observation and the decision that medical necessity for admission cannot be made at that time.
- The maximum time frame to place a patient in observation is 48 hours. Twenty-three hours is the unwritten limit and the guideline recommended when monitoring observation.

ROLES OF THE CASE MANAGEMENT TEAM

It takes all members of the care team to develop and implement the transition plan. As the coordinator of the patient's care, the case manager assumes the ultimate responsibility for the transition plan. Social work and nursing are the two other disciplines that are critical to the transition planning process.

Case Manager's Role

There are many elements to the role of the case manager in transition planning. There are 10 areas where case managers can positively affect the transition plan.

1. Establish a trusting relationship.
2. Be the liaison between the patient, the patient's family, and the health care team.
3. Decrease fragmentation across health care settings.
4. Ensure quality health care along the continuum.
5. Personalize care in an impersonal setting.
6. Provide early identification of all patients with simple and complex discharge planning needs.
7. Identify all issues required to establish a workable plan.
8. Evaluate opportunities to manage patient care in less costly settings.
9. Make sure discharge planning needs are met for all patients.
10. Bridge the gap between acute hospitalization and postacute needs.

The interpersonal component of the case manager's role is perhaps more critical to transition planning than any other role component. Patients and families must have confidence that the case manager has the patient's best interest as his or her primary concern. Case managers must be able to integrate the implications of the patient's clinical status with the anticipated discharge date and the psychosocial variables associated with the patient and the episode of care. Case managers are expected to plan for transition on all patients. The ability to identify simple and complex discharge needs will help to focus the case manager's efforts and allocate more time to the complex multidimensional patient. Evaluation of all levels of care and settings will provide the case manager with opportunities to furnish the patient and family with every appropriate option. The key to effective transition planning is the coordination of care that facilitates utilization of the appropriate continuum-of-care services offered to the patient. Through access to these services, the patient's ultimate care experience is improved.

In summary, the case manager is responsible for

- assessment of the patient's clinical, psychosocial, and financial presentation (synthesis and analysis)
  1. identification of treatment options in collaboration with the physician and the health care team
  2. identification of appropriate levels of care and care setting alternatives
- coordination of care
  1. reinforcement and clarification of the plan of care
  2. initiation and follow-up of referrals and consults
  3. coordination of transition to posthospital care
- serving as the primary contact with the payer for complex clinical transitions
  1. coordinating and negotiating insurance benefits with the treatment and transition plan
- assisting with ongoing patient and family education and reinforcement of discharge instructions
- promoting quality of care and clinical best practice
- evaluating effectiveness of the transition plan
- managing costs
  1. Ensuring timely ordering, sequencing, and scheduling of procedures and treatments
  2. limiting duplication of services
  3. ensuring program consistency
- negotiation with
  1. patient and family
  2. multidisciplinary team
  3. payers
  4. postacute care providers and community services
- documentation of
  1. the transition plan and level of care
  2. discharge plan summary
  3. delays in care and discharge (variance tracking and reporting)
  4. communication with patient, physician, and other care providers

Social Worker's Role

The social worker's role is to assist the case manager with complex cases where the patient and the family require psychosocial and crisis intervention. The social worker's primary role is to promote patient and family adaptation to the disease process or disability. Second, the social worker should work alongside the case manager to assist with transition planning, implementation, and evaluation.

The social worker's role encompasses, but is not limited to, the following:

- Express concern with the patient's ability to cope and adapt to physical, psychological, and social changes resulting from illness or injury.
- Conduct timely psychosocial assessment interviews.
- Provide counseling for problems related to the environmental needs, family and interpersonal conflict, and physical and /or mental illness.
- Intervene in crisis situations to resolve the crisis and use negotiation skills.

Nurse's Role

The nurse has the opportunity to interface with the patient and family from a pure clinical perspective. Nurses play an integral role in transition planning due to the very nature of their role at the bedside. They provide ongoing clinical support through clinical assessment, bedside care, and clinical and disease-related teaching. The case manager depends on the nurse to complete the following functions so the case manager can effectively coordinate and communicate the transition plan.

- Identify case management needs that will be critical to the transition plan based on clinical assessments.
- Participate in interdisciplinary meetings.
- Collaborate with case managers to complete the comprehensive assessment of health care needs.
- Provide patient education.
- Assist with patient and family discharge/transition instructions.

CONCLUSION

The critical elements to successful transition planning are the case manager's proactive involvement in the patient's care. Case managers become the focal point in the care being delivered and are the conductor of the plan. If the plan is carefully crafted, the team understands the big picture and the ultimate outcome desired. Case managers establish relationships that are built on trust and mutually accepted patient and family goals. Case managers bear the responsibility of being the clinical and fiscal advocate for the patient, provider, and payer. They are rewarded through the satisfaction experienced by all the constituents served.

SUGGESTED READINGS

Acute Health Division, Department of Human Services, Victoria, Australia. "Post Acute Care Program." http://hna.ffh.vic.gov.au/ahs/quality/pac3.htm (5 September 2000). Accessed 15 February 2001.

K. Bower, *Case Management by Nurses* (Kansas City, MO: American Nurses Pub., 1992).

Discharge Direct. "Interpretive Guidelines." http://www.dischargedirect.com/regulations/guidelines.asp (4 April 2000). Accessed 20 March 2001.

Institute for Clinical Evaluative Sciences. "Early Discharge Planning Strategies." http://www.ices.on.ca/docs/macro1.htm. Accessed 15 February 2001.

"M&R Care Guidelines: Inpatient and Surgical Care." http://www.mnr.com/pdf/isc.pdf. Accessed 10 April 2001.

Chapter 13

Postacute Services

Sara Atwell

TAKE THIS TO WORK

1. In response to industry changes and new regulatory and reimbursement requirements, postacute services have refocused their core businesses, service delivery, and relationships with the markets in which they serve.
2. Case managers have had to proactively anticipate discharge needs and understand postacute admission criteria and the effects of regulatory changes on patients as well as on acute and postacute providers.
3. Just as level-of-care criteria are the drivers for movement from the intensive care unit to telemetry, the case manager needs to understand unique criteria for each postacute venue.

Historically, postacute care referred to the health care services that a patient received following an acute care episode of care. These services consisted of basic nursing care and therapy services provided after hospitalizations in other institutional settings, such as nursing homes, and at home. With the transformation of postacute services in the early 1980s, an increasing number of patient care services that were previously provided in the hospital setting are now being provided in postacute environments. As a result, the level and intensity of services provided in postacute settings have increased. The continuum of services available to patients in need of continued skilled and basic nursing and therapy services has quadrupled in the past decade. The continuum of postacute services spans high-intensity long-term care such as subacute, skilled nursing, and acute rehabilitation services to assisted living and residential housing with outpatient therapy and basic nursing offerings (Exhibit 13–1).

The passage of the Balanced Budget Act (BBA) in August 1997 created one of the greatest turning points in American health care. It was Congress's solution to uncontrollable Medicare spending and misutilization of postacute venues. The goal of the BBA was to reduce overall Medicare reimbursement and change provider incentives for utilization of postacute services.

The BBA has affected the level of care and intensity of services in postacute venues. Due to the change in reimbursement, postacute services have changed market strategy, patient focus, and intensity of service. Acute care providers continue to rely on postacute venues to meet necessary and appropriate patient outcomes, needed length-of-stay (LOS) reductions, and timely discharge needs.

Exhibit 13–1 Key Components of the Postacute Care Continuum

- **Subacute care facility/program**—A level of care that is less invasive and costly than acute care, yet is more intensive, sophisticated, and of shorter duration than traditional nursing home care. It is outcome-oriented treatment provided immediately after, or in some cases instead of, hospitalization. Subacute care is provided in a variety of settings including acute care hospitals, prospective payment system-exempt rehabilitation hospitals/units, skilled nursing facilities, and in the home.
- **Skilled nursing facility (SNF)**—A residential health care facility that, under the supervision of a physician, provides nursing and aide services on a 24-hour-a-day basis. Room and board, therapies, medical social services, and other health-related services and social activities are also provided. SNFs are either hospital-based or free-standing.
- **Prospective payment system-exempt rehabilitation hospitals and units**—Rehabilitation hospitals and rehabilitation distinct-part units within acute care hospitals provide intensive physical, occupational, and speech therapy to patients with functional disabilities. Medicare requires that at least 75 percent of patients served must receive care for one or more of 10 specified conditions related to neurological and musculoskeletal disorders and burns. In general, beneficiaries treated in these facilities must receive at least three hours of therapy daily during their stay.
- **Long-term care hospitals**—Medicare-participating hospitals with an average length of stay exceeding 25 days that are not otherwise classified as rehabilitation or psychiatric hospitals. These facilities provide a wide range of services to a variety of patients, but often specialize in services such as physical rehabilitation, chronic respiratory care, and pain or wound management.
- **Swing-bed program**—A Medicare program that allows acute care hospitals to use designated "swing beds" for either acute or skilled nursing facility (SNF) care. To be certified as a swing-bed provider, a hospital must be located in a rural area.
- **Adult homes**—Long-term residential services provided to functionally impaired persons who are no longer able or willing to remain in their own home. Such services include room and board (residents have their own room), housekeeping, personal care, social activities, meals, case management, assistance with medication, and safety supervision. Other services such as nursing, therapy, or additional personal care services may be arranged through licensed or certified home care agencies.
- **Enriched housing**—Residential programs consisting of independent apartment-type living arrangements in which functionally impaired individuals primarily age 65 and over are provided with room and board and other support services such as assistance with housekeeping, shopping, meal preparation, personal care activities, and 24-hour emergency coverage. Other home care services may be arranged for through licensed or certified home care agencies.
- **Assisted-living facilities**—Programs providing health, residential, and supportive services to persons who could be eligible for nursing home placement but who may be safely cared for in this setting. In addition to the services of an adult home or enriched housing program, skilled nursing; physical, occupational, and speech therapies; personal care or home health aide services; personal emergency response services; and medical supplies and equipment may also be provided.
- **Continuing care retirement communities (CCRCs)**—An all-inclusive, lifetime contract that guarantees a living environment and continuum of care for adults who are Medicare eligible. Residents pay a substantial entrance fee and monthly fees to live in a CCRC. Services include independent living units, meals, nursing facility services, home care services, and social and recreational activities. The community must provide access to physician services, rehabilitation services, and prescription drugs. Other services such as enriched housing or assisted living may also be available within the community.
- **Comprehensive outpatient rehabilitation facilities (CORFs)**—A Medicare-certified program operated exclusively for the purpose of providing diagnostic, therapeutic, and restorative services to outpatients. CORFs are physician supervised.
- **Adult day health care (medical model)**—Outpatient programs usually run by nursing homes that provide supervision, medical and psycho-

continues

Exhibit 13–1 continued

logical care, and social activities to older persons residing in the community who cannot be alone or who prefer to be with others during the day. Other services may include nutrition, social services, rehab therapy, nursing care, dental care, medication administration, and other ancillary services as needed.

- **Adult day care (social model)**—Similar to the medical model, these are outpatient programs that provide socialization and activities, supervision and monitoring, personal care, and nutrition, but no medical care. These services are provided by nursing homes and community organizations, such as senior centers, to functionally impaired individuals living in the community.
- **Respite care**—The provision of short-term stays (less than 42 days per year) in a SNF or substitute home care services for the purpose of providing family caregivers or other informal supports with temporary relief from the responsibility of providing care to impaired individuals in the home.
- **Certified home health agency (CHHA)**—A Medicare-certified organization that provides nursing, aide services, durable medical equipment/supplies, therapy, and medical social services to persons who require these services in the home.
- **Licensed home care services agencies (LHCSAs)**—Organizations that are not Medicare-certified but that may provide nursing, aide services, medical equipment, and/or therapy services to persons who require these services in the home.
- **Personal care**—Aide-level service that provides assistance with activities of daily living (bathing, dressing, eating, toileting), instrumentals activities of daily living (shopping, meal preparation, laundry), and health-related tasks (e.g., monitoring temperature, preparing special diets).
- **Hospice care**—A Medicare-certified program that provides palliative care services to terminally ill Medicare beneficiaries with a life expectancy of six months or less. Services include nursing care, medical social services, physician, counselor, home care aide and homemaker services, medical equipment and supplies, therapies, and bereavement counseling for families. Care can be provided in a variety of settings, including inpatient and at home.

Care management is perhaps the most promising large-scale health care strategy that offers a potential for significant cost savings while improving the quality of patient care. The key to care management, however, is successful patient management across the continuum, extending across all care venues, from ambulatory, acute care, and postacute care settings. Ideally, care management is the process that eliminates fragmentation and provides an integrated delivery system with its cohesiveness. Case management programs are key to early discharge disposition identification, appropriate resource utilization, facilitation of clinical best practice, and appropriate utilization of postacute services (Figure 13–1).

Case managers must understand postacute reimbursement, admission criteria, and the provision of services in each postacute venue of care. The remainder of this chapter will outline postacute admission criteria for skilled, subacute and intermediate nursing care; home health care; rehabilitation; and long-term acute care hospitals (LTACHs). Where applicable, BBA implications that affect discharge and admission to postacute services are also provided.

POSTACUTE ADMISSION CRITERIA

Skilled Nursing Facilities (SNFs)

Skilled nursing facilities (SNFs) provide 24-hour/7-day nursing services for convalescent patients. In an SNF, registered nurses, licensed practical nurses, and nurse aides provide services prescribed by the patient's physician. Emphasis is on medical nursing care with restorative nursing care and physical, occupational, speech, and therapeutic recreation therapies provided. SNFs can be hospital based or free-standing. There are state licensure and federal certifi-

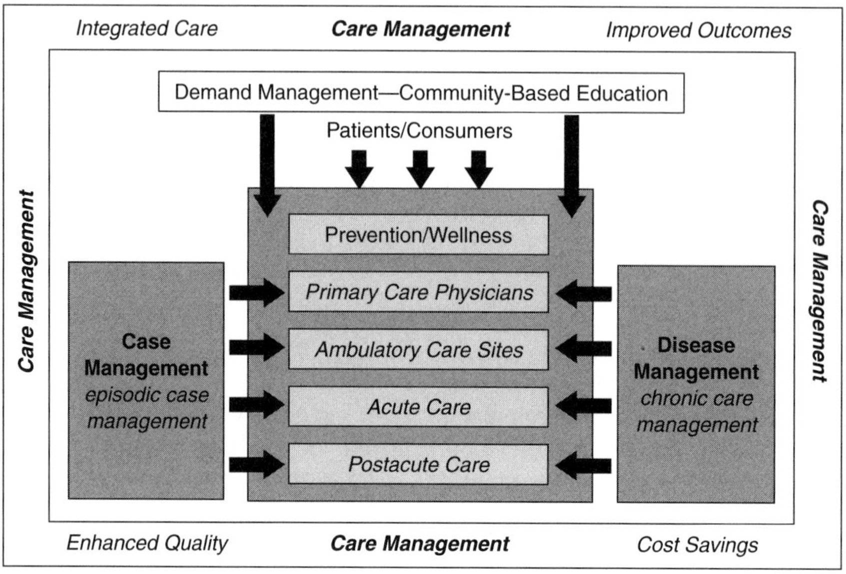

Figure 13–1 Continuum of Care Management Graph

cation requirements that allow for eligibility to participate in both Medicare and Medicaid programs. Patients for skilled nursing services must require:

- intermittent physician monitoring
- nursing and/or aide services on a 24-hour basis
- continuous skilled services daily that are medically reasonable and necessary
- a relatively short LOS of 30–100 days (can receive up to 100 days of prorated Medicare coverage for skilled nursing care)

Skilled services provided

- are expected to be restorative in nature
- are expected to result in improvement over a reasonable period of time (Patients/residents must show steady improvement due to skilled intervention.)
- require interventions performed by a licensed professional (e.g., a nurse or a physical, occupational, and/or speech therapist). These services include but are not limited to wound management, requiring daily dressing changes; parenteral and enteral feeding; intravenous (IV) therapy; physical, occupational, and speech therapy; and tracheostomy management.

Subacute Care

Subacute care blends the sophisticated technology of hospital care with the lower cost operations of an SNF. This, in effect, reduces the cost of care while increasing the severity and intensity of service delivered. Subacute units are operated under the skilled nursing license, thus all patients must meet, at a minimum, skilled nursing criteria. Subacute units typically provide a wider range of medical rehabilitative and therapeutic services than a traditional SNF and tend to meet the needs of patients that have greater medical and rehabilitative complexities.

The following indicators profile subacute patients:

- require an average of four direct nursing hours per patient day

- require intermittent physician contact, an average of three days per week
- are stable but complex, and require medical and/or rehabilitative intervention
- have an expected LOS of 5 to 20 days

Typical patient populations seen in subacute units are

- complex medical patients (patients with chronic conditions and comorbidities)
- congestive heart failure
- high-level stroke
- orthopaedic—total joint replacement
- postcoronary artery bypass graph with complications
- renal failure
- trauma
- diabetes mellitus with complicating factors

A typical process for referring skilled and subacute patients to SNFs is provided as Figure 13–2. This process will vary depending on your postacute network, influx of managed care and payer expectations, and the operational issues of the provider.

BBA Implications for SNFs

The prospective payment system (PPS) for SNFs effective July 1998 is based on RUG-III, a 44-group classification system. The RUG-III classification system classifies patients into homogenous groups according to health and functional characteristics and the amount and type of resources used. Unlike hospital diagnosis-related groups (DRGs), which classify patients on a per discharge basis, RUG III was developed to classify patients on a per diem basis. This per diem is ultimately meant to cover all routine, ancillary, and capital-related Part A costs, as well as the cost for most Part B services incurred during a Part A stay. This has significant effects on reimbursement for SNFs.

To operate effectively under the PPS, SNFs now must operate as efficiently as possible, closely managing patient care utilization, data quality, and costs. According to the Health Care Financing Administration (HCFA), 99 percent of Medicare-certified SNFs have experienced an average revenue reduction of between 17 and 19 percent. This has significantly impacted the types of patients and the services provided in SNFs. SNF providers are being more selective with admissions. They are hand-picking patients to more closely match the current patient complement within the facility/program and require the acute provider to verify that the patient meets specific criteria before the patient is considered for placement. Many facilities now perform on-site assessments of potential admissions in order to ensure that criteria are met and that patients will fall within the set per diem, positively affecting the SNF's revenues.

Case managers will need to be proactive with SNF/subacute placement so as to avoid unnecessary delays in the patient's plan of care and the acute discharge.

Intermediate/Extended Care Nursing Facilities

Intermediate or extended care facilities provide care for older adults who are too ill or disabled to live independently but who are not ill enough to require hospitalization. These facilities provide regular medical, nursing, social, and rehabilitative services in addition to room and board for people who are not capable of independent living. Intermediate nursing facilities provide basic medical services short of the need for 24-hour skilled nursing care. These facilities must meet state licensure as well as federal certification requirements and are reimbursed by state Medicaid programs and through private funding.

Intermediate nursing facility patient admission criteria include the following:

- require minimal physician monitoring
- are unable to provide self-care/activities of daily living and do not have a capable or willing caregiver to perform care
- are unable to remain in their residence safely
- do not require skilled services by a licensed professional on a daily basis
- require minimal nursing care

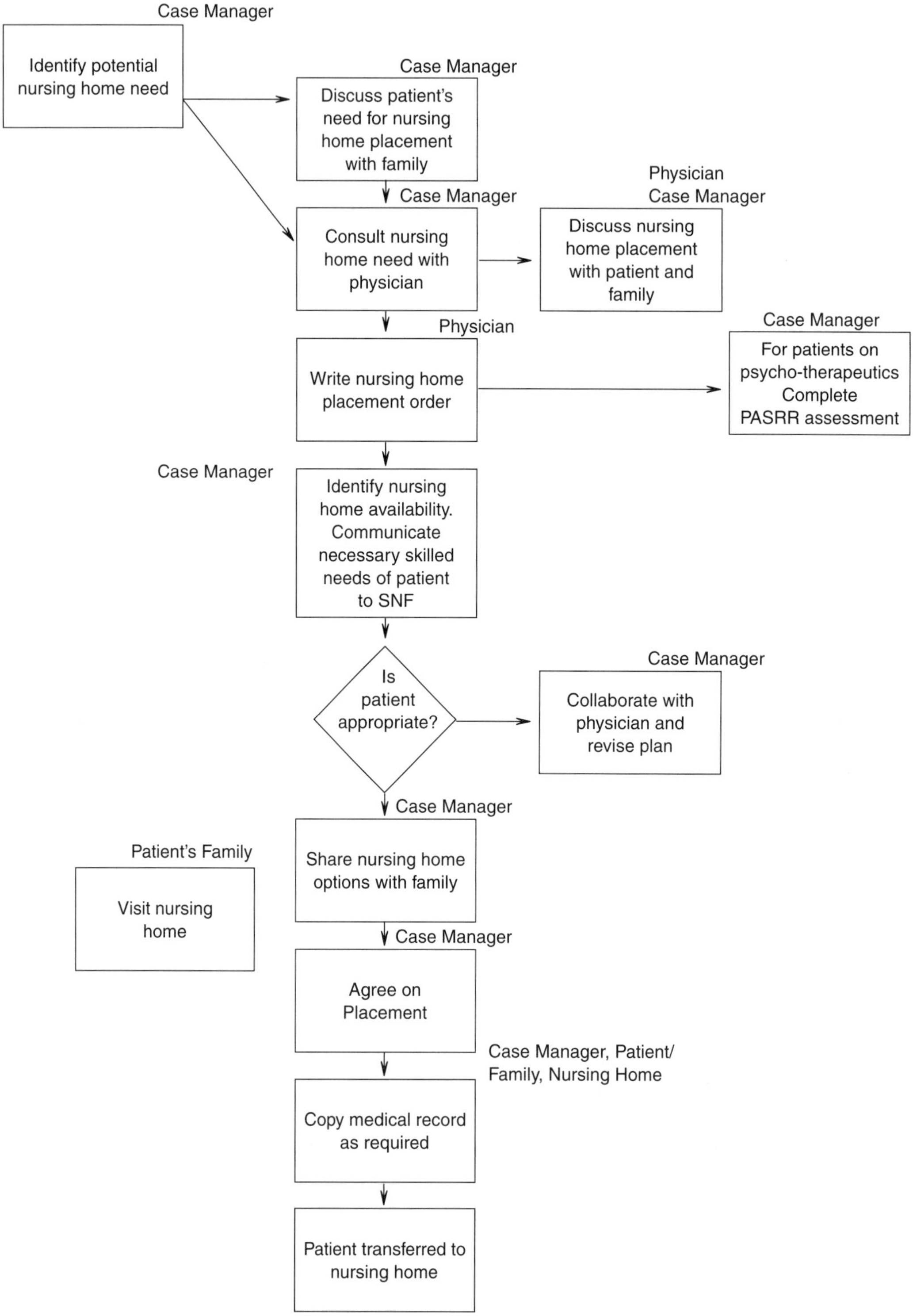

Figure 13–2 Nursing Home Placement Process Flow

Home Health Care

Home health care covers a broad range of services and provides continuous or intermittent care to persons recovering from illness or persons who are chronically or terminally ill. Medicare and home care participating third-party payers cover intermittent home care services. Continuous care services, often referred to as private duty care, are seldom reimbursed by Medicare or third-party payers.

A patient is eligible for Medicare home health if the following criteria are met:

- The care is ordered by a physician.
- The patient is homebound. Homebound is defined as
    1. bedridden, ambulatory with assistive devices, chair bound, ambulatory with restrictions, and partial weight bearing
- The need for care is intermittent.
    1. daily home visits with an end site in mind
    2. one to four visits per week
    3. more than one visit per day

The intermittent, homebound patient must possess/need one of the following items to be considered skilled:

- nursing assessment
- diabetic care—insulin Intramuscular (IM)/ Intravenous (IV)
- tracheotomy care
- ostomy care
- chest physiotherapy
- bowel/bladder training
- venipuncture
- decubitus care/training
- wound care/training
- catheter insertion/care

BBA Implications for Home Health

Prospective payment for home health care was implemented October 1, 2000. The change from cost-based reimbursement to a flat rate per 60-day episode, based on the patient's acuity, the case mix index, and the weight index (determined by the OASIS documentation tool), will drastically change home health care revenues. Flat rate reimbursement will change under the following conditions: patients with low utilization, less than four visits per episode, significant changes in the clinical condition, partial episodes that occur due to a return to the acute care setting and readmission to home care, and outlier patients who fall beyond the expected episode of treatment. Home care agencies are in the process of reevaluating their focus of care and service line offerings. Appropriate and early identification of home care needs is imperative. More so than ever before, the integration of home care with other postacute services is essential in providing comprehensive care to the patient.

Inpatient Rehabilitation

Rehabilitation is extended and intensive restorative therapy services are provided on a regular basis to persons with traumatic or disabling conditions. Rehabilitation services typically include physical, occupational, speech, and vocational therapies. Other services provided in rehabilitation venues of care include psychology, recreation therapy, respiratory therapy, nursing, social services, and case management. Inpatient rehabilitation is typically provided in three care delivery venues: acute rehabilitation hospitals and/or distinct part units, skilled nursing facilities, and LTACHs. Case managers should use the criteria described in the following paragraphs to determine the appropriate site for inpatient rehabilitation.

Acute Rehabilitation

Acute inpatient rehabilitation hospitals and/or distinct part units are required by Medicare to deliver three hours of therapy and must have 75 percent of their patients fall into one of 10 rehabilitation diagnostic categories. The rehabilitative diagnostic categories are trauma, orthopaedics, arthritis, stroke, spinal cord injury, amputee, complex medical, pain management, brain injury, and transplant.

When assessing a patient for acute rehabilitation, ask the following questions:

- Is the patient medically stable?
- Does the patient have impaired immobility and/or functional self-care deficits and is he or she able to tolerate and/or progress toward a total of three hours of therapeutic activity per day?
- Is the patient and/or the patient's family motivated and able to learn?
- What are the duration and coverage of benefits?
- Is there a responsible party who is able to sign documents prior to and during admission?

Criteria to consider prior to admission to an acute rehabilitation program are presented in Exhibit 13–2.

Subacute Rehabilitation

Subacute medical rehabilitation units focus on short-term (average LOS 25–30 days) rehabilitation for patients with medical complexities and rehabilitation needs. These patients generally require four to four-and-one-half nursing hours per patient day and therapies that extend up to three hours per day. Subacute medical rehabilitation units tend to provide rehabilitation to patients who have other medical issues that won't allow them to meet the three-hour-per-day therapy requirement of acute rehabilitation programs. The medical complexities often include wound management, IV therapies such as antibiotics and hyperalimentation, and respiratory therapy intervention.

LTACHs

LTACHs are Medicare PPS-exempt hospitals. They are reimbursed per Medicare discharge as opposed to prospectively on the basis of DRGs. LTACHs provide intensive medical and rehabilitation services to patients who continue to require inpatient care. These patients often have multisystem failures that require intensive monitoring and gradual rehabilitative intervention. One of the distinguishing factors of an LTACH is that it must maintain an overall average LOS of greater than 25 days. Consequently, LTACH patients have greater medical and rehabilitative complexities that require longer term intervention than that seen in acute rehabilitation programs, acute inpatient care, and subacute and SNFs.

Basic criteria used to assess LTACH patients include the following:

- The patient requires daily physician monitoring.
- The patient is medically complex, requiring an acute inpatient hospital with an expected ALOS of 26 days.
- The patient requires long-term telemetry.

Exhibit 13–2 Acute Rehabilitation Criteria

Medical Stability
All diagnoses determined; all currently controlled
Rehabilitation diagnoses defined
Current treatments defined
Infections under treatment/limitation defined
Organ systems stable

Functional Capacity
Patient able to tolerate total of three hours of therapy daily
Functional deficits defined
Mobility skills defined
Organ system support capabilities defined
Apparent motivation to achieve functional capacity

Support System
Final destination defined
Family/other support system defined
Caregivers defined

Insurance Coverage Defined
Limits of in/out coverage
Limits of durable equipment coverage
Limits of pharmaceutical coverage

- The patient is on a long-term multiple antibiotic regimen.
- The patient is multiple-trauma, requiring long-term inpatient intervention.
- The patient is ventilator dependent, with weaning potential or anticipated discharge to home.
- The patient requires rehabilitation therapy but may not withstand a minimum of three hours/day.

There are multiple benefits to LTACHs. These benefits, when experienced within an integrated delivery system model, can benefit both the patient and the providers of care.

- Reimbursement resembles cost-based reimbursement. This reimbursement is set within a specified amount.
- The Tax Equity and Fiscal Responsibility Act (TEFRA) capped after the base year. TEFRA is based on the severity of illness and intensity of service provided to LTACH patients within the facility.
- The health care system's continuum of care is extended.
- There are no limitations on the types of patients admitted, provided they meet the aggregate 25-day length of stay.
- Services and resources are able to be cross-utilized within the health care system's continuum of services.

BBA Implications for LTACHs

An extension for the implementation of PPS for LTACHs has been granted (as of August 2000). A per discharge payment based on PPS DRGs is expected to be implemented by October 2002. This will affect the types of patients and the services currently provided in LTACHs. Integrated delivery systems will have to rethink how they use this postacute environment and advantages they bring to the system.

HOSPITAL TRANSFER RULE

The Hospital Transfer Rule has changed the way specific patients are discharged to the postacute environment. As of October 1998, 10 DRGs are paid a per diem as opposed to the defined PPS rate when they are discharged prior to the Medicare geometric mean. When transferred from an acute care hospital to another acute care hospital or a postacute care provider (e.g., a PPS-exempt hospital/distinct part unit, SNF, or home health agency), these DRGs are paid under the transfer payment methodology, which is

Table 13–1 Ten Acute Care Transfer Diagnosis-Related Groups

DRG	*Description*	*Geometric Mean**	*Average Payment***
14	CVA	4.9	$4,874.49
113	Amputation, excluding upper limb & toe	9.8	$10,897.39
209	Major joint procedure	4.9	$9,158.17
210	Hip & Femur procedure w/cc	6.1	$7,488.65
211	Hip & Femur procedure w/o cc	4.7	$5,141.81
236	Fractures of Hip & Pelvis (medical)	4.1	$3,008.58
263	Skin Graft & Debridement w/cc	8.8	$8,290.61
264	Skin Graft & Debridement w/o cc	5.4	$4,416.93
429	Organic Disturbances & Mental Retardation (medical)	5.2	$3,578.48
483	Tracheostomy except for face, mouth, & neck diagnoses	33.9	$65,784.91

**Federal Register,* May 8, 1998
**St. Anthony's DRG Guidebook, 1998

twice the per diem for the first day and the per diem for each subsequent day. DRG 209, 210, and 211 are exceptions. The transferring hospital is paid 50 percent the first day and 50 percent the remaining days (Table 13–1).

Case management of these DRGs will require an understanding of the reimbursement and the effects to the acute provider when discharging/transferring early.

SUGGESTED READINGS

U.S. Department of Health and Human Services, Health Care Financing Administration. "Health Care Financing Administration: The Medicare, Medicaid, and SCHIP Agency." http://www.hcfa.gov. Accessed 14 February 2001.

"Feds Create Recipe for Managed Care," *ACHA's Provider Magazine,* June 1998, 29–31, 32, 33, 36–41.

H. Gill, "How Impending Transfer Issue Will Affect Hospitals and Post Acute Care Providers," *Post Acute Strategy Report 3*, no. 8 (August 1998).

CHAPTER 14

Home Health Care

Peggy H. Rodebush, Laura L. Waltrip, and G. David Baker

TAKE THIS TO WORK

1. For home health follow-up, consider the following:
   - Is this patient a risk for a complication or relapse?
   - Does the treatment plan include new or changed medications and/or treatments that require teaching and monitoring?
   - Is the patient capable of self-care? Is there an able and willing caregiver who requires teaching and monitoring?
2. Communicate early with patient, family, and physicians regarding ongoing treatment options.
3. Document level-of-care requirements and any specialty service or equipment needed.
4. For Medicare patients, document homebound status and the need for intermittent skilled nursing and/or therapy, which could be addressed in the patient's home.
5. Obtain physician orders for transition to the selected home health agency.
6. Investigate payer coverage and obtain a preferred provider list, if any.
7. Assist the patient and his or her family in the selection of their preferred home health provider.
8. Remember: The ultimate goal of home health is to promote independence with care.

How often are patients sent home from a physician's office or clinic, emergency department (ED), or hospital with prescriptions and follow-up instructions, only to return a short time later with no improvement or in worse condition? How many health care providers are puzzled and frustrated by patients who are noncompliant or simply unable to carry out instructions? Without a good understanding of patients' home environment, lifestyle, and family support system, providers are lacking the complete picture necessary for successful medical management.

Home health care has matured and evolved to become a critical component of medical management. It is used successfully in pre- and postacute

Source: Reprinted from P.H. Rodebush, L.L. Waltrip, and G.D. Baker, Home Health Care, in *The Managed Health Care Handbook, 4th Edition,* P. Kongstvedt, ed., pp. 480–495, © 2001, Aspen Publishers, Inc.

care settings and is vital in the existing environment of cost-efficiency pressures and quality measurement through the continuum of care. There are many different types of home health care, including medical and nonmedical care, intermittent and continuous care, custodial and skilled care, and formal and informal care. The limits of each of these categories are usually not driven by the medical needs of the patient, but by the financing mechanism available for payment of the services provided. For example, Medicare, as the predominant home care payer, has traditionally consisted of multiple medical disciplines within a highly coordinated plan of treatment. The complete team, if medically necessary, comprises a registered nurse (RN), physical therapist (PT), licensed practical nurse (LPN), occupational therapist (OT), speech therapist, social worker, and home health aide (HHA).

The limits of care are frequently set in the federal code that authorizes payment for the care and describes the conditions that must be met by providers to participate in the federal programs. The goal of the Medicare program is to improve the health and functional status of patients. Medicare approves payment for this care only as long as progressive improvement can be shown and in some specific chronic cases that require skilled nursing follow-up on a long-term basis (such as monthly urinary catheter change).

Older persons receive most home care because of the age criteria of Medicare and older persons' higher health care needs. There is an increasing number of non-Medicare, younger patients receiving home care services, however. This growing younger market is an extension of the improving clinical capabilities of home care providers and the increasing number of third-party payers that recognize home care as a viable medical alternative or adjunct to more expensive acute and subacute care.

WHAT IS HOME CARE?

Home care encompasses a broad range of medical, social, and support services. It involves the delivery of health care at home typically to persons who are disabled, chronically ill, terminally ill, or recovering.

Care may be intermittent or continuous. Continuous care is frequently referred to as "private-duty care" because it is seldom reimbursed by Medicare or third-party payers. This type of care is typically offered by organizations other than those providing intermittent care designed for the capitated Medicare program and for third-party payers who stipulate intermittent care. Continuous and intermittent home care differ in the duration of time for care delivery. Private-duty care is usually for service unit increments longer than 1 hour or service units that are billed relative to the number of hours or shifts spent delivering care. A service unit for intermittent home care is described as a patient visit.

Both continuous and intermittent care have complex and support care components. Continuous care may range from RN support for ventilator-dependent patients to companions for older people or confined persons. Intermittent care requires highly skilled professionals who can work independently in the home, under a physician's orders, with typically much stronger problem-solving and technical skills than the same professionals would have in many inpatient medical settings. Likewise, HHAs provide intermittent support care, such as bathing, assistance in moving about the home, and meal preparation.

HISTORY OF HOME CARE

Care provided to a member of a household by a recognized health care practitioner or member of the household has been in existence for centuries and preceded institutional care. It started as a local phenomenon focused on the neighborhood, village, or town in which the ill person lived. As practitioners' ability to care for the ill improved, the level of the care provided in the home evolved with it.

Health care focused outside the home began to develop as the involvement of religious and academic organizations in health care increased and formal medical education evolved. As these organizations began to serve ill people, larger, more complex health care organizations began to emerge, providing hospitals where higher levels of care were developed and could be provided.

Home care in the modern sense existed as a cottage industry until the early 1980s, when a lawsuit concerning excessive paperwork and unreliable payment policies led to a revision in the Medicare home health payment policies. With the favorable ruling from that lawsuit in 1986, which clarified expanded coverage for beneficiaries, the Medicare annual benefit outlay and the number of agencies grew significantly until 1997 and 1998. The period of growth and expansion was fueled by a growing demand for care at home, as well as recognition that complex medical care could be safely provided in the home, with patient satisfaction frequently increasing. With expansion, the share of the health dollar devoted to home care grew (see Figures 14–1, 14–2, and 14–3).This increase in expenditures received great scrutiny from the federal government and resulted in changes to reimbursement practices. The implementation of the Balanced Budget Act (BBA) of 1997 resulted in severe reimbursement restrictions that continue to have a dramatic impact on the home health care industry. As of 1999, the industry was experiencing a sharp decline in the number of agencies serving patients: in 1997, there were 10,570, but in June 1999, there were only 8,613 (see Figure 14–4). The shrinking numbers of providers has created growing concern that not all those who need home care services will get them, especially in rural areas.

INDICATORS AND PREDICTORS OF HOME CARE DEMAND

There are multiple factors contributing to the evolution and growth of the home care market, including

- demographic shifts (resulting in a greater proportion of older people in the U.S. population)
- the shrinking hospital system (because of cost containment pressures)
- decreased availability of informal caregivers (producing a need for more formal caregivers)
- improved home care technology

Demographic Shifts

The first major factor contributing to the evolution of the home care market is the much-discussed "graying of America." The number of persons reaching retirement age and Medicare eligibility age is increasing and is predicted to grow exponentially in the next few decades. Americans' life expectancy has increased from

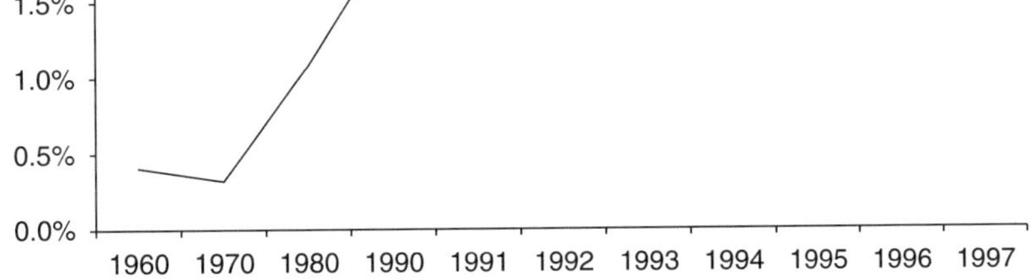

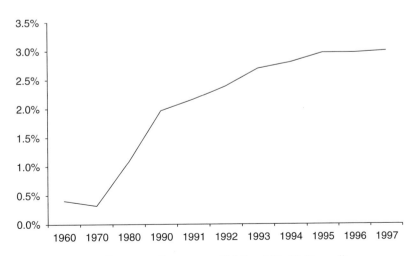

Figure 14–1 Home Care Expenditures as a Percentage of National Health Expenditures.

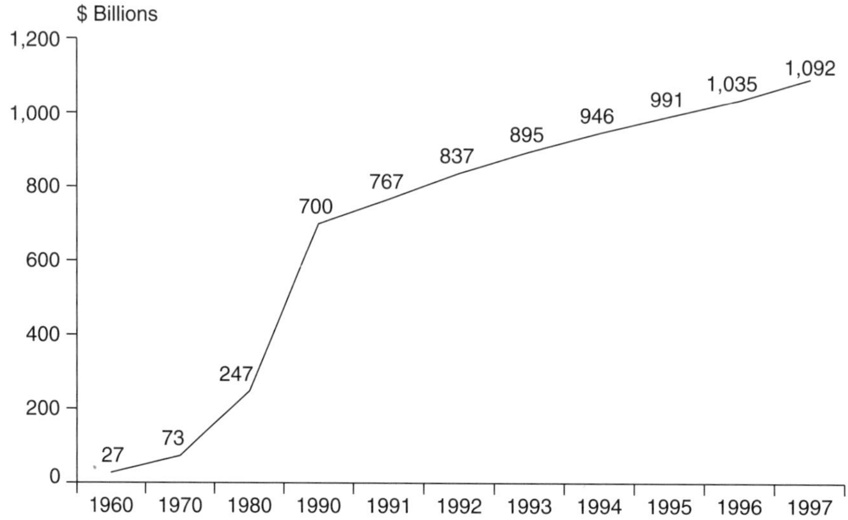

Figure 14–2 National Health Expenditure Trends.

age 63 in 1940 to age 82 today. By 2100, it is projected that the United States will have 20.1 million residents over 85 years old, 50.6 million over 75 years old, and 89.9 million over 65 years old (Figure 14–5).[1] This growing aged population continues to put tremendous pressure on the health care system.

The Shrinking Hospital System

The hospital industry continues to struggle with an excess of acute care beds in many markets as well as continued pressures to reduce costs and generate positive net income. As a result, hospitals have continued to experience mergers, acquisi-

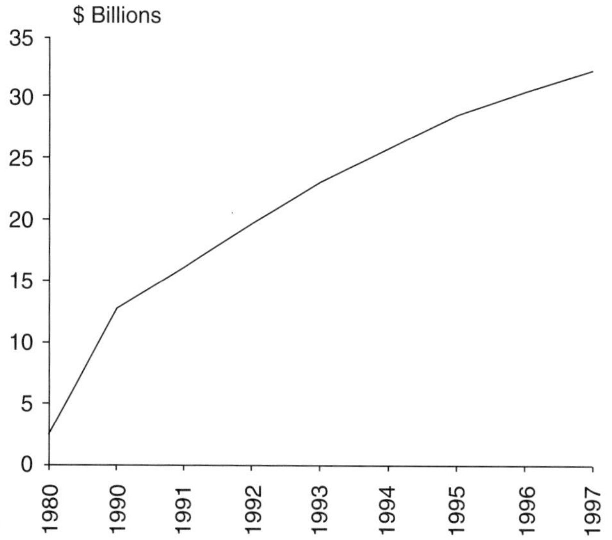

Figure 14–3 Home Health Care Expenditure Trends.

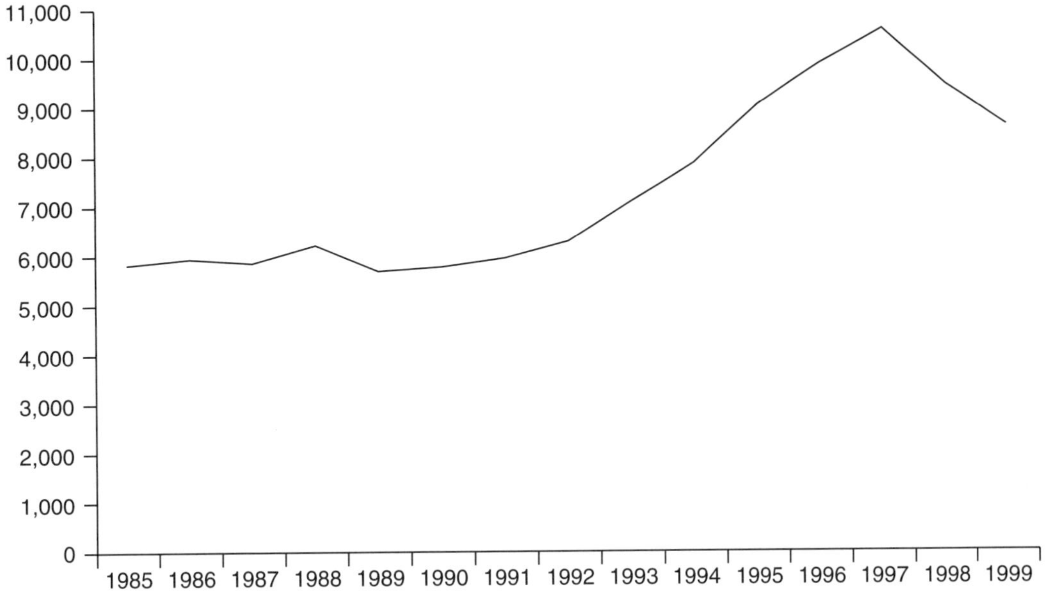

Figure 14–4 Number of Home Health Agencies from 1963 to 1999. *Note:* The numbers in the table in the text cannot be replicated by NAHC. Both the Office of the Actuary and NAHC recognized the numbers above as accurate home health agency totals. Figures for 1999 are through June 4, 1999.

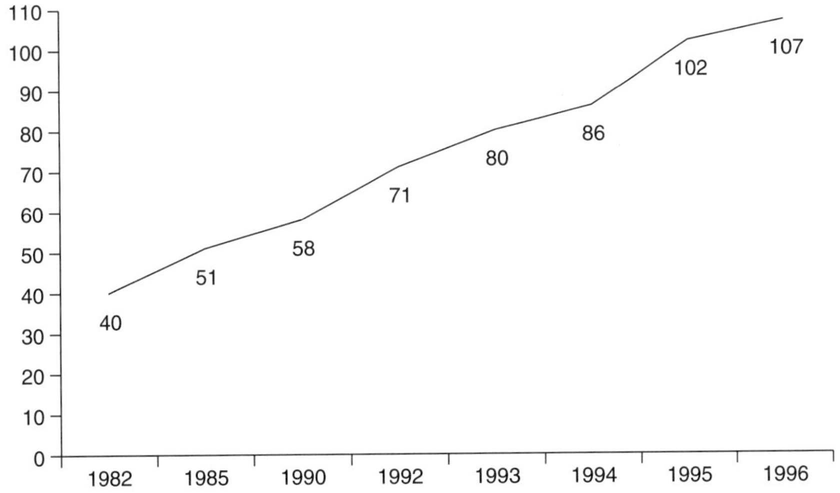

Figure 14–5 Number of Home Health Patients Served per 1,000 Medicare Enrollees.

tions, and consolidations, and to downsize. Meanwhile, the number of acute care hospitals and the acute care length of stay continue to decline (see Table 14–1 and Figures 14–6 and 14–7). Many of the patients still need some level of care following hospital discharge. Increasingly, the home care industry has experienced the "sicker and sooner" discharge for acute care, with many patients being referred to home care agencies. With less costly care available through home care and with sicker

Table 14–1 Inpatient Beds Trends

Year	*Total Hospitals*	*Average Beds per Hospital*	*Beds per 100 Enrollees*
1975	6,707	1,132	51.5
1980	6,780	1,152	46.9
1995	6,414	1,074	29.4
1996	6,376	1,056	28.4
1997	6,293	1,037	27.0

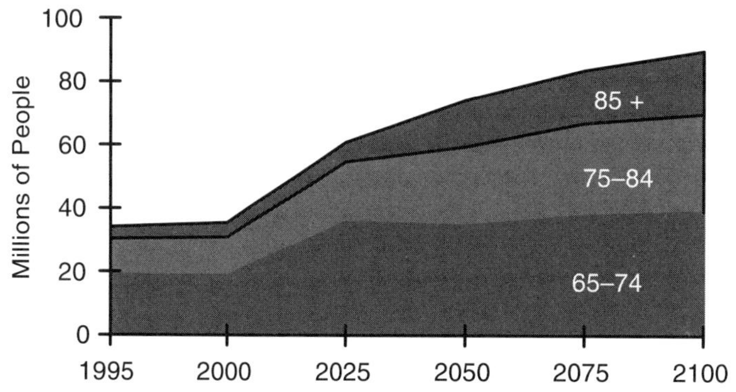

Figure 14–6 Persons Aged 65 and Older in the United States.

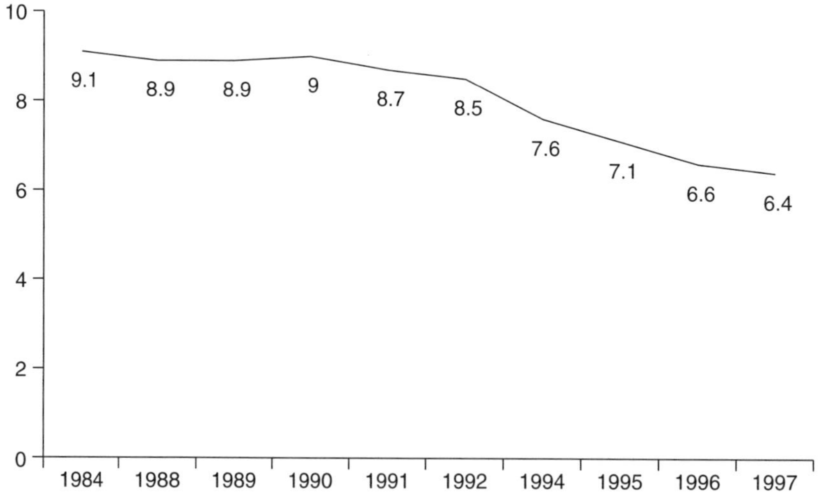

Figure 14–7 Trends in Medicare Average Length of Stay (in Days).

patients being discharged sooner, the home care industry has moved forward to fill this void.

Decreased Availability of Informal Caregivers

It is estimated that 9 to 11 million people need home care services. Many of these people will receive care from family members, friends, or others. These "informal caregivers" are not compensated.[2] Due to the breakdown of the nuclear family, the increased mobility and dispersion of extended families, and the fact that many would-be informal caregivers work outside the home and are themselves in need of assistance, there are fewer informal caregivers available. The gap created by the loss of informal caregivers will necessitate a shift to the formal caregiver, and this shift will contribute to the growth in demand for home care services.

Improved Home Care Technology

Telemedicine companies have entered the market in recent years with technology appropriate for the home setting. Their products have evolved from large, robotic machines to smaller, more streamlined monitoring devices. The equipment placed in patients' homes has been extremely expensive in the past. However, recent reductions in the costs of telephone technology and computer hardware and software have made equipment more affordable. For example, adult working children may now have visual contact with aging parents through advances in telephone equipment and resources. This regular contact may be enough to provide peace of mind and prevent placement of a parent in a long-term care facility.

HOME CARE SERVICES AND DISCIPLINES

The home care market is segmented due to the unique nature of the various services as well as differing reimbursement mechanisms for each service type. A single patient can receive care from one or several service areas. ***Home care services can generally be divided into the following four groups:***

1. traditional nursing services
2. infusion services
3. medical equipment and supplies
4. respiratory services

Traditional Nursing Services

Traditional nursing services form the largest category of home care services. When most people think of home care, they envision traditional services, which include care provided by RNs, LPNs, HHAs, certified nursing assistants, and medical social workers (MSWs). In-home rehabilitation services, frequently grouped with traditional nursing services, are performed by licensed or registered therapists, including PTs, OTs, dietitians, and speech-language pathologists (SLPs).

Infusion Services

Home infusion services are often viewed as a component of traditional care. Infusion services require a higher skill level of nursing, a pharmacy component, and a safe, clean home environment. Types of infusion therapy conducive to home administration include continuous or intermittent chemotherapy, parenteral nutrition support, antibiotics, hydration, and pain control. These services have experienced rapid and sustained growth, and in the past 10 years, their fees and quality of service have been scrutinized. In 1996, infusion services in the United States were a $6 billion market.[3]

Medical Equipment and Supplies

Home medical equipment and supplies are generally nonclinical items that consist of durable medical equipment (wheelchairs, walkers, hospital beds, and activities-of-daily-living [ADL] equipment and supplies) and other disposable medical supplies. In 1996, the U.S. medical equipment market was $1.5 billion.[3]

Respiratory Services

Home respiratory services, often viewed as the clinical component of home medical equipment and supplies, consist of home oxygen and respiratory therapy services. This U.S. market was $4.5 billion in 1996.[3]

HOME CARE PROVIDERS

Formal home care services are offered by a multidisciplinary mix of medical and nonmedical professionals.

Nurses

Nurses include RNs and LPNs. These medical professionals provide skilled services—including assessments, injections, intravenous therapy, psychiatric care, wound care, education, disease management, and case management—that certain patients may need. RNs have received 2 or more years of formal education and training and are licensed to practice in individual states. LPNs have 1 year of specialized training. They are also licensed in individual states and must operate under the supervision of an RN.

Physical Therapists

PTs perform treatment to restore loss of mobility and strength caused by physical impairments. They may also be involved in the treatment and management of complex wounds. These professionals may use specialized equipment to conduct these therapeutic treatments. An important aspect of therapy is the education of the patient and other health care professionals in proper physical techniques to alleviate pain and prevent initial or future injury. A licensed physical therapy assistant may also provide services under the direction of a PT.

Occupational Therapists

OTs provide treatments similar to physical therapists' but focus on improving the patient's performance of ADLs. ADLs include eating, drinking, dressing, bathing, and performing other routine household duties. An OT often must address the physical, social, and emotional needs of the patient. A certified occupational therapy assistant may also provide services under the direction of an OT.

Speech-Language Pathologists

SLPs provide care to diagnose, restore, and improve the speech and swallowing function of patients having dysfunction due to stroke or injury. SLPs work to improve the communication function of these patients by using specialized tools and techniques. These therapists also work with patients suffering from problems with breathing and swallowing.

Respiratory Therapists

Respiratory therapists provide care related to the treatment of patients with pulmonary and respiratory dysfunction. This care frequently involves the use of specialized equipment, including ventilators, oxygen concentrators, liquid oxygen dispensing systems, nebulizers, continuous positive air pressure apnea monitors, and other respiratory support equipment and supplies.

Medical Social Workers

MSWs assess and help improve patients' psychological and social difficulties. MSWs counsel patients with illnesses or disabilities and their families, helping them understand the resources available to them. These resources include public and private agencies that may temporarily assist the patient and patient's family, providing food, shelter, funds to pay bills, clothing, and so on. Frequently, the MSW will assist in completing the required documentation and coordinating the support needs of more acutely ill patients.

Pharmacists

Pharmacists provide technical and advisory services for home infusion services. Pharmaceutical products must be prepared, and supplies and deliveries must be coordinated with the ordering physician, the nurse, the patient, and often the patient's family. Pharmacy technicians may be utilized under the supervision of a pharmacist. One of the most important roles for the pharmacist is to provide education to patients and other staff members regarding medication administration and compliance and monitoring for adverse side effects. Home care patients, even those not on infusion drugs, are often on a large number of medications. Pharmacists can often assist in evaluating the home medication management process and for that reason, are often included in multidisciplinary case conferencing.

Dietitians

Dietitians offer nutritional monitoring and education to those patients needing dietary support services as part of their treatment regimen. Nutritional counseling continues to be critical for management of most chronic conditions, such as diabetes and cardiac disease. It is also required to appropriately manage the medically complex pediatric population.

Home Health Aides

HHAs frequently provide the majority of services in traditional home care agencies. These caregivers may have specialized training and are not licensed by the state, though many states require a certification process. HHAs assist patients with a large variety of support services, including ambulation, bathing, toileting, personal care, and dressing. Under Medicare, these services must be provided under the guidance of an RN.

Nonmedical home caregivers, including HHAs, homemakers, and companions, are an important component of the service mix. HHA services are reimbursed by Medicare as long as a medical plan of treatment is in effect. Some Medicaid programs have waivers that pay some costs of HHA or homemaker services for the very frail or low-income ill under certain conditions. However, most types of home care services, although they improve the person's quality of life and play a major role in raising health status and safety, are not reimbursable by third-party payers.

Homemakers

Homemakers provide support services in the form of general household duties, including meal preparation, laundry, light housekeeping, and shopping. They usually do not participate directly in the care for medical needs.

Companions

Companions are frequently called "sitters." These individuals provide a physical presence and safety net for those patients who should not be left at home alone. These caregivers do not provide medical care and are generally viewed as custodial.

Volunteers

Volunteers provide a vast number of services to the home care patient. Their involvement is determined by their individual capabilities and the needs of the patient. They are used extensively in hospice programs for bereavement care. These professionals operate from a variety of organizations, including home care agencies, hospices, staffing (private-duty) agencies, registries, medical and supply companies, and pharmaceutical and infusion services companies. These organizations may operate independently, vertically through common ownership with hospitals or skilled nursing homes, or horizontally with other home health agencies through partnerships or common ownership.

Physicians

Although they are last in this discussion and receive the smallest share of home care funds, physicians are the gatekeepers for most home care services. In both traditional Medicare and commercial payment scenarios, the physician goes uncompensated for medical supervision of all home care services unless payment is handled indirectly under a full-risk arrangement. The physician is responsible for initiating the plan of treatment and all changes, which can be numerous under Medicare, given the progressive rehabilitation requirement and the generally frail condition of the Medicare population. Additionally, physicians may conduct visits to the patient's home, although this is not common.

Physicians do work closely with home care service providers to determine patient needs and which mix and frequency of services best meet those needs. Care plans for Medicare patients under a physician's care must be reviewed every 62 days, or more frequently, as the patient's medical needs change. The home care provider usually reviews these Medicare plans of care as part of a multidisciplinary approach to meeting the patient's needs. In many cases, physician time involvement for home care patients approaches (and sometimes exceeds) that for acute hospitalized patients.

REGULATIONS GUIDING HOME CARE

Home care service providers that participate as Medicare providers are subject to Title 42 of the Code of Federal Regulations. This section of the code describes the Conditions of Participation that home health agencies must comply with to become Medicare-certified agencies and to provide care to Medicare and Medicaid recipients. These regulations establish minimum requirements for management and patient care. These regulations, which have undergone numerous changes, were initially based on the belief that any reasonable and appropriate caregiver could understand medical instructions and administer progressive rehabilitative care.

Medicare-certified home care services were loosely regulated in the past. The Health Care Financing Adminstration (HCFA) allowed state regulatory agencies to serve as approval authorities for entry and continued participation in the Medicare system. These approvals came in the form of annual state surveys performed by state employees using a combination of local, regional, and national regulations, more often than not subjective and incorrectly interpreted by providers and regulatory agencies alike. The surveys usually lasted 1 to 3 days and consisted of nonstatistical sampling of medical charts for audits, limited visits to patient homes, and reviews of policies, procedures, and other documents. The results of these surveys were discrepancy lists; the agency had a certain amount of time to develop a correction plan and forward it to the regulators. The agency might then be subject to a reinspection.

These regulations were relatively toothless in the past. However, recent legislation has imposed substantial criminal and other penalties for fraud and abuse of the Medicare system. This new breed of regulations includes the Operation Restore Trust (ORT) initiatives, surety bond regulations, and the BBA of 1997. Additionally, numerous rulings and mandates from HCFA, the Department of Health and Human Services, fiscal intermediaries, and even the president have substantially altered the way home health agencies currently operate and will operate in the near future.

Certification of a Medicare agency is the responsibility of HCFA. However, most state health departments have attained "deemed status" to conduct on-site surveys and reviews of agencies in their state. Thus, a single review team applies the higher standards or the combined federal and state standards, making Medicare and Medicaid reimbursement possible. In many states, agencies cannot bill commercial carriers without state (and often, therefore, federal) certification and licensure.

If providers do not desire to participate in the Medicare and Medicaid programs, they are subject to existing state requirements. The majority of states do not have specific requirements for nonparticipating providers. Frequently, however, private third-party payers require an agency to be Medicare certified in order to care for their beneficiaries and receive reimbursement.

For patients to qualify for home health coverage under the Medicare system, the following four conditions must be met:

1. The physician must have determined a medical need for home care and developed a plan of care.
2. The care described in the plan of care must be for intermittent skilled nursing, therapy, or speech services.
3. The patient must be homebound.

4. The home health agency delivering care must be certified to participate in the Medicare program.[4]

Once these four conditions are met, Medicare will generally approve the following types of services:

- skilled nursing care on an intermittent or part-time basis, but not full-time
- HHA services on an intermittent or part-time basis, but not full-time
- PT, based on medical necessity
- SLP, based on medical necessity and reasonableness
- OT, based on medical necessity and reasonableness (OT can be provided in the absence of any other skilled care.)
- medical social services
- medical supplies
- medical equipment (Medicare Part B generally pays for 80 percent of the approved amounts, and the patient is responsible for the remaining 20 percent.)[4]

The length of time that care may be delivered is based on the medical reasonableness and necessity of the care to be delivered. Limitations do exist on the number of days and hours of care that may be received.

Part-time care is defined by Medicare as

- 28 hours a week of skilled nursing and HHA care
- services provided 7 days a week if they are provided for fewer than 8 hours per day
- allowable increase to 35 hours if Medicare agrees that the patient's condition merits the change

Intermittent care is defined by Medicare as

- 28 hours per week of skilled nursing care and HHA care, with an increase to 35 hours a week if the patient's condition merits the change
- services provided 6 days a week
- in some cases, nursing and HHA services provided for a maximum of 8 hours a day, 7 days a week, for 21 consecutive days, with a defined extension beyond 21 days for extreme cases[4]

These limitations do not apply to therapy services, which may be provided for as long as they are deemed medically responsible and necessary.

The indemnity, health maintenance organization (HMO), and, more recently, large self-insured employer sectors have developed a broader understanding of the value of medically necessary home care. Initially, approvals for reimbursement were on a case-by-case exception basis, led by nurse case managers who arranged for complex long-term care, such as intravenous antibiotic therapy, in the home. The main driver was cost, with the added benefit of customer satisfaction. As these sectors became more creative, programmatic handling of home care began (e.g., supporting earlier discharge of new mothers and babies with one or two home visits and follow-up telephone calls). Hospitals initiated these efforts to differentiate themselves and increase margins under case rate contracts.

Commercial HMOs also followed the path of Medicare HMOs in seeking procedure-specific (e.g., lumbar laminectomy) or disease-specific carve-outs. Programs focused on specific disease states require highly skilled professionals. Successful implementation of the programs hinges on close working relationships of the discharge planning teams, which include inpatient and home care program coordinators, payer case managers, and physicians.

FINANCING HOME CARE SERVICES

Health care expenditures have significantly increased in the past 30 years, and the source of payments has undergone a fundamental shift. Private funds were far and away the primary payer source in 1960. In 1997, federal, state, and local funds represented just less than half of total expenditures (see Figure 14–8). Expenditures for home health care services have increased astoundingly since 1980. Home health care has been one of the fastest-growing segments of Medicare system expenditures, until the recent slowdown. It has grown from 2.9 percent of all

Medicare payments in 1980 to more than 9 percent in 1997. Figure 14–8 shows the growth in home health care expenditures nationally.

Home care services are paid for by a variety of payer sources, from public or private organizations to patients or responsible parties. There has been a shift in home care payer types. In 1980, federal funds accounted for 37 percent of home care payments (Figure 14–9). Private funds, including private health insurance and other private sources, contributed 38 percent. By 1997, federal funds had risen to 48 percent, an 11 percent increase. Medicare represented 83 percent, $12.8 billion, of those federal funds. (The federal fund figures recently declined slightly, from $15.5 billion in 1996 to $15.4 billion in 1997. Medicare's portion declined from $13.2 billion in 1996 to $12.8 billion in 1997.) By 1997, private source funds had declined to 23 percent, a 15 percent decrease from 1980. During the same period, out-of-pocket reimbursement remained the same at 22 percent, and state and local funds contributed 4 percent in 1980 and 7 percent in 1997, a 3 percent increase.

Public third-party payers constitute the largest sector of funding sources. These payers include Medicare, Medicaid, the Department of Defense, the Maternal and Child Health Bureau, the Department of Veterans Affairs, Indian Health Services, Social Services Block Grant programs, workers' compensation programs, and other community service organizations.

Though federal programs continue to be the predominant funding source for home health care services, the changes in the reimbursement system made by the BBA of 1997 had a fundamental, lasting impact on home care providers. The BBA contained many provisions designed to reduce the cost of home health services. An interim payment system (IPS) for Medicare was created effective October 1, 1997. Medicare reimbursement changed to the lowest of actual allowable costs, per visit cost limits, or agency per beneficiary annual limits (annual unduplicated Medicare admissions multiplied by the agency per beneficiary limit). IPS established the per beneficiary annual limit based on a mix of agency-specific costs and census region costs.

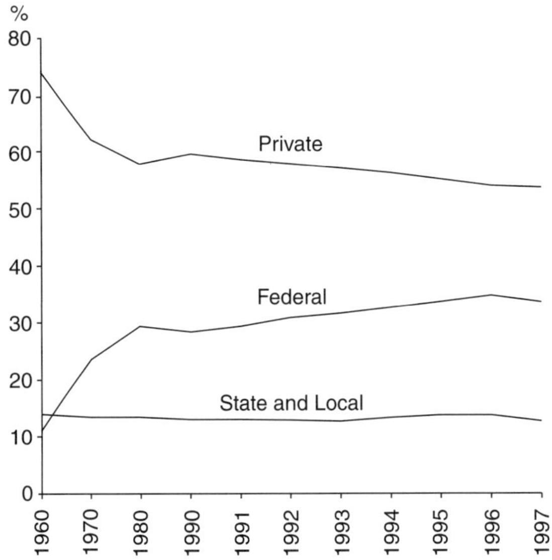

Figure 14–8 National Health Expenditures by Payer Type.

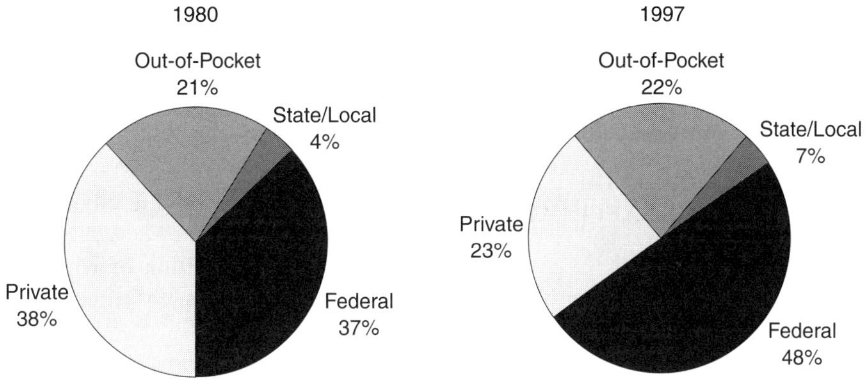

Figure 14–9 Home Health Care Payer Types.

The cost was defined from Medicare cost reports filed in 1994.

Additional provisions and clarifications to the BBA were approved by Congress in 1998.

- All agencies below the national median rate would be adjusted based on a formula blending the agency-specific rate and the national median rate.
- Agencies above the national median rate would receive no change.
- New agencies (agencies starting prior to October 1, 1998) would receive 100 percent of the national median rate.
- "New, new" agencies (agencies starting after October 1, 1998) would receive a per beneficiary rate of 75 percent of the national median rate.

Other provisions also illustrate the intent of HCFA to reduce overall expenditures and discourage the growth of new agencies.

- A prospective payment system (PPS) became fully effective as of October 1, 2000. This will replace the IPS. HCFA is developing the unit of service (reportedly based on episodes of care) and how to apply a case mix adjuster. HCFA had expected to have industry case mix data from Outcomes and Assessment Information Set (OASIS) data. With the OASIS implementation postponed, HCFA reportedly will use limited OASIS demonstration project data.
- Nine census region geographic areas were created.
- A transfer provision from hospitals to skilled nursing facilities and home care agencies was created for 10 diagnosis-related groups and will involve partial reimbursement under certain circumstances.
- Cost limits by discipline were reduced on average 15 percent effective October 1, 1997.
- Cost limits by discipline were further reduced by 15 percent effective October 1, 2000, regardless of the implementation of PPS.
- Venipuncture, an important qualifying skilled service, was no longer funded by HCFA.
- Provisions were established for proration of annual episodic rate between providers.
- Billing will be based on the site of service, not the location of the billing office or parent corporation, thus preventing agency offices in a higher-reimbursement urban setting from billing for services in a lower-reimbursement rural setting.
- Sequential billing was implemented but then eliminated as of July 1, 1999.

- Visits will be reported in 15-minute increments.
- Periodic interim payments were eliminated October 1, 2000.

RECENT LEGISLATION AND REGULATORY ISSUES AFFECTING HOME CARE

There has been continuous scrutiny of home health care related to fraud and abuse of the reimbursement system. The focus has been primarily on the Medicare reimbursement system, with its incentives and opportunities for fraud and abuse. ORT has been successful in detecting this fraud and abuse. The Secretary of Health and Human Services stated at one point in early 1998, at the height of ORT activities, that 40 percent of all Medicare home health care claims were fraudulent. The statement was reportedly based on results of sample claims audits. This statement and others like it created controversy and mistrust for lawmakers and, to some extent, the public. The ORT program was expanded from 5 to 12 states and eventually the whole nation. In late 1997, the ORT program introduced wedge audits as another tool in its review of home care. These quick-hit, limited-focus audits have been particularly injurious to the home care industry. In fiscal year 1997, the Department of Health and Human Services identified $1.2 billion for recovery in collections, fines, settlements, and restitution. This represented a sixfold increase over 1996. Criminal and civil prosecution cases totaled 1,340 in fiscal year 1997, and more than 2,700 providers were excluded from participation in federal and state programs. The home care industry has continued to struggle with this sustained level of scrutiny and investigation, with many providers going out of business due to demands for payback of overpayments as a result of ORT-related audits.

The BBA of 1997 contained additional provisions to fight fraud and abuse in home care, including the following:

- new penalties of $50,000 per violation for providers paying kickbacks for referrals
- requirements that providers disclose Social Security numbers and employer identification numbers so that past offenders may be screened out
- requirements for surety bonds from home health agencies
- a clearer definition of what qualifies as skilled services, to prevent unnecessary visits
- authority to deny payment to providers that bill in excess of what other providers bill for similar services

Surety bonds have been put on hold as a requirement for home health agencies, but the requirement is likely to be reinstated in the near future. Other actions by HCFA have included the following:

- Home health agencies are being asked about related business interests before admission as a Medicare provider. This will help determine if there are any previous instances of fraud and abuse and will also help to prevent unauthorized billings through nonexistent or nonapproved companies.
- Home health companies must have provided care to at least 10 patients requiring skilled services before being allowed to provide care to Medicare beneficiaries. At least 7 of those patients must be receiving care at the time of the survey for approval to receive a Medicare provider number.
- Claims review has increased to 25 percent of claims submitted. HCFA has set aside $10 million to perform audits, such as the compliance audits and wedge audits. This is nearly double past expenditures.
- Fiscal intermediaries have hired medical directors to advise claims processors and providers on medical necessity of care.

The provisions outlined herein and the effects of continued fraud and abuse activities have fundamentally changed the home health care industry.

MEASURING QUALITY IN HOME CARE SERVICES

The federal government and the home health care industry are aggressively pursuing initiatives to measure and improve the quality of home care services. Two rulings announced in March 1997 have affected the home health care industry. The first ruling revises Medicare's Conditions of Participation to include

- a requirement that HHAs be subject to criminal background checks
- the expansion of existing HHA qualifications to include only HHAs who have completed nurse aide training or competency evaluations
- active involvement of patients in the planning and conduct of their care through discussions between care providers and patients about expected outcomes of care
- a requirement that home care agencies coordinate all the physician-ordered care for patients

The second regulation requires that home health agencies use the OASIS. This standardized system is designed to monitor patients' condition, levels of function, and satisfaction. This system requires that each new patient receive a standardized assessment within 48 hours of admission. This assessment is designed to determine the patient's care and support needs. It is updated continually to monitor and track changes in the patient's condition. This continuous assessment would end upon discharge of the patient from the home health agency. Home health agencies are required to evaluate the OASIS assessments, track and submit this information, and incorporate changes in their quality improvement programs. These data sets can also be used by inspectors and surveyors to standardize the agency surveys and to identify improvement opportunities related to patient care and satisfaction.

The Joint Commission on Accreditation of Healthcare Organizations (Joint Commission) also monitors home health care organizations through a comprehensive quality survey process utilizing home care–specific standards. The most recent version of standards was published for 1999. The accreditation process is voluntary and conducted in three-year cycles. For home health organizations that are hospital based or affiliated with health systems, the three-year accreditation cycle generally coincides with that of the rest of the health system. The Joint Commission also conducts random, unannounced surveys on approximately 5 percent of accredited agencies.

EXAMPLES OF ADVANCED CLINICAL PRACTICES IN HOME CARE

Leading home care practices are not well documented, yet there are examples of wide variations and innovations. For instance, West Coast agencies have been successful in managing post–total hip replacement care in 6 to 8 visits with outcomes similar to those realized from 8 to 12 visits on the East Coast. Many managed care organizations (MCOs) are utilizing experienced home health clinicians to conduct health risk assessments (HRAs) in the home setting. The accuracy and completeness of the HRAs have been found to be enhanced when done in the home setting, especially when screening for high-risk members.

Recognizing the high incidence of psychosocially driven ED visits, a very large southern home health agency has become creative in working with a number of hospitals to manage their Medicare risk ED visits. It has developed a triaging program that identifies patients before processing at the hospital and refers them to an adult day care program with after-hours homemaker care to effectively decrease ED visits and their related admissions by 25 percent.

An example of a procedure-specific clinical process that has been developed by another southern agency for post-lumbar laminectomy using a combination of accelerated postoperative teaching and two home care follow-up visits reduced inpatient hospital stays from 5 or 6 days to 2 days.

The increasing number of frail elderly requiring medical management has led to the establishment of "home hospital" programs in a number of academic settings throughout the country. Typically, these services are overseen by a geriatric service line or a medical center's own home health agency. Patients are maintained at home, even through acute episodes, through a multidisciplinary approach that includes home visits by physicians and other geriatric clinicians, thereby minimizing the complications often seen when the frail elderly enter an institution.

Disease state case management companies have entered the market with a home care model that combines in-home environmental assessments and routine visits with up to daily telephone contact to maximize treatment compliance in chronic diseases such as congestive heart failure. These companies have shown the ability to significantly reduce ED visits, admissions, and overall costs associated with diseases such as congestive heart failure and asthma.

Academic medical centers focusing on medical and/or technological research have been turning to and testing telemedicine approaches. Some MCOs, seeking cost-effective alternatives, have begun to invest in telemedicine as a way to closely monitor patients' conditions without costly home visits or office visits. A 1996 study done by a West Coast MCO found that "video visits" averaged 18 minutes per patient, whereas in-person evaluations took an average of 45 minutes plus travel time. A successful telemedicine approach, however, typically involves a combination of actual home visits and telephone contacts.

It is unclear at this time what influence the Internet and Web-based access to information (good and bad) will have on the dynamics of home health care. Some agencies are already utilizing resources available on the Internet for patient education purposes. It will be increasingly important for providers to be aware of the information patients may be accessing in their homes, and to monitor for confusion or conflicting approaches to health care at home.

REFERENCES

1. Health Care Financing Administration, U.S. Department of Health and Human Services, Bureau of Data Management and Strategy, *HCFA Statistics*, publication no. 03394 (Washington, DC: Author, 1996).
2. Health Care Financing Administration, press release, January 13, 1998.
3. K. Schworm and E. Gruenwedel, "The Industry's Facts and Figures," *HomeCare* (July 1997): 36.
4. Health Care Financing Administration—Medicare and Medicaid, U.S. Department of Health and Human Services, *Medicare and Home Health Care*, publication no. 10969 (Washington, DC: Author, 1996).

CHAPTER 15

Hospice and End-of-Life Care

Anne C. Dye, Peggy H. Rodebush, and Geri Hempel

TAKE THIS TO WORK

1. Identify patients with documented, progressive terminal diagnosis with anticipated life expectancy of six months or less.
2. Document patient's preference for palliative versus curative treatment.
3. Communicate effectively with the patient, family, and physician regarding ongoing treatment options when identifying hospice as an option.
4. Investigate payer coverage and obtain a preferred provider list, if any.
5. Document level-of-care requirements and any specialty services or equipment needed.
6. Obtain physician orders for transition to the selected hospice.
7. Obtain patient notice of election of the hospice benefit and physician certification of terminal illness prior to enrolling the patient in a hospice program.
8. Use palliative treatment protocols, rather than curative techniques, for a hospice patient hospitalized for conditions unrelated to the terminal diagnosis.
9. Identify community and volunteer resources for the hospice patient and family members.
10. Identify an interdisciplinary team to treat all dimensions of health: physical, psychological, emotional, and spiritual.

MEDICAL MANAGEMENT AND END-OF-LIFE CARE

Introduction

The main focus of health care in the United States during the past 50 years has been the aggressive treatment and eradication of disease and illness to prolong life. Overall, that approach has proven to be very successful. During the past 50 years, experts have created vaccines to eliminate such communicable diseases as polio and smallpox, developed noninvasive surgical interventions, and perfected open-heart surgery so it is now routine. Partly because of these medical and public health advances, the population in the United States has increased rapidly. The number of older adults in particular has grown and will be likely to continue to grow at a tremendous

---

Source: Reprinted from A.C. Dye, P.H. Rodebush, and G. Hempel, Hospice and End-of-Life Care, in *The Managed Health Care Handbook, 4th Edition,* P. Kongstvedt, ed., pp. 508–520, © 2001, Aspen Publishers, Inc.

rate. In fact, the population aged 65 and over is expected to increase by 35 percent between 1996 and 2015 (Figure 15–1).These demographic changes, an attempt to contain costs, an increasing need for individuals to take control over their own health care, and changing attitudes about death and end-of-life care have influenced medical management decisions over the past 10 years.

Clinicians now face an array of chronic illnesses that progress to terminal phases. These illnesses may be classified by site of care (e.g., acute care facility, nursing home, home, hospice), by disease (e.g., congestive heart failure, cancer), or by intervention (e.g., cardiothoracic surgery, diagnostic radiology). However, dying patients experience illness in a much more fragmented way than dying patients once did. They get care from a number of provider sites, with multiple medical specialists attending to illnesses that cannot be cured. It is a challenge to standardize pain management across providers, and quality of care and outcomes are not adequately measured. According to the Center to Improve Care of the Dying:

> End-of-life care often falls to physician specialists focused on rescue (e.g., oncologists, cardiologists) when multi-disciplinary teams attentive to nursing and social issues could provide more effective and more reliable supportive care. All the evidence suggests that patients and their families have little ability to reshape care to better meet their needs compared with the influence of provider supply and established care patterns.[1]

U.S. health care advances and research are respected throughout the world. However, in the zeal to become the world's greatest healers, U.S. health care providers have failed to sufficiently educate and prepare health care professionals to provide end-of-life care. It is not enough to teach our health care professionals how to identify and

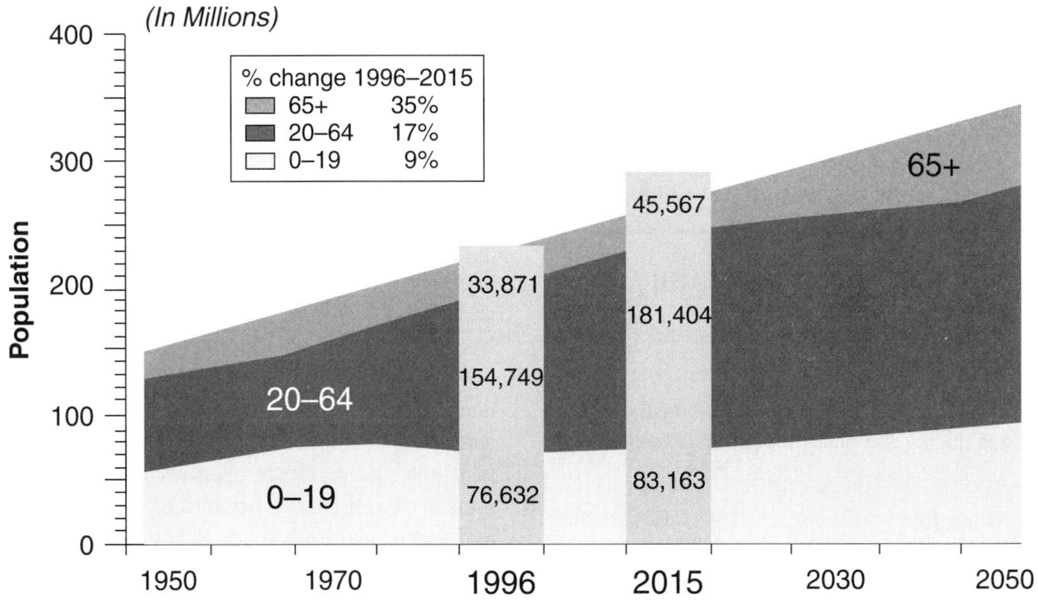

Figure 15–1 Actual and Projected Population Growth, 1950 to 2050.

refer terminally ill patients to appropriate palliative care providers. Every health professional who deals directly with patients or families needs to know how to deal both compassionately and competently with the seriously ill and dying patient. Palliative and end-of-life care needs to be incorporated into the traditional care delivery model and into managed medical care.

Most people agree that whenever possible, a person should be able to die at home, surrounded by family. However, some health care providers have trouble understanding what the patient and family want and how to assist them during the end-of-life process. It is critical for health care providers to understand that the patient and family members want to be treated with compassion and dignity, to receive support and care, to have adequate pain control, to avoid becoming victims of technological advances, to know when everything that can be done has been done, and to be assured they will not be abandoned by the health care system when the end of life is near.

Given the likelihood that end-of-life care will be given by a variety of health care providers, it is important that there be an interdisciplinary approach to the process. *To effectively manage the end-of-life process, the health care team must take the following steps:*

- *Reduce fragmentation of care.* Develop certainty regarding who should care for people with terminal illness, and work from an established plan. Initiate advanced care planning discussions within 24 hours of a patient's admission to a facility or home care, and document the plan in the patient's medical record.
- *Communicate effectively and compassionately with the patient and family.* Assess providers' own feelings, attitudes, and expectations surrounding death, and consider patients' cultural and spiritual diversity. Begin bereavement assistance and support before the patient dies.
- *Assess and treat all dimensions of health.* To improve the quality of life for the terminally ill patient, assess the patient's physical, psychological, emotional, and spiritual well-being.
- *Identify ways to obtain resources.* Assist the patient and family in identifying and accessing all available community resources.
- *Develop and/or adopt standardized tools.* Use standardized tools to assess symptoms experienced by the patient at the end of life. Based on the information obtained from the assessment, develop a plan that provides for intervention and symptom management. Develop pain and symptom management protocols.
- *Collaborate with an interdisciplinary team.* The care provided to the patient should be coordinated and available around the clock, and providers should be sensitive to diversity issues as well as the patient's and family's needs. Each member of the health care team should make a specific contribution, but others should offer assistance. For instance, pain management is generally in the realm of the physician, but other members of the team should be able to provide insight into pain management as well.
- *Reduce fear and anxiety.* Both pharmacological and nonpharmacological protocols should be developed to manage the patient's symptoms and reduce his or her stress.

It is the health care provider's obligation to help terminally ill patients receive the support and care that they deserve, and it is the obligation of the health plan's medical management function to assist in the process. Americans are not dying well. The Study to Understand Prognoses and Preferences for Outcomes and Risks of Treatment found there is still too much unwarranted aggressive treatment against patients' wishes. Despite advances in pain relief, too many people are still dying without adequate pain control. There is still not enough communication between physicians and patients; many patients (or their families, when appropriate) are never asked about treatment preference. We can and should do better.[2]

Hospice care represents a comprehensive solution that fits many different models of medical care management. It is a mode of care for the terminally ill patient that may or may not encompass facility-based care.

THE BASICS OF HOSPICE CARE

Philosophy

Hospice is a remarkable treatment modality. It often combines state-of-the-art pain management techniques and pharmacology with counseling, personal care, and (when desired) spiritual support to provide comfort to individuals entering the last months of their lives. Because hospice is focused on care for the terminally ill, it encompasses areas not typically considered part of medical management or the health care continuum. Hospice professionals are called on to aid patients and families in understanding the meaning of their lives, and deaths; to reconcile themselves to death as the natural end to life; and to fulfill last wishes when possible.

As defined by Flexner, hospice is a "medically directed, nurse coordinated program providing a continuum of home and inpatient care for the terminally ill patient and family. It employs an interdisciplinary team acting under the direction of an autonomous hospice administrator."[3] It is also a philosophy of care that accepts death as a natural part of life, seeking neither to hasten nor prolong the dying process, and existing solely to support the terminally ill person and family through the last stages of life. The primary objective of hospice is to provide supportive care and counseling to the dying patient and family. The clinical goals of hospice are oriented toward palliative care, with pain management and symptom control, not curative therapy, as the primary focus of treatment.

Senator James Randolph, in establishing National Hospice Week (SR 170, March 18, 1982), described hospice well: "Hospice is a place, people, and a philosophy. It is a system of care that seeks to restore dignity and a sense of personal fulfillment to the dying. The focus is on the patient and the family, rather than on the disease—and the aim is not to extend life, but to improve the quality of life that remains."

The first hospice in the United States opened its doors in 1974. It began as a grassroots reaction to the depersonalization of care and treatment for the dying patient. Early supporters of hospice recognized a need to isolate the terminally ill patient from the treatment-based philosophy of the acute care setting. Today, hospice has developed into an integral component of the health care continuum.

The majority of hospices in the United States today are designed to provide care in patients' homes. Although services may be provided in a variety of settings and facilities, the home setting is a main component of the hospice philosophy. Providing care in this nontraditional health care setting also helps to contain the costs of care. Care for a terminally ill patient in the hospital setting is expensive, and hospice provides a cost-effective alternative to the high-technology, labor-intensive acute care setting. But more important, the home setting provides the greatest comfort to the dying patient.

Structure and Organization

Hospices in the United States come in all shapes, sizes, and reimbursement models. Programs are located in office buildings, physician offices, and even churches. These programs may have contractual arrangements with other facilities to provide inpatient care. They may be freestanding with their own inpatient unit or may be affiliated with a hospital or an extended care facility. A program may be for-profit or not-for-profit. Currently in the United States, most hospices are not-for-profit. The staffing model may be all paid staff, a combination of paid staff and volunteers, or all volunteer. Volunteers in an all-volunteer model work cooperatively with agencies and other programs to provide the necessary services.

Regardless of the structure of the hospice, standards have been established by both regulatory agencies and the National Hospice Organization (NHO) that serve as the guiding principles for care of patients and families. These standards include requirements that care be available 7 days a week, 24 hours per day, with integrated inpatient and home care services available. Volunteers are used to assist with the patient and family during both the dying process and the bereavement process. An interdisciplinary team guided by a medical director plans and provides the care. The family members and anyone important to the patient participate in hospice care, working closely to support the patient during the final days.

FINANCING AND REIMBURSEMENT

Medical Coverage for Hospice Services

Hospice care is financed through several mechanisms: Medicare, Medicaid, private insurance, private pay, donations, and grants (Figure 15–2). Although reimbursement for hospice services increased dramatically in recent years, Medicare remained the primary payer, representing 68 percent of hospice revenues, or $1.2 billion in 1994.[4] Medicaid hospice expenditures grew as well, totaling $197.6 million in fiscal year 1994, an increase of 53 percent over the $128.9 million spent in fiscal year 1993.[5]

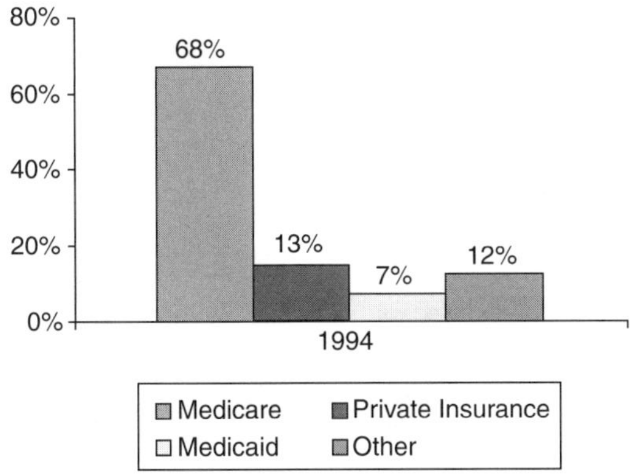

Figure 15–2 1994 Hospice Revenues by Payer. *Note:* "Other" indicates donations, grants, and private pay.

The Medicare Benefit

The Medicare hospice benefit is available under Part A of Medicare. Medicare reimburses Medicare-certified hospices on a per diem basis by level of care, including routine home care, inpatient care for acute symptom management, continuous care, and respite services for durations of not longer than 5 days per episode. Persons electing hospice must have a terminal diagnosis with a life expectancy of 6 months or less, as certified by a physician. Care is provided in a variety of settings, including inpatient facilities and homes.

Persons electing to use their hospice benefits under Medicare must select this benefit in lieu of traditional Medicare reimbursement for all treatments related to their terminal illness. Services provided include skilled nursing, physician services, home health aides, social workers, home medical equipment, palliative medications, laboratory testing, volunteer services, and bereavement counseling. These services are available 24 hours a day.

Managed Care

The key factors affecting hospice's success within a managed care environment include demonstration of quality, evidence of cost-effectiveness, and willingness to share financial risk.[6] Providers are developing strategies to address these factors, as increasing numbers of hospice programs have begun to compete for managed care contracts. For example, in Baltimore, Maryland, hospice services for patients with acquired immune deficiency syndrome (AIDS) covered by Medicaid are included in an AIDS care capitation program designed by Johns Hopkins AIDS Service, Johns Hopkins HealthCare LLC, the Maryland Department of Health and Mental Hygiene, and health maintenance organizations (HMOs) in Maryland.[7]

Eighty-two percent of managed care plans offered hospice services as part of their benefit package in 1993.[8] Managed care organizations (MCOs) such as Kaiser Permanente, Group Health Cooperative, and AvMed continue to recognize the value of hospice and operate their own hospice programs that serve Medicare, Medicaid, and private clients. However, there is little information published on the managed care dollars spent providing hospice services. Additionally, hospice is still a carve-out for Medicare HMOs, and patients have to disenroll from Medicaid HMOs to receive Medicaid hospice benefits.

SIZE OF THE U.S. HOSPICE INDUSTRY

Agency Characteristics

In 1995, the overall revenues for the hospice market were estimated at $2.8 billion, with Medicare revenues at about 68 percent, or $1.9 billion (unpublished data, A.C. Dye, Ernst & Young, 1997). According to the NHO, there were approximately 3,200 operational or planned hospice programs in all 50 states and Puerto Rico as of April 1998. The Health Care Financing Administration (HCFA) reported that 1,857 Medicare-certified hospice programs provided hospice services to 309,336 Medicare patients in 1995.[9] The average length of stay (ALOS) for these patients was 59 days. Home health agency–based hospices made up 27 percent of the hospice market, and not-for-profit hospices represented 72 percent of the hospice industry (Figure 15–3).[4]

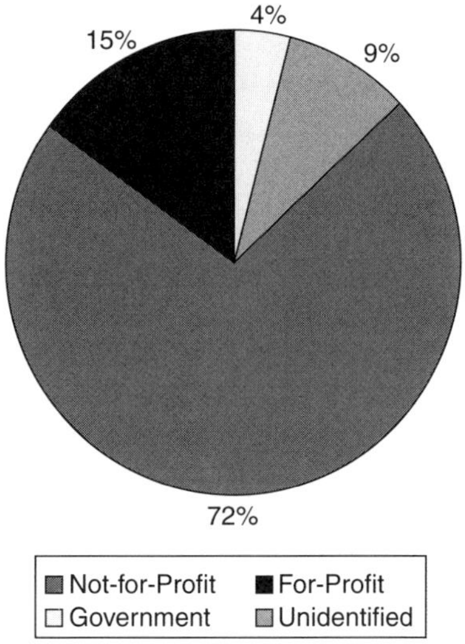

Figure 15–3 1995 Ownership Status of Hospice Programs.

Patient Information

In 1995, approximately one out of every seven individuals who died in the United States from all causes (not just terminal illness) received care from a hospice program.[4] HCFA statistics show that hospice patients are more likely to be older, married, and living with their spouse.[10] The most prevalent diagnoses at admission were related to cancer (71 percent), diseases of the heart and circulatory system (9 percent), and respiratory conditions (6 percent).[10] The number of hospice patients is expected to more than double between 1990 and 2000 (Figure 15–4).

Still, too few terminally ill persons receive care from hospice services. According to the Hospice Association of America, patients who received care other than hospice often died in the hospital instead of in the comfort of their own homes. Just 13 percent of hospice patients were admitted to the hospital two months prior to their death, compared to 41 percent admitted from other care providers during the same period of time.[11]

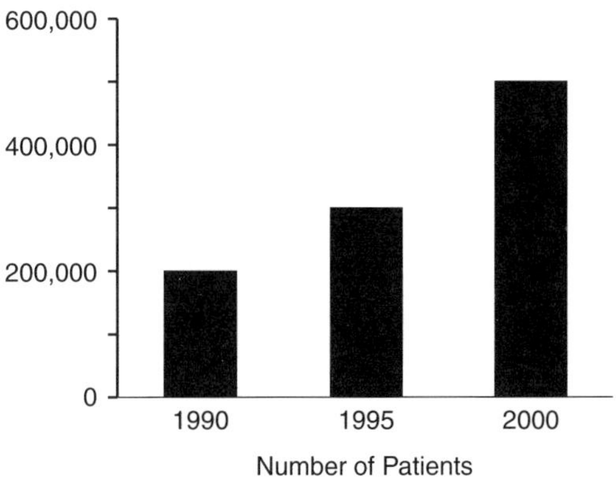

Figure 15–4 Hospice Patient Growth, 1990–2000. *Note:* 2000 figures are projections.

Growth Projections

The number of Medicare-certified hospices more than doubled between 1990 and 1995, largely as a result of the 1989 congressional mandate to increase reimbursement rates by 20 percent (Figure 15–5). The provider that emerged with clear market dominance was VITAS Healthcare Corporation. Fiscal year 1998 revenues for VITAS were about $220 million; the second largest hospice, VistaCare, reported revenues of only about $75 million for the same period. It is expected that, with the aging of the baby boomer population and the increasing acceptance of hospice, the number of hospice programs will increase rapidly. The House Ways and Means Committee projected an average annual growth rate for hospice at 25 percent through the year 2000.[12]

MAJOR POLICY ISSUES

Ethics

Hospice began as a philosophy of care inspired by volunteer activity. As a philosophy, hospice is straightforward. It accepts death's inevitability and seeks to support the dying person and his or her family and friends through palliative symptom control, counseling, and support. Challenges arise when this philosophy is translated into a program of care that receives third-party reimbursement. The hospice must justify the terminal diagnosis of the population served, provide care and services at a lower cost than most programs oriented toward cure, and be responsible for providing many nontraditional services, such as spiritual support, anticipatory grief counseling, and bereavement care.

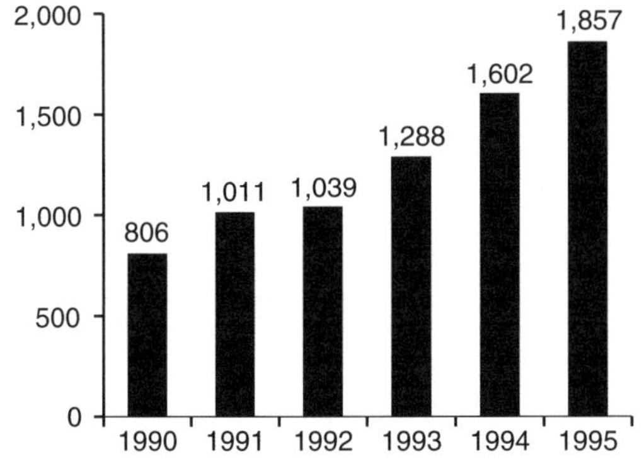

Figure 15–5 Medicare-Certified Hospice Growth by Year.

Any health care program that limits resources and aims to serve a select group of people must provide justification for the allocation of benefits. Traditionally, the allocation of benefits has been the responsibility of the government, third-party payers, or charities, and not the responsibility of the provider. The Medicare regulations established for hospice have set criteria that the hospice must observe for patient selection and restriction of treatment modalities. However, it is the providers' responsibility to define which services a patient receives and which resources are used in caring for him or her.

By its very nature, hospice has the potential to involve ethical and moral dilemmas. The NHO has issued a code of ethics to guide the staff of hospice and palliative care programs through issues such as physician-assisted suicide, confidentiality, removal of artificial nutrition and hydration, and pain control.[13] In order to address these issues, hospices should support the development of internal ethics committees. Ethics committees are a key component in any health care organization and can assist in establishing baseline criteria regarding organizational policy for service provision, patient population, questions regarding suicide and assisted suicide, responsibility for resource conservation and allocation, and responsibility for care for those patients who do not qualify for services. As consumers of health care become more educated regarding the hospice philosophy and hospices develop a major role in the health care continuum, hospice ethics committees will play a vital role in how the medical community provides comfortable, compassionate, and palliative care to the terminally ill.

Legal Issues

In recent years, health care providers have been faced with a growing awareness of and concern regarding the legal and regulatory issues surrounding the industry. Hospice providers may be at a particular disadvantage because of the type of care they provide. Legal issues may arise from a variety of areas, including, but not limited to, malpractice, wrongful death, negligence, and nontreatment. The fact that a hospice is believed to provide a valuable service does not necessarily protect it from potential legal issues. To succeed, a hospice needs to understand the situations that could lead to litigation and have safeguards developed to minimize exposure to liability.

One of the most important safeguards a hospice can have to reduce its exposure to legal issues is a quality improvement program. Properly implemented, a quality improvement program will provide the hospice with tools for continuous improvement throughout the organization, thus reducing potential liability issues. Equally important is a risk management program designed to reduce liability exposure and foster an awareness within the organization regarding legal liabilities. Although risk management programs must be tailored to individual organizations, the following basic elements should be included:

- continuing review of insurance to determine adequacy of coverage
- ongoing review of the physical premises and equipment to discover and correct defects
- ongoing personnel performance appraisals and revision of hospice policies so that those policies reflect adequate quality of care measures
- maintenance of systems for investigating adverse incidents to prepare a defense and to develop procedures for avoiding future occurrences
- support of grievance procedures to handle patient and family complaints, solve problems, and prevent litigation[14]

Care Provision

The advent of Medicare certification in 1983 created extensive requirements with which hospice programs must comply to be eligible for federal reimbursement. Currently, Medicare requires hospice programs to be responsible for providing certain core services—including skilled nursing, social work, and counseling—performed by noncontract employees. Noncore services may be provided by contract employees and include physician services, home care aide/homemaker services, physical therapy, speech therapy, occupational therapy, volunteer services, and bereavement counseling. Additionally, the hospice is required to provide all medications, laboratory work, medical equipment, and supplies that relate to the terminal diagnosis.

Although the Medicare program dictates the scope of services to be provided, the hospice defines how and to what extent services will be provided. Following an in-depth admission process, the hospice admits the patient into the program. Next, during an interdisciplinary team conference, a plan of care is established outlining the services the patient will receive. The care plan is then modified based on the patient's needs throughout the course of care. Services may be provided in the home or in an inpatient setting.

The hospice recognizes the special needs of the terminally ill patient, and all programs and services are developed to meet those needs. Although hospice programs may provide services in different ways, there are certain fundamental guidelines in developing the care delivery model. These guidelines distinguish hospice from other programs. Hospice care is

- exclusively for the terminally ill
- focused on the patient and family
- provided to the family through the bereavement period
- provided by an interdisciplinary team
- medically directed
- available 24 hours a day, 7 days a week
- a service that uses volunteers as an integral part of the program

SERVICE MODELS

Hospices may be licensed in several ways, depending on the affiliation of the provider. It is important to model potential cost report and other financial implications before choosing the licensure category for newly licensed programs. Additionally, there are criteria that must be satisfied for each licensure classification.

The Government Accounting Office classifies hospice providers into the types discussed below. There are specific advantages and disadvantages to each model. The community or organization must address all planning issues prior to determining which hospice type is best.

Free-Standing Hospice

The free-standing hospice is a separate facility providing both inpatient and home hospice services. Inpatient services may be provided by the hospice or contracted with a local hospital or nursing home. The considerable start-up costs for a free-standing hospice and the continued operating expenses require aggressive financial planning.

Hospital-Based Hospice

Hospital-based hospice programs are a distinct unit of a hospital that provides inpatient hospice services, also known as a palliative care unit. The program may provide home hospice services through its own hospital-based hospice or through a contracted arrangement with a free-standing program. The hospital unit generally requires remodeling of the physical plant to adapt to the hospice concept. A hospital-based program may have less autonomy than a free-standing program. However, it does have increased access to hospital resources and the medical community. The hospital-based hospice is guided by the governing board of the hospital, and the mission and philosophy of the hospice are generally those of the hospital.

Reimbursement is generally provided through the Medicare hospice benefit and other third-party payers. Due to the hospital affiliation, there may be an enhanced opportunity for inclusion of the hospice in managed care contracts.

Hospice Affiliated with an Extended Care or Skilled Nursing Facility

Some hospice programs are a distinct part of a skilled nursing facility (SNF) or an extended care facility (ECF). Home hospice arrangements are generally provided through a community-based or a facility-based hospice. Many patients in a nursing home have a terminal illness, and the hospice provides the opportunity for the patient and family to take advantage of additional services. The hospice improves the continuity of care offered to the nursing home patient.

The mission and philosophy of the hospice complement those of the ECF or SNF. The hospice is governed by the facility board. Reimbursement is provided through the traditional Medicare hospice benefit and some limited third-party payers. A facility-based hospice may have some opportunities for recruitment of staff and volunteers, depending on the reputation of the facility in the community.

Hospital-Based Hospice Home Care

This type of hospice is a hospital-based home health agency that provides hospice services. Inpatient services are provided either through the hospital's separate part or through a contracted arrangement with an ECF or SNF.

In this arrangement, the mission and philosophy of the hospice complement those of the home health agency and the hospital. The hospice may function as a semiautonomous program of the home health agency. If the inpatient unit is with the hospital, continuity of care is enhanced through the availability of the various programs. This arrangement provides patients with the opportunity to transfer among programs easily. There is the potential, however, for home care and hospice programs to compete for referrals with common hospice diagnoses such as cancer and to question when to refer patients from curative treatments in home care to more palliative hospice programs.

Reimbursement is provided through the Medicare hospice benefit and other third-party payers. The hospital-based hospice has an improved opportunity to obtain other third-party contracts due to the affiliation with the home health agency and the hospital.

Community-Based Home Health Agency Hospice

Part of a community-based home health agency, this type of hospice requires an agreement with a facility to provide inpatient services. The mission and philosophy of the hospice complement those of the home health agency, and the governing board of the agency provides the direction for the hospice. The hospice could function as a semiautonomous program that enhances the services offered through the home health agency. The home health–based hospice can provide services to a patient through a terminal care program of the home health agency prior to admitting the patient to the hospice. Reimbursement of the hospice is generally through the Medicare hospice benefit and other third-party payers.

HOSPICE COST AND STAFFING

The budget structure for hospice is unlike that for many other levels of care, primarily because reimbursement is both per diem and all-inclusive of services provided for the terminal illness. But as with other levels of care, there are direct costs such as employee salaries and fringe benefits, transportation, equipment, and supplies. Indirect costs include public relations, fund-raising activities, volunteer recruitment and training, staff education, and space considerations. Key statistics to include when developing the budget for a hospice include the following:

- *Average daily census.* The average daily census is the number of patients that the hospice will care for on a daily basis.
- *Average length of stay (ALOS).* The ALOS is the average number of days a patient will stay on service. The most expensive time during the course of care for a hospice patient is during the admission process and when the patient is actively dying. If patients are admitted to service late in the course of illness, the costs to the hospice will be high. Also, if patients are admitted for a short period of time, the true value of the hospice for the patient and the family is not recognized.
- *Payer mix.* The Medicare hospice option pays a per diem rate. The average daily home rate was approximately $96 as of 1998. Many MCOs may pay a per diem rate or break out the services.
- *Staffing ratio.* Critical to determining the staffing ratio are the ALOS and the level-of-care needs of the patient. If a hospice's ALOS is less than 30 days, the level of care is greater, and therefore the staffing needs will be higher than those for a hospice whose ALOS is greater than 60 days. Patients referred to the hospice who are close to death require more visits and services than patients who stay on the program longer. The NHO indicated that for programs with an ALOS of 60 days, approximately 34.5 visits are made. They were distributed as shown in Figure 15–6. The NHO recommends the staffing plan shown in Table 15–1.

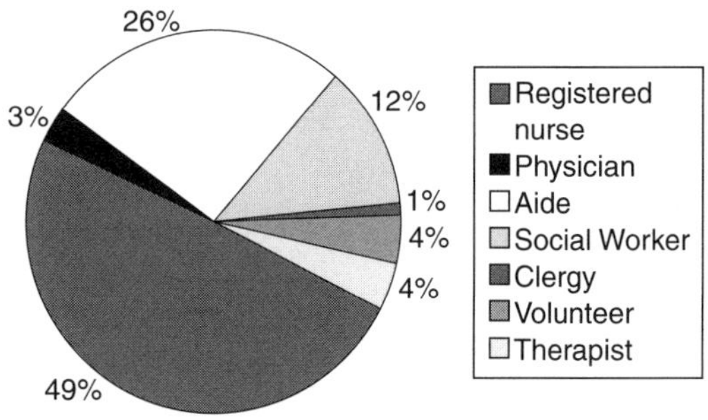

Figure 15–6 Distribution of Staff Providing Visits for Programs with ALOS of 30 Days.

Table 15–1 Hospice Staffing Recommendations

Discipline	*Daily Census*	*FTEs**
Registered nurse	8–12	1
Social worker	20–30	1
Chaplain	40–60	1
Home health aide	12–15	1
Volunteer coordinator	60–80	1

*FTE = Full-time equivalent

- *Expenses per patient per day for major costs.* The hospice is required to provide all supplies, equipment, drugs, and treatments directly related to the terminal diagnosis. To accurately determine the cost of operating the hospice, the cost of medical supplies, equipment, drugs, and treatment must be monitored. Typical productivity standards are shown in Table 15–2.

SPECIALTY PROGRAMS

Hospice care continues to be a relatively new field of practice in the U.S. health care system. There are many innovative programs that serve the terminally ill in unique and caring ways. Examples of these programs are described below.

Zen Hospice Project Residence Program

This program operates a four-bed hospice residence. The primary goal of the program is to provide care and support to patients with terminal illnesses in a homelike setting. The residence is a restored Victorian home with high ceilings, fireplaces, and a patio and garden. Services are available to people with AIDS, cancer, and other life-threatening illnesses. Family and friends are encouraged to visit and actively participate in the patient's care. Medical services are provided 24 hours per day, 7 days per week, through a collaboration with Visiting Nurses and Hospice, a program of the California Pacific Medical Center.

Table 15–2 Hospice Provider Productivity Standards

Discipline	*Average Visits per Day*
Registered nurse	3.7
Licensed practical nurse	4.2
Social worker	2.5
Home care aide	4.5

Hospice in Nursing Homes

Florida's Panel for the Study of End-of-life Care reported that in 1997, Florida hospice programs served 46,608 patients, just under 2,000 of which were in nursing homes. While end-of-life care alternatives to the traditional hospice model are being piloted in nursing homes through mechanisms such as Robert Wood Johnson Foundation grants, at least one hospice provider has developed hospice services specifically designed to address the nursing home population. VITAS Healthcare provides long-term care (LTC) teams that are dedicated to the care of terminally ill nursing home patients. In addition, it provides assistance to the LTC facility in state surveys, palliative care education for staff, and bereavement support for families and facility staff.

Pediatric Hospice Programs

The death of a parent or a loved one is devastating. However, nothing is more traumatic for a family than the loss of a child. Pediatric hospices are being developed nationwide to provide support and services to this special population. The family of a pediatric patient may be more likely than other families to use the services of a pediatric hospice during both the dying process and the bereavement process. These hospices are designed especially to provide the necessary support and services.

Disease State Management Protocols

Several hospices have begun to provide disease-specific care to terminally ill patients.

VITAS Healthcare has developed an emergency response plan for chronic obstructive pulmonary disease (COPD) hospice patients. The plan is designed to provide immediate intervention in respiratory crises and to decrease emergency department visits and hospitalizations. The Hospice of North Central Florida, in cooperation with 6 other hospices around the country and under direction from Dr. Joanne Lynn of the Center to Improve Care of the Dying, is piloting disease management protocols for COPD and congestive heart failure (CHF). The program focuses on CHF and COPD patients nearing the end of life (the last 2 to 3 years). The goals of MediCaring are to improve care at the end of life by developing appropriate, optimal, cost-effective services that blend the best of palliative care with the best of medical and disease management and to propose sustainable service, financing, and regulatory reform in Medicare through a national demonstration project involving health care provider organizations nationwide (including hospices, large group practices, Medicare MCOs, and the Veterans' Affairs Health Care System).

Florida Palliative Home Care Program

The Florida Palliative Home Care Program is a new Medicare-certified home health agency developed by five hospices serving 16 counties in Florida. It offers care to chronically ill preterminal patients and provides a hospicelike range of care to those not yet eligible for the hospice benefit. It is thought that this model will also increase the LOS in hospice for this patient population, as patients will be discharged to the participating hospices earlier than from more traditional home health, community, or acute care providers.

Hospice Care of Rhode Island AIDS Case Management Program

Hospice Care of Rhode Island, a partner of the Lifespan Healthcare System, developed an AIDS hospice program using Ryan White Title II funding in the early 1990s, primarily as a response to increasing mortality rates for this population. Recently, it has implemented a case management program in collaboration with the Miriam Hospital Clinic, as treatment advances in recent years have increased the chronicity of the high-risk AIDS population in its service area. It is hoped that this program will avert hospitalizations and improve quality of life for and management of preterminal AIDS patients as they approach hospice-appropriate stages in the disease process.

FUTURE INTEGRATION AND AFFILIATION STRATEGIES

Utilization of hospice care services has increased tremendously in the past 10 years, primarily as a result of the implementation of the acute care prospective payment system in 1982 and the move to increase Medicare hospice reimbursement rates in 1989. Concern about escalating costs and overutilization of services has shaped current reimbursement trends in both the public and the private sectors. Accordingly, the market is beginning to change dramatically as network and provider consolidation continues and strategic integration and affiliation trends accelerate. The next 5 years will see a dramatically changed business and health care environment within the postacute care industry. The key challenge for hospice care providers will be to develop and implement effective strategies to address these changing factors in an environment increasingly dominated by managed care, including:

- probable shift of Medicare from fee-for-service prospective payment reimbursement structures to Medicare HMO products (a trend that slowed in 1998 and 1999 but is likely to pick up again)
- selective managed care contracting strategies
- vertical integration strategies for postacute care providers (e.g., nursing homes, rehabilitation centers, home health providers, and hospice providers as integrated service lines)

- increasing need for disease management product line development
- strong information technologies that bridge service lines

It is clear that hospice will continue to provide needed care to the terminally ill and that it will remain an important service to individuals and families, including those in managed care programs. It is equally clear that it will become more integrated with other modalities of care and that the need for hospice will increase for the foreseeable future. Hospice and end-of-life care can no longer be dealt with on a case-by-case basis, but must be fully integrated, just as case management and disease management are.

REFERENCES

1. Center to Improve Care of the Dying, http://www.gwu.edu/~cicd/. Accessed 2 November 1999.
2. L. Snyder, "Die Hard: End-of-Life Care in America," *Pennsylvania Medicine* (July 1996): 10–11.
3. J.R. Flexner, "The Hospice Movement in North America—Is It Coming of Age?" *Southern Medical Journal 72* (1979): 248–250.
4. National Hospice Organization, *Fact Sheet* (Arlington, VA: Author, 1996).
5. Hospice Association of America, *Hospice Facts and Statistics* (Washington, DC: Author, 1996).
6. M. Michal, *Managed Care: The Characteristics of a Successful Hospice,* http://www.rbvdnr.com. Accessed October 1997.
7. M. Kusinitz, *Johns Hopkins To Announce AIDS Capitated Care Program,* http://hopkins.med.jhu.edu/newsmedia/press/1997/january/1997.htm. Accessed January 1997.
8. Lewin-VHI, Inc., *Hospice Care: An Introduction and Review of the Evidence* (Arlington, VA: National Hospice Organization, 1994).
9. K. Beebe, *Hospice State Summary* (Washington, DC: Health Care Financing Administration, Bureau of Data Management and Strategy, Office of Health Care Information Systems, 1996).
10. National Center for Health Statistics, *An Overview of Home Health and Hospice Care Patients: Preliminary Data from the 1993 National Home and Hospice Care Survey; Advance Data from the Vital and Health Statistics of the Centers for Disease Control and Prevention,* publication no. 256 (Washington, DC: Author, 1994).
11. P. Lemkin, "Hospice: Can It Work within Managed Care?" *Caring* (August 1997): 22–28.
12. House Ways and Means Committee, *1996 Green Book* (Washington, DC: Author, 1997).
13. American Health Consultants, Tips for Deciding about a Hospice Ethics Committee, in *The 1996 Hospice Manager's Resource Bank* (New York: 1997).
14. M. Richards, *Medical Risk Management: A Preventive Legal Strategy* (Gaithersburg, MD: Aspen Publishers, Inc., 1982).

Chapter 16

Community-Based Case Management

Sharon E. Brodeur

TAKE THIS TO WORK

1. *Case management assessments* address home conditions, family support, psychosocial factors, and lifestyle issues, as well as presenting symptoms, medical history, lab, and other test results.
2. *Disease state management* programs are organized programs with the goal of managing a population with a specific diagnosis (e.g., diabetes, asthma, congestive heart failure).

   Disease state management programs include individual and/or group education, demand management, and regular contact initiated by either the patient or the program to monitor adherence to treatment recommendations and health status.
3. *Health risk assessments* are completed by the member or patient either "online" or on paper and allow for the identification of individuals who have complex or serious medical conditions.
4. *Multidisciplinary teams* involved in providing case management include the physician, registered nurse, and social worker.
5. *Referral* to case management may be based on diagnosis, high utilization patterns, health risk assessment results, or claims review.
6. *Risk stratification* is a method of classifying members who have been determined to need community case management, according to the expected intensity of case management needs and the anticipated time required to meet the treatment goals established by the case manager and the member. For example:
7. *Demand management programs* are usually nurse-operated call centers that rely on physician-developed and peer-reviewed computerized clinical algorithms to guide the discussion between the caller and the nurse.
   - Level One: Acute short-term
   - Level Two: Chronic short-term
   - Level Three: Acute long-term
   - Level Four: Chronic long-term

Until recently, the practice of medicine emphasized the management and cure of acute illness. Within the past decade, however, medicine has increasingly focused on the provision of care for patients with chronic illness. Recent reports have underscored the high social and economic costs of chronic diseases. More than 90 million Americans live with chronic illnesses, which account for 70 percent of all deaths in the United States and one third of the years of potential life lost before age 65. The medical care costs of people with chronic diseases account for more than 60 percent of the nation's medical care costs.[1] In 1990, chronic diseases accounted for $600 billion of the annual $1 trillion costs of medical care in the United States.[2] The United States cannot effectively address escalating health care costs without addressing the problem of chronic diseases.[3] Community case management can be an effective intervention to assist patients with chronic illness to maintain their health, avoid hospital admissions, and reduce emergency room utilization. In addition, community case management is used to assist patients after medical events, such as strokes, trauma, or surgery, who may not have been able to be discharged without assurance that care would be coordinated in the community.

INCENTIVES TO ESTABLISH COMMUNITY CASE MANAGEMENT

In order for a community case management program to demonstrate a return on investment for the parent organization, there must be an economic incentive to keep patients out of the hospital. Health care organizations that are paid a per diem rate or on an indemnity basis for each admission will not have a financial interest in preventing admission. However, integrated delivery systems or managed care organizations (MCOs) operating under a capitated contract will have an economic incentive to develop programs that reduce hospital utilization. Hospitals that have a high percentage of Medicare admissions or a high proportion of Medicaid or uninsured patients may also be able to document cost savings as a result of implementing a community case management program.

Documentation of both clinical and financial results demonstrates that patients enrolled in a community case management program are admitted to the hospital less frequently and use the emergency room less often than patients who are not enrolled in a program.[4] In addition, not only are clinical and financial results indicative of the success of these programs, but programs usually produce high satisfaction scores among participants. With the aging of the baby boom generation, the challenges of managing chronic illness will be key to containing health care costs in an increasingly cost-sensitive environment. Programs that manage patients outside of the hospital setting and increase the ability of individuals to effectively manage their own care are demonstrating the ability to control costs while at the same time they increase patient satisfaction.

DEFINITION

Although case management has been defined in many ways, for the purpose of this book, the Case Management Society of America (CMSA) definition will be used. CMSA defines case management as "a collaborative process which *assesses, plans, implements, coordinates, monitors, and evaluates* options and services to meet an individual's health needs through communication and available resources to promote quality cost-effective outcomes."[5] This definition identifies critical components of the case management process (italics) that will be explored in this chapter. In addition, mechanisms to identify patients who will benefit from community case management will be discussed. Figure 16–1 provides an overview of the case management process.

Case management is provided in a variety of health care settings, including acute inpatient, rehabilitation, home care, behavioral health, and the community. Each of these settings may define the role of the case manager differently, although the core components and activities remain the same. For example, the acute care case manager or care coordinator frequently monitors the use of resources on clinical pathways, whereas case managers in behavioral health programs may provide targeted counseling inter-

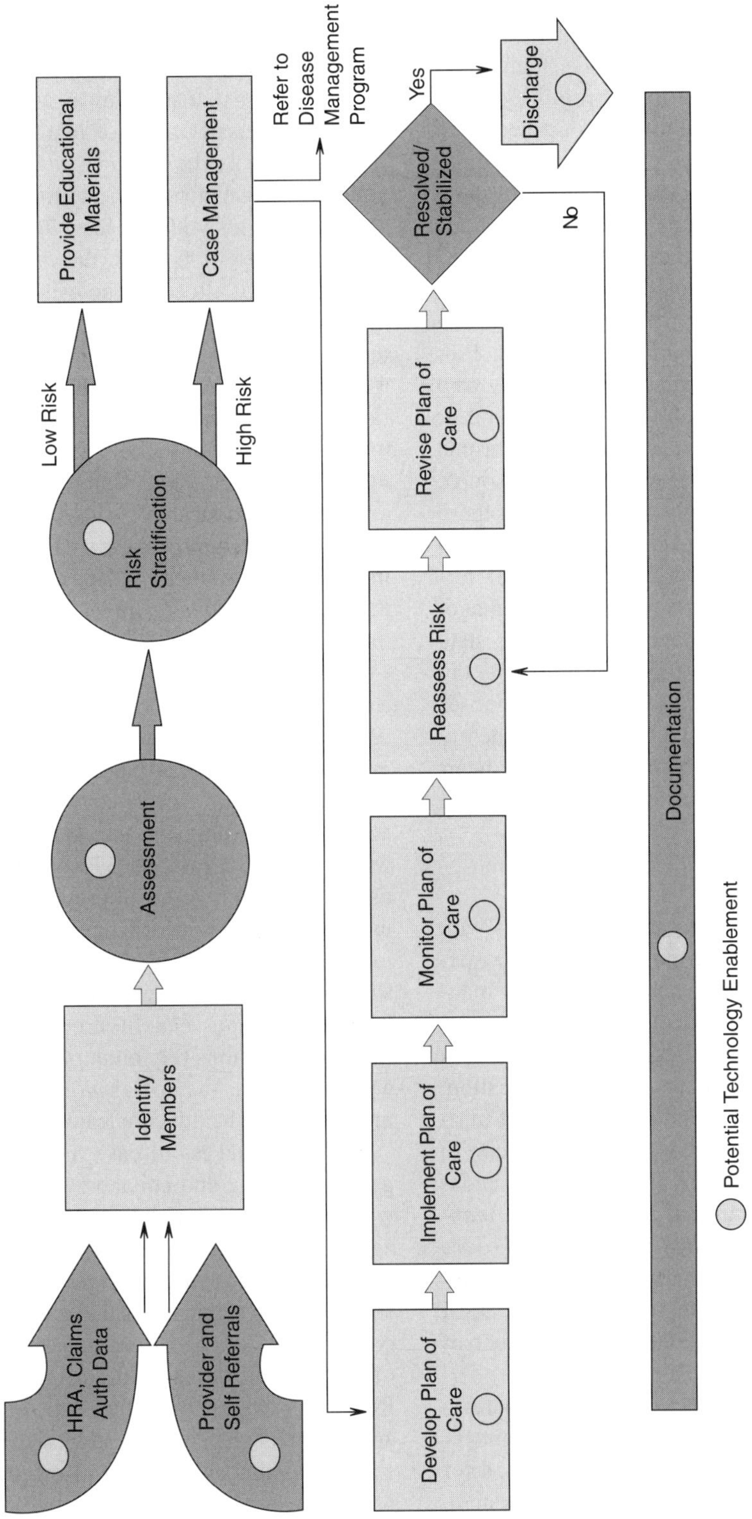

Figure 16–1 Community Case Management Process

vention. Acute care case managers focus on ensuring an appropriate length of stay in the hospital, whereas the community case manager's goals are oriented toward keeping the patient healthy and out of the hospital or emergency room. Both are concerned with monitoring quality, although the acute care setting may have a designated outcomes manager who assumes primary responsibility for these activities.

In most organized health care systems, approximately 20 percent of the members or subscribers use 80 percent of the resources. Predominant in this 20 percent are the elderly who are diagnosed with chronic illness and/or comorbidities. In addition, children with chronic illnesses, such as asthma, are also high resource users. MCOs increasingly are identifying these high resource users and developing interventions to reduce unnecessary utilization of services. In addition to community case management, MCOs are also developing disease state management (DSM) programs targeting the needs of high-cost population groups. Diagnoses for which DSM programs are most frequently developed include diabetes, congestive heart failure (CHF), and asthma.

DSM Programs

DSM programs are organized programs with the goal of managing a population with a specific diagnosis. Although community case management is one component of DSM programs, DSM programs also include organized interventions, such as individual and/or group education, demand management, and regular contact initiated either by the patient or by the program to monitor adherence to treatment recommendations and health status. *Community case management may be provided to patients who are not candidates for DSM programs.* Community case management is both a component of DSM programs and an intervention independent of such programs.

As the health care system has become increasingly fragmented and complex, case management has been identified as a useful method for helping patients navigate through the system. Case managers act as advocates and educate their patients about how to use the services offered by a variety of health care settings and providers. Some experts portray a variety of frameworks for classifying case management. The first of these is the *brokerage* framework, in which case managers advocate for their patients and link patients with services. In the *social entrepreneurship* framework, the case manager is responsible for allocating budget dollars to services and determining the most cost-effective alternative for providing needed services. Case managers in managed care and payer organizations use this model most frequently. A third model focuses on the involvement of a *multidisciplinary team*, which arranges, delivers, and monitors care provided for specific clients.[6,7] Current approaches to case management incorporate all of these frameworks and identify the case manager as someone who can fulfill multiple roles.

The multidisciplinary team, including the physician, registered nurse, and social worker, has advantages because it ensures the input of complementary disciplines in planning and delivering care. Patients who receive community case management are coping with the challenges of living with a chronic disease. Social workers add expertise to the team in terms of providing family and individual support, identifying underlying behavioral issues, providing crisis intervention and short-term counseling, and arranging for eligibility within various benefit structures. Although most organizations rely on nurses to function as case managers, the social worker is a critical member of the health care team.

Key to a successful case management program are strong and collaborative relationships with physicians. The best community case management programs encourage and facilitate partnerships between case managers and physicians so that the physician trusts the case manager and comes to rely on the case manager's knowledge of the patient's condition and medical needs. Regular communication between the physician and case manager can both address the time constraints of the physician and ensure that the patient's care is well coordinated. Some case management programs place case managers in the office of physicians who have large numbers of patients in the case management program. Other programs rely on regular case conferences and phone contact between the physician and case manager. Strong relationships between nurses in the physician's office and community case managers will also achieve the goal of maintaining close contact regarding the patient's needs. An office nurse and the case manager together can resolve a patient's pressing issues without even involving the physician. Physicians who have learned to use a case manager effectively will find that it optimizes their time and their office staff's time because the patient is not forced to depend on the physician's office to solve all problems in coordinating care.

COMPONENTS OF COMMUNITY CASE MANAGEMENT

Identification and Referral to Community Case Management

Patients who may benefit from community case management are identified by diagnosis, frequent hospital admission or readmission, high utilization of the emergency room, or through health risk assessment (HRA) data. MCOs use claims data to identify members with a pattern of high utilization and with diagnoses that may trigger a referral. However, because this identification is retrospective, health care systems also rely on referrals from case managers based in the emergency room, hospital-based case managers, and physicians.

Diagnosis as Trigger

In designing a community case management program, specific diagnoses are identified as triggers for referral to case management. The trigger diagnoses are dependent on the demographics and high-volume, high-cost diagnoses of the enrolled population. For example, an MCO that has enrolled a young commercially insured population might not refer pregnant women for case management. However, most Medicaid programs enroll all pregnant women in case management and specifically target women who have high-risk pregnancies. The diagnoses listed in Exhibit 16–1 may trigger a referral to community case management.

Not all persons diagnosed with the above illnesses will require ongoing community case management. Some patients will benefit from short-term case management immediately after discharge from the hospital, but will have sufficient resources and ability to manage their own health care needs without a case manager. Other individuals may require extensive intervention until they are stabilized, and still others may benefit from enrollment in a DSM program. The decision is affected by both the nature of the patient's condition and the patient's ability to adhere to self-care programs.

Utilization as Trigger

The second category of triggers for referral to community case management is based on utilization. This information is generally garnered from claims data. Therefore, early referral is dependent on the organization's ability to generate reliable data that are tracked and trended so that utilization patterns are identified. By the time these data are analyzed, the organization may have already generated high costs related to overutilization. Therefore, claims data are usually used in conjunction with other referral mechanisms. Exhibit 16–2 lists utilization data that trigger referral to community case management.

Again, not all patients who are triggered for referral to community case management will require services over an extended period of time. The referral to case management will result in assessment by a case manager who will determine the need for ongoing services.

HRA is Trigger

The third mechanism for triggering a referral to case management is an HRA. Health care systems may design their own HRAs, purchase an HRA tool, or contract with a commercial vendor to administer surveys. Most large payers now include HRAs on their Web sites for members to complete. These HRAs may be general in nature and provide an overview of health status or may

Exhibit 16–1 Diagnoses that Trigger Referral to Community Case Management

Acquired immune deficiency syndrome (AIDS)
Alzheimer's disease
Amputations
Amyotrophic lateral sclerosis (ALS)
Asthma
Birth trauma
Bleeding disorders
Brain tumor
Cardiovascular accident (CVA)/stroke
Cerebral hemorrhage
Cerebral palsy
Chronic obstructive pulmonary disease (COPD)
Chronic renal failure
Congestive heart failure (CHF)
Cystic fibrosis
Diabetes (newly diagnosed, poorly controlled, gestational)
Failure to thrive
Guillain-Barré
Head injury/traumatic brain injury
High-risk pregnancy
Hip fracture
Huntington's disease
Leukemia
Liver disease
Metastatic cancer
Multiparity (twins, triplets)
Multiple congenital anomalies
Multiple sclerosis
Multiple trauma
Muscular dystrophy
Osteomyelitis
Parkinson's disease
Premature infant
Pyelonephritis
Respiratory dependency—any cause
Scleroderma
Sickle cell disease
Spina bifida
Spinal cord injury
Stab/gunshot wound
Transplants (organ, bone marrow)
Tuberculosis

Exhibit 16–2 Utilization Data that Trigger Referral to Community Case Management

High claim—greater than $20,000
Multiple medications—5 or more in a 3-month period
Multiple outpatient surgeries—3 or more in 1 year
Multiple providers
Multiple skilled nursing facility admissions—2 or more in 1 year
Multiple ED visits—3 or more in 6 months
Multiple hospitalizations—2 or more in 1 year
Hospice care
Home health care—duration more than 2 weeks

be targeted to assessing risk in members with specific diagnoses, such as heart failure. HRAs are completed by the patient and are only as accurate as the patient's information and perceptions of his or her health status.

The Health Care Financing Administration (HCFA) requires MCOs to conduct an HRA on new Medicare members within 90 days of the effective date of the member's enrollment. The MCO is free to choose the form of the initial assessment. However, regardless of the form, the assessment must be of sufficient adequacy to allow for the identification of those beneficiaries who have complex or serious medical conditions. In addition, most state Medicaid agencies that enroll recipients in managed care plans contract with an enrollment broker to conduct the enrollment process and administer a short HRA prior to enrolling the member in a plan. The results of the survey are provided to the managed care plan when the Medicaid member is enrolled.

HRAs are scored and the resulting profile is used to refer patients into DSM programs, ensure the provision of health education materials, and determine which patients would benefit from contact by a case manager. HRA data are used to identify diagnostic triggers or risk factors indicating a need for community case management. For example, the Medicaid HRA asks the member if she is pregnant, determines prior history related to pregnancy, and determines whether the member has any symptoms of a problem pregnancy. This information is transmitted to the MCO that can then enroll the member in a prenatal case management program. Similarly, HRAs that screen for cardiac risk factors can be used to trigger a referral to a case manager for assessment and eventual enrollment in a DSM program.

Assessment and Risk Stratification

Assessment

When a member is referred to case management, an assessment is conducted to determine if the patient needs services and what level of services is required. Assessments are disease specific and address home conditions, family support, psychosocial factors, and lifestyle issues, as well as presenting symptoms, medical history, and lab and other test results. Assessments provide the case manager with sufficient information to determine the patient's current health, related history, and family and psychosocial factors, and identify which factors are enablers or barriers to maintaining health and adherence with treatment recommendations. Most assessments are initially administered over the phone, although in some cases, a home visit will provide important information in assessing a patient's needs. The home visit is particularly useful if a patient is diagnosed with an illness that may be exacerbated by home conditions, such as asthma, or if the member does not respond well to telephone intervention. Medicaid members, for example, may benefit from a home visit to determine whether there are sufficient resources to adhere to the treatment recommendations and to begin to establish a trusting relationship between the case manager and the member.

The ultimate goal of the assessment is to determine the patient's current medical status, begin to identify and prioritize needs, and stratify the patient's health risk. For example, a patient with asthma who does not know how to use a peak flow meter, lives with two cats despite allergic triggers for asthma attacks, and admits to being non-adherent with medication would be referred for case management and, possibly, enrollment in an asthma DSM program. On the other hand, a member with well-controlled asthma who is adherent with treatment recommendations and well educated regarding appropriate interventions may require less support following the assessment.

Risk Stratification

Risk stratification is a method of classifying members who have been determined to need community case management according to the expected intensity of case management needs and the anticipated time required to meet the treatment goals established by the case manager and the member. A formal risk stratification also provides case management supervisors with data on intensity of service needs in staff caseloads, thus assisting with caseload leveling. One method of stratifying patients by risk is outlined below:

- *Level One: Acute, short-term.* Members with an acute condition that is anticipated to be short-term in nature.
  - *Example:* Member with a postoperative wound infection with an expected two to three weeks of wound care and skilled nursing; expected to meet criteria for discharge within approximately four weeks.
- *Level Two: Chronic short-term.* Members with a chronic condition that is anticipated to be short-term in nature.
  - *Example:* Member with Crohn's disease who recently underwent a colostomy and may need colostomy teaching and care; expected to meet criteria for discharge within 60 days. (Given the patient's chronic condition, the case may be reopened in case management based on a reassessment of member needs.)
- *Level Three: Acute, long-term.* Members with an acute event that may have longer term sequelae.
  - *Example:* Member with an acute stroke with left-sided hemiparesis and dysphasia; will require rehabilitation and multiple therapies for an extended period of time.

- *Level Four: Chronic, long-term.* Members with a chronic condition with ongoing longer term needs.
  - *Example:* Member who is post-transplant and will require care on an ongoing basis; may be stabilized and meet criteria for discharge from case management but may be periodically reopened as needed.

Risk stratification is used in assigning cases to case managers. A case manager's caseload may range from 20 to 40–45 depending on the severity of the patients' risk and how frequently contact between the case manager and the patient is required. Case managers may be generalists or specialists, although excellent assessment skills are important for a case manager, and most programs strive to hire community case managers who have significant clinical expertise with the patient population with which they are working.

Patients receiving case management are reassessed on a regular basis (e.g., every 30 days) to determine if the patients' needs and condition have changed. Key to maximizing the financial benefits of community case management is the ability to ensure that cases are closed and patients are discharged when it is clinically necessary. Cases that are kept open for longer than 60 days because the patient is determined to be in need of support should be evaluated to ascertain if the case manager is really providing essential services. Even if cases are closed, they can be reopened if the patient's needs change, and patients should be encouraged to contact the case manager if they have a need for additional services. Patients who have established a positive relationship with a case manager will usually take the initiative to make a telephone call if their needs change.

PROVIDING CASE MANAGEMENT

Developing and Implementing the Plan of Care

As in any other health care setting, the plan of care provides a guide for documenting the patient's needs, identifying goals and objectives, documenting planned interventions, and monitoring progress. The case manager will identify the patient's needs based on the nursing assessment and physician's orders and, in developing the plan of care, will incorporate all of the patient's health care needs: medical, psychosocial, financial, and supportive. The value of relying on a multidisciplinary team is apparent in developing the patient's plan of care because the case manager, the social worker, and the physician all play a key role in identifying needs and developing necessary interventions.

The case management team will implement portions of the patient's plan of care and coordinate services implemented by others. For example, the physician and/or case manager may identify a need for a transplant patient to receive health teaching regarding the importance of diet, daily weights, and adherence to antirejection medication. The case manager will provide the teaching, coordinate a referral to a nutritionist if needed, and then monitor the patient to ensure that he or she is following the physician's medical advice. The social worker's role includes the provision of individual and family counseling to assist the patient and family to address the many challenges of coping with chronic illness. The case manager will also coordinate services such as home care, durable medical equipment, rehabilitation, financial assistance, and community support services.

The case manager must be prepared to assume multiple roles in coordinating care for the patient. For example, a patient who needs outpatient rehabilitation but has no means of transportation to the rehabilitation facility will need to have transportation arranged. At the same time, it is important that the case manager avoid encouraging overdependency on the program. To this end, if the patient is able to assume responsibility for arranging his or her own transportation, the case manager's role is to monitor that these arrangements are made as necessary. The ability to know when to assume responsibility for arranging care and when to encourage the patient to arrange his or her own care is one of the unique and important personal characteristics that community case managers develop. The relationship between the patient and the case manager is unique in that the case manager has to be both a care provider and a coach; he or she may provide support for the patient, yet, at the same time, challenge the patient's tendencies to become too dependent.

Although it may be easier to assume responsibility for providing and arranging care, the case manager must always keep in mind that the ultimate goal is to enable the patient to care for his or her own needs and thus encourage independence. At the same time, the case manager may have patients within the caseload who are a challenge in terms of adherence to care and who may seek to manipulate the system. The experienced case manager will learn to assess not only the patient's physical condition, but also the patient's personal characteristics for coping with illness, and coordinate care accordingly.

Monitoring and Evaluating Services

Once a plan of care is established and implemented, the case manager's role is to monitor the patient's status and services to ensure that services are being delivered as needed and to reassess the patient's condition if it is stabilized or as new needs develop. Monitoring the patient's care can frequently be accomplished through telephonic case management with either the case manager or the patient initiating a phone call to determine the patient's current health status, answer questions, and evaluate service provision. Telephonic case management is more efficient than face-to-face case management because the case manager can work from one central location and the patient does not have to leave his or her home. The case manager may establish a regular time to check with patients each week or more often if necessary. Case management computerized systems include prompts so the case manager will know when a patient phone call is due, as well as provide a notes screen to track the patient's progress on his or her plan of care.

Monitoring the plan of care incorporates the oversight of the provision of medical, psychosocial, financial, and community services, as well as monitoring the patient's current physical status and adherence to his or her treatment plan. Monitoring is directly related to ascertaining the patient's progress in achieving identified goals and objectives on the plan of care. Just as hospital-based case managers start planning transition to the next level of care immediately on admission, the community case manager begins the implementation of the patient's plan of care "with the end in sight." That is, the case management goals should enable the case manager to determine when the patient is ready for discharge from the program.

Discharge

As the patient's needs stabilize and he or she demonstrates the ability to coordinate and manage his or her own care, the case manager's contacts will become more infrequent. This is an indicator that the patient is becoming ready for discharge from the program. When it is clear that the goals and objectives of the plan of care have been achieved, the case manager should prepare the patient for discharge. Further, if some of the goals and objectives have not been met, and it is clear that they are never going to be met, the patient may also need to be discharged from the program. Prior to discharging the patient from the program, the case manager will contact the physician to discuss the patient's discharge. If the physician disagrees with the discharge, the plan of care should be modified to incorporate revised goals and objectives. If the physician signs off on the discharge, the case manager will contact the patient to accomplish the discharge.

On occasion, some community case managers may find it difficult to discharge patients in a timely manner. However, in order to maximize case management resources, and to foster the patient's independence, it is important that any barriers to discharge, including the case manager's personal resistance, be addressed in a supervisory relationship. Case management policies should clarify when discharge from case management will occur and relate discharge to the patient's achievement of the goals identified in the plan of care or a determination being made that some goals will not be achieved. The provision of ongoing support is not usually a cost-effective role for case managers to assume. That is, it would be cost prohibitive for case management to become case "maintenance." Patients who are managing chronic illness may be given the case manager's business card and encouraged to contact the case manager if they develop new needs or encounter difficulty with services being provided.

Demand management programs can address a patient's ongoing needs for a resource to ensure that health-related questions are answered. In most cases, discharge can be achieved within 60 days. The exception to this is when a patient is coping with a terminal chronic illness that is not well controlled and may become acute at any time, such as patients diagnosed with acquired immune deficiency syndrome (AIDS) who are not well controlled with medication. It is important that the community case managers providing services for this type of population learn to hand the case off to other case managers. For example, if the patient is cared for in a hospice program, the hospice nurse will assume responsibility for coordinating all of the patient's care and the community case manager can assume a secondary role of backing up the hospice nurse. Again, the patient can be readmitted to community case management if there is a need for resuming service.

Community case managers are uniquely positioned to effectively evaluate the provision of services to their patients. Integral to arranging services is the acquisition of information regarding the accessibility and effectiveness of medical and community services used by their patients. Data obtained from community case managers regarding the lack of services in the community and barriers to accessing services can be extremely useful both informally and formally. Administrative contacts with entities that present barriers to service can result in changing systems of care in the community. Data regarding the lack of services can be used by community planning agencies and integrated health care delivery systems that are concerned with addressing gaps in services. Case managers should be encouraged to communicate problems in arranging services for their clients in order to clarify which problems are systemic in nature and may be receptive to change.

PRIMARY DISEASE AND DEMAND MANAGEMENT INITIATIVES

DSM programs have proliferated over the past five years with vendors across the country offering programs for chronic diseases such as CHF, asthma, chronic obstructive pulmonary disease, AIDS, and depression. Managed care companies and integrated delivery systems may choose to purchase DSM programs from a vendor or to develop and operate their own programs. Demand management programs help patients to manage their illness and are a critical component of disease management programs. "Over the past 10 years, demand management has emerged as an effective strategy for managing the delivery of health care. For many MCOs, the centerpiece of demand management initiatives is the nurse call center."[8(p.22)] Demand management programs usually consist of nurse-operated call centers that rely on physician-developed and peer-reviewed computerized clinical algorithms to guide the discussion between the caller and the nurse. Demand management programs provide a possible alternative for patients who may otherwise go to the emergency room or contact the physician after hours.

Nurses who staff call centers answer questions patients have concerning their health care, provide health education, and direct patients to the most appropriate level of care. As the nurse and caller work through the algorithm together, the nurse documents the conversation in the computer system. Ultimately, the patient determines what route of treatment will be chosen. Most call centers operate either 24 hours a day 7 days a week or during peak calling hours, including nights and weekends. The goal of demand management programs is to help patients to manage their symptoms and to differentiate between medical concerns that require emergency room care and those that can be managed with home remedies or a next-day appointment with the physician. Nurses in demand management programs operate in close collaboration with physicians and, after a telephone call with a patient, communicate the nature and outcome of the call to the caller's primary care physician. Some nurse call centers also schedule appointments for patients who need to be seen by their physician.

Demand management programs frequently include a health education library that enables callers to obtain additional information about specific health concerns by listening to tapes in the library. Internet technology also enables patients with computers to access health information over a Web site. Web sites may include e-mail provisions so that the patient can communicate with a nurse via e-mail. Web sites may combine an HRA for specific diagnoses with educational materials related to the diagnosis.

Telephone triage systems depend heavily on the utilization of appropriate technology. A telephone system that routes callers to available staff in the order of their call and a computerized system for reviewing patient, payer, and demographic information as well as medical history are important components in a demand management program. Call center technology also enables documentation of a caller's intent when first contacting the advice line, and at the end of the call, thereby enabling the program to collect data on emergency department visits that have been averted. Links between primary care physician offices and the call center enable computerized transmission of the nature and outcome of calls to the physician's office.

"Payers and consulting organizations report average annual savings of $50 to $240 per member using telephone triage."[9(p.49)] However, in addition to achieving cost savings through telephone triage programs, published patient satisfaction surveys indicate a high degree of satisfaction with demand management programs. Demand management programs complement community case management programs and continue to be a source of advice and information for a patient who is no longer in need of case management.

REFERENCES

1. The Robert Wood Johnson Foundation, *Annual Report 1994; Health, United States* (Washington, DC: U.S. Superintendent of Documents, U.S. Government Printing Office, 1994).
2. C. Hoffman et al., "Persons with Chronic Conditions: Their Prevalence and Costs," *Journal of the American Medical Association 276*, no. 18 (1996): 1473–1479.
3. Centers for Disease Control and Prevention Web Page. http://www.cdc.gov. Accessed 21 July 2000.
4. D. Grandinetti, "New Groups Are Profiting from Case Management," *Medical Economics 75*, no. 15 (1998): 69–83.
5. M. Newell, *Using Nursing Case Management to Improve Health Outcomes* (Gaithersburg, MD: Aspen Publishers, Inc., 1996).
6. D. Lee et al., "Case Management: A Review of the Definitions and Practices," *Journal of Advanced Nursing 27,* no. 5 (1998): 933–939.
7. V. Beardshaw and D. Towell, "Assessment and Case Management: Implications for the Implementation of 'Caring for People,'" *King's Fund Briefing Paper 10* (1990).
8. W.D. Lynch and J.H. Otis, "Stop! In the Name of the Bottom Line," *Managed Healthcare 10,* no. 3 (2000): 22–28.
9. M. Sabin, "Telephone Triage Improves Demand Management Effectiveness," *Healthcare Financial Management 52,* no. 8 (1998): 49–51.

SUGGESTED READINGS

D. Albertson, "Getting the Big Picture on Disease Management," *Employee Benefit News 13,* no. 8 (July 1, 1999).

D.W. Bulger and A.B. Smith, "Message Tailoring, An Essential Component for Disease Management," *Disease Management Health Outcomes 5,* no. 3 (March 5, 1999): 127–134.

E.L. Cohen, *The Outcomes Mandate: Case Management in Health Care Today* (St. Louis: Mosby, 1999).

S.A. Musich et al., "Costs and Benefits of Prevention and Disease Management," *Disease Management Health Outcomes 5,* no. 3 (March 5, 1999): 153–166.

M. Newell, *Using Nursing Case Management to Improve Health Outcomes* (Gaithersburg, MD: Aspen Publishers, Inc., 1996).

S.K. Powell, *Case Management: A Practical Guide to Success in Managed Care* (Philadelphia: Lippincott Williams & Wilkins, 2000).

CHAPTER 17

Communications between the Hospital-Based Case Manager and the Payer

Barbara Gray and Kathryn W. Bradshaw

TAKE THIS TO WORK

1. The effective case manager must have *exceptional* communication skills.
2. Consider working with a mentor to further develop your communication skills.
3. Understand the level of information required and be prepared to be responsive.
   - Report information in a format preferred by the payer.
   - Be proactive in communicating relevant information.
4. When negotiating, understand the hospital's reimbursement structure and the payer's incentives and offer win/win alternatives based on cost benefit analyses.
5. Be persistent, be positive, be collaborative—alternatives developed in collaboration with the payer are often superior and increase buy-in to the proposed solution.
6. Understand what makes your payer contact successful and the information payers need to do their jobs efficiently and effectively.

Why does the subject of communications between the hospital case manager and the payer warrant its own chapter? There are at least three reasons.

1. To perform his or her job successfully, the hospital case manager must work effectively with his or her payer contacts.
2. Perhaps the single most important success factor in working effectively with the payer is exceptional communication skills.
3. Being an exceptional communicator is not easy.

The perceptive hospital case manager views the payer as his or her client—in effect, the hospital case manager works for the payer, not the other way around. The most successful case managers understand that the payer is not only a client, but is also a relationship. And not just any relationship, at that. The hospital case manager–payer relationship could be viewed as a type of arranged marriage, where neither party has the benefit of choosing his or her work partner and both have the task of "making it work." Sometimes their goals are consistent, sometimes not, and often the other party is poorly understood. The successful hospital case manager will understand this dynamic and realize that the onus is on him or her to bridge these gaps and derive successful outcomes from the relationship.

Consider that the number one complaint in marriages is ineffective communication. It stands, then, that the key to success in making the arranged hospital–payer relationship work is effective communication. The successful hospital case manager draws on the same communication skills that are successful for him or her in the clinical settings (i.e., when dealing with patients, their families, physicians, and other clinicians and hospital staff). To further develop his or her communication skills, the case manager may wish to identify a mentor within the case management department or take advantage of the abundance of communication resources that offer books, seminars, and personal coaching on the art of successful communication. For the purpose of this chapter, we offer three observations that are universal and particularly applicable to the case manager.

1. The best communicators care about people.
2. The best communicators are proactive.
3. The best communicators initially endeavor to learn about the other party's needs.

The means by which the hospital case manager communicates with his or her payer counterpart can be an important asset—or detriment—to the working relationship. There are several methods by which the case manager will be required to communicate with payers (e.g., verbal, fax, electronic). Certainly, it's important that the information is sent effectively no matter what the medium. At the same time, understanding the pros and cons of various contact methods will assist the hospital case manager in capitalizing on the advantages and working through the disadvantages, thereby furthering the working relationship with his or her payer counterpart. Table 17–1 summarizes the advantages and disadvantages of the various payer contact methods. *Approach is everything.*

WHAT INFORMATION TO COMMUNICATE

Most payers request the same essential information relative to patient demographics, initial "baseline" reviews, and concurrent or ongoing reviews. Some payers request more detailed clinical information relative to the patient's admission. In some instances, payers may even ask for information that may not be directly related to determining medical necessity for the patient's admitting diagnosis, treatment, or continued stay, such as glycohemoglobin on a diabetic admitted for bypass surgery. *The key: Understand your payer contact and the level of information that may be requested, and be prepared to be responsive to the requests.*

Demographic Information

Basic demographic information is required by all payers. Typically, this information includes the patient's

- full name
- current address
- date of birth
- Social Security and/or insurance numbers
- phone numbers
- emergency contact

Initial Reviews

Many payers require a complete review of systems to establish the patient's baseline information. Some payers request only information that is directly applicable to the admitting diagnosis/procedure. Standard initial review information typically includes the following:

- comprehensive patient history, including significant comorbidities
- diagnosis, reason for admission, and/or events leading to admission

Table 17–1 Payer Contact Methods Advantages and Disadvantages

Method	*Advantages*	*Disadvantages*	*Helpful Hints*
Phone			
Case manager direct contact	Personal relationship and trust development	Case manager time spent "holding" for payer	Use updated payer grids to ensure that you have correct insurance information and phone numbers
	Concurrent exchange of information	Payer contact staff member may not have authority to certify (i.e., may require a callback)	Report accurate and timely information
	Firsthand information is communicated w/decreased risk of inaccuracies	Must have ready access to chart in order to communicate additional information	Work collaboratively with payer and involve payer in the patient's progression of care; communicate barriers to discharge as soon as possible
	Minimizes callbacks to payer to communicate additional requested information	Reduces time case manager can spend facilitating care and proactively/concurrently managing resource utilization	Know your payer contact staff and their • criteria used for approval • limitations w/ certification process • time constraints
	Receive number of days certified or denial at time of call		Schedule specific times for follow-up if necessary and be on time
	Concurrent management of potential denial		Clearly document with whom you spoke and the date and time of the call
			Know your patient's full benefit package
			Be prepared to discuss alternative solutions and complete a cost benefit analysis for each solution

continues

Table 17–1 continued

Method	*Advantages*	*Disadvantages*	*Helpful Hints*
Centralized payer contact	Personal relationship and trust development	Lack of firsthand communication of information w/ increased risk of inaccuracies	When using a centralized payer contact office, case management staff must provide all utilization review information
	Concurrent exchange of information	May increase callbacks to payer to communicate additional requested information	Batch calls whenever possible; consider incorporating into contract negotiations
	Receive number of days certified or denial at time of call	Concurrent management of potential denial will likely require discussions between payer staff and case manager in charge of the case, warranting additional calls	Establish internal pager system for provider-based payer contact staff to alert case manager of denial
	Allows case manager to spend more time with patient, enabling proactive management of resources and care facilitation	Lack of immediate accessibility to chart to provide additional information requested	Payer contact staff must be well versed in medical terminology and should have utilization review or medical records experience
	Payers may be more willing to batch calls, saving time for all parties involved		To be maximally successful, program must be fully developed, well organized, and consistently followed (e.g., detailed policies, procedures, and protocols that specify responsibilities, accountabilities, and time frames)

continues

Table 17–1 continued

Method	*Advantages*	*Disadvantages*	*Helpful Hints*
Fax			
	Minimizes case manager time spent "holding" on phone	Lack of access to fax machines (e.g., may not be located in patient care areas, direct patient care issues may take precedence)	Recommended only if payer is willing to use established criteria as foundation for approval (i.e., InterQual or payer developed)
	Information may be more focused and/or better organized, as case manager has the opportunity to review and edit report before sending	May require rework if need to document in multiple places	Consider reviewing documentation policies, procedures, forms, etc., to reduce need for redocumentation and ensure that payer requirements relative to fax formats are met
		Lack of concurrent approval (i.e., requires callback from payer)	
		Method not as conducive to building relationships, understanding unique payer criteria, and being current on any changes in policies, procedures, etc.	Need to define the time frames/deadlines that must be met by both the provider and the payer for fax communication to be effective
		May require additional administrative time relative to filing fax sheets, confirmation sheets, following up to ensure fax received, etc.	Evaluate this communication method relative to internal costs/benefits and individual payer acceptability/receptivity
		Some payers prefer real-time, one-on-one discussions	
Electronic			
	Eliminates need for duplicative communication and documentation (e.g., concurrent reviews can "build" on baseline information readily available)	Systems still under development, and will take time for "bugs" to be worked out, both technically and operationally	Perform test cases prior to "go live" of electronic submission and ensure risk management department has approved process

- prior tests/procedures and results
- level of care and substantiating treatment
- initial diagnostic workup ordered (labs, tests, and procedures)
- admission vital signs (and baseline if available)
- admission lab and diagnostic test results
- medications (including type, dose, and route) and intravenous fluids—especially those requiring intensive care monitoring
- expected discharge date
- treatment plan
- scheduled date and time of tests/diagnostics/procedures
- consults ordered (some payers will also request the time ordered)
- special monitoring devices (i.e., telemetry, intracranial pressure, pulmonary capillary wedge pressure)

Continued Stay Reviews

Payers vary in the type and level of information they require as part of a continued stay review. In general, most payers will request only that information that is directly pertinent to evaluating medical necessity for the admitting diagnosis/procedure. Some payers are beginning to focus less on medical necessity and more on care coordination; for these payers, discharge planning and treatment plan information will be more pertinent than clinical information that demonstrates medical necessity.

To the extent possible, case managers should report information in a format that is preferred by the payer. In some instances, payers may provide the hospital case manager with a preferred format, or be willing to develop a communication tool together with the hospital. If developing a continued stay review form, keep it as simple and user friendly as possible. A sample payer review form is presented in Exhibit 17–1.

One of the responsibilities of the hospital case manager is to prevent denials for medical necessity. To be successful, the hospital case manager must be as proactive as possible in communicating relevant information. For uncomplicated cases, it is generally advantageous to communicate the anticipated date of discharge. This allows the hospital case manager to identify potential payer issues relative to length of stay and/or medical necessity, and to discuss those issues early on in the patient stay. Similarly, if the hospital case manager anticipates delays in discharge because of comorbidities, complications, or other factors, communicating this as soon as possible maximizes the time to problem solve and develop alternative solutions that may prevent denials.

NEGOTIATIONS

At some point in his or her tenure, the hospital case manager will need to negotiate with the payer contact on one or more issues related to continued stay, medical necessity, discharge planning, or benefits exception. To be successful in negotiating the preferred outcome (e.g., approval for continued hospital stay, extension of benefits, etc.), the hospital case manager must be well prepared prior to the discussion. The most successful case managers

- Understand how the hospital is being reimbursed (e.g., case rate, per diem, percent of charges).
- Understand the payer's financial incentives.
- Understand how the patient's benefit package may impact the payer's decisions.
- Come with alternatives (two or more is far better than one).
- Prepare cost benefit analyses, using credible data.
- Offer alternatives that are win/win—for the patient, the payer, and the hospital.

The successful negotiator solicits input from the decision makers. For the hospital case manager, this means getting the payer's involvement in developing creative solutions to difficult or complex patient situations. Alternatives developed in collaboration with the payer are often superior to those developed independently by either party, and the payer's investment in the process increases buy-in to the proposed solution.

Exhibit 17–1 Sample Insurance Review Form

PRIMARY INSURANCE:________________________

SECONDARY INS:________________________

CM, RN INITIALS:________________________

ADMISSION/REVIEW DATE:____________________

Addressograph

CASE MANAGEMENT NOTES

Reason for Admission ________________ Surgery: Date:________	Failed Outpatient Treatment Yes No If Yes Explain: Pertinent Medical History:
Clinical Findings:	Treatments: Medications: Abx Heparin Insulin Analgesics Thrombolytics Chemo w/IV Antiemetics IVF____________________ Other Medications:
Imaging/ECG:	Treatment Plan:
Laboratory:	Expected Discharge Date: ____/____/____

The successful negotiator also understands that, if at first you don't succeed, *don't give up.* In the event that the two parties cannot come to consensus initially, the seasoned hospital case manager works to better understand the decision maker's process and incentives, and offers one or more alternatives that provide a better win–win. This is when a respectful, trusting relationship will be exceptionally important to the tone and productivity of the hospital–payer discussions. Finally, the successful hospital case manager goes into discussions with a positive attitude—cooperation often begets cooperation.

MAKING IT WORK

The successful hospital case manager understands his or her payer contacts, the world they live in, and their pressures and constraints. They

Exhibit 17–2 Top Ten Ways To Please Your Payer

1. **Be on point.** Provide pertinent, concise information that clearly communicates medical necessity.
2. **Provide the information they want.** Minimize the need for the payer to request additional information.
3. **Act as a care coordinator, not a clerk.** Use your clinical decision-making skills and judgment to proactively develop and coordinate a discharge plan for your patient.
4. **Be informed.** Know your patient's medical condition prior to contacting the payer.
5. **Be available.** Ensure that your case management staff are readily accessible for callbacks from the payer.
6. **Be collaborative.** Consistently work with payers to develop mutually beneficial solutions, involving/seeking input from the payer regarding discharge planning for complex cases (consider that the payer may have managed similar issues and provide innovative solutions that support the patient and save you time).
7. **Be timely.** Demonstrate respect for the payer's time and workload through timely communications.
8. **Be trustworthy.** Be forthright with your payer regarding your patient's medical condition, recognizing that although you may have different perspectives, you share the same goal: providing efficacious, high-quality care for your patient.
9. **Don't shoot the messenger.** Understand the boundaries of authority with whom you are working and appreciate the parameters within which the payer contact works.
10. **Treat the payer contact as an individual.** Recognize that payer staff are human, too.

understand what makes their payer contacts successful and the information they need to do their jobs efficiently and effectively. They treat their payer contacts as people, not barriers. In an effort to better understand these issues, we interviewed several leading national payers regarding how hospital case managers can help make the hospital–payer relationship work. The top 10 suggestions from payer representatives are summarized in Exhibit 17–2.

SUGGESTED READINGS

B.A. Glanz, *The Creative Communicator* (New York: McGraw-Hill, 1993).

D. Walton, *Are You Communicating?* (New York: McGraw-Hill, 1989).

PART V

Information Technology Support for Case Managers

CHAPTER 18

The Case Manager's Guide to Hospital Cost Accounting Systems

Timothy J. Rowell and David W. Plocher

TAKE THIS TO WORK

1. For your role in efficient patient care, your hospital's charges are far less important than costs.
2. Cost definitions may vary slightly from one chief financial officer to the next, but generally, your largest impact on various efficiencies will be on direct variable cost (DVC), through general length of stay and intensive care unit length of stay reduction.
3. Secondary impact will be obtained by attention to intubation duration, parenteral therapy duration, supplies, and drugs.

Key measures of the success for a case management program include the clinical, emotional, and financial results for the patient population it manages. With the increasing emphasis on financial measures, it has become essential that case managers be comfortable with financial concepts, processes, and systems. To assist managers in improving financial results, hospitals have invested in sophisticated cost accounting systems to measure, track, and control the elements of care at multiple levels and from multiple viewpoints. These systems are designed to assist clinical managers in

- setting budgets and performance goals
- measuring progress against these budgets and goals
- assessing the impact of alternative treatments or care decisions
- identifying occurrences and causes of high-cost cases
- validating the results achieved through the implementation of new plans of care
- communicating with finance and administration in a common, measurable way about these results

However, if the cost accounting system is not introduced with sufficient training and explanation, the cost accounting system outputs can seem like more of a barrier than the enabling tool they are intended to be.

This chapter will provide some general cost accounting concepts and background, relate these concepts to the case manager, discuss typical outputs of a cost accounting system, and share some words of advice on successfully using these concepts and tools.

COST ACCOUNTING CONCEPTS AND WHAT A CASE MANAGER SHOULD KNOW ABOUT THEM

Cost accounting concepts have been used successfully in industry by manufacturing organizations to understand the cost in producing their products, to manage and control costs, and to improve profits. A hospital is not an assembly line and a patient is not a product; however, the health industry has seen that it can apply these concepts to its world and has, in fact, successfully applied these tools to care for its patients and manage its resources in a cost-effective and medically responsible way. We will review some of these concepts and relate them to the case manager role. First, we will work on understanding cost.

A High-Level Cost Definition and Different Views of Cost

The total cost for an organization can be summarized as the sum of the labor and nonlabor resources, in monetary terms, required to produce an organization's final product or service. In a hospital (as in a manufacturing organization), these costs can be viewed on a departmental/functional basis or on a patient/service line basis.

- In a *departmental or functional view* of costs, a hospital's total cost is the sum of its labor and nonlabor costs for all of its departments, such as nursing units, laboratory, radiology, dietary, housekeeping, finance, and administration. Department directors manage according to information in this view.
- In a *patient or service line view* of costs, a hospital's total cost is the sum of the labor and nonlabor costs in caring for all patients in a service line, over all service lines, such as orthopaedics, cardiology, obstetrics, psychology, or general surgery. Service line directors, medical directors, and case managers manage costs according to information in this view.

Hospital cost accounting systems track and report information to support both of these views. Additionally, different managers within the hospital often address the same elements of cost but use different views and different means of addressing them. For example, a nursing director may address nursing costs by taking actions to reduce the number of worked hours per patient day in a patient care area, whereas a case manager would do so by reducing the number of patient days for patients in an area or service line. The implication here for case managers is that they are generally addressing cost from a patient (per case), a diagnosis-related group (DRG), or a service line viewpoint; and that the costs they are managing are another manager's departmental costs.

The Elements of Cost and How To Impact Them

The cost of an organization can be viewed (in a simplified way) as a cost equation involving a number of cost elements. This same equation can be used to "drill down" and view costs at varying levels of detail, in support of an organization's varying objectives. For example, for hospital vice-presidents managing at a hospitalwide level, the total cost of a hospital could be summarized as

Cost (Hospital) = # Admits × [(labor hrs/admit × labor rate/hr) + (nonlabor units/admit × nonlabor cost/unit)]

Drilling down, for service line directors viewing the cost of a service line or one of the DRGs within our service line, our total cost could be summarized as

Cost (DRG) = # Admits (DRG) × [(labor hrs/admit x labor rate/hr) + (nonlabor units/admit × nonlabor cost/unit)]

Drilling down again, for case managers controlling the costs of a given patient population or (in this case) of a given patient or case, the total cost for that case could be summarized (again, in a simplified way) as

Cost (Case) = # Days × [(labor hrs/day × labor rate/hr) + (nonlabor units/day × nonlabor cost/unit)]

We could continue to drill down to the various treatments, tests, and activities that make up an inpatient day, but will conclude our illustration here. The point is that in each of these situations, the manager can be thought of as working with a cost equation that has a number of variables or elements of cost, and can reduce cost by favorably impacting any of these cost elements. In the last situation, examples of how the case manager can favorably impact the cost of providing care for a given patient or group for each of the cost elements are

- *# Days*—any activity to reduce the number of patient days (read length of stay [LOS]) or to reduce the number of days in more expensive settings, such as days on a critical care unit. Activities can include making sure key treatments or procedures occur at optimal times to facilitate recovery, avoiding unnecessary days early and late in a stay, and coordinating necessary postacute care.
- *Labor hours per day (or per test or exam for diagnostic areas or per procedure for treatment areas)*—any activities to reduce the number of hours required to provide care for a patient, such as the use of time-saving equipment or technologies, alternate care models and staffing ratios, or alternative levels of supervision or administrative support.
- *Labor rate per hour*—activities to impact the overall cost per hour, including adjusting the clinician skill mix, controlling the use of overtime, or reducing reliance on contract employees.
- *# Nonlabor units*—activities to reduce the use of drugs or supplies, including eliminating unnecessary tests, challenging standing orders, or reducing the frequency of particular tests or treatments.
- *Nonlabor cost per unit*—activities to impact the overall cost per unit, such as substituting generic or less expensive drugs/supplies or standardizing on the use of particular drugs/supplies.

Again, the descriptions presented above are a simplification of the actual hospital cost accounting by using one broad equation to represent what are actually hundreds of component units, costs, and rates; they were presented to illustrate a few points.

- The cost of patient care can be impacted by addressing a number of elements of cost, including number of units (or utilization) and cost per unit (or productivity), including labor hours per unit, labor rates, and nonlabor per unit costs.
- Cost accounting systems estimate, measure, and track these elements of cost and report them in detail and summary form to support a manager's understanding and control of them.
- Department directors more typically manage the productivity or cost per unit elements of cost, their responsibility being to deliver high-quality services in the most cost-effective and efficient way (low cost per unit).
- Case managers more typically manage the number of units or utilization elements of cost, their responsibility being to facilitate the decisions around timing, frequency, and occurrence in a patient's treatment regimen.
- Cost improvements related to utilization-related improvements are often difficult to realize unless they are coordinated with departmental improvement efforts. This final point leads to a discussion of types of cost, which is the subject of the next section.

Types of Cost and Which Types Can Be Impacted by a Case Manager

As is apparent in the concepts thus far, cost accounting is interested in modeling costs, particularly costs per unit of service, such as per day, per meal, per test, per surgery minute, and so on. Cost accounting systems categorize costs in a number of ways to explain or model how costs behave or change in relation to factors such as time, level of activity in a unit of service, or closeness of an activity to a unit of service. We will briefly describe two such categories—fixed versus variable cost and direct variable versus indirect variable costs—followed with a discussion of their implications for the case manager.

- *Fixed costs* are costs that remain constant over a relevant range of activity and relative time frame. These are often judgment calls, but costs considered fixed in a hospital setting include capital-related costs such as building or equipment depreciation and interest, certain costs of maintaining the physical plant and facilities, and some management and administrative costs. These types of costs will remain relatively stable, regardless of the level of census or volume of tests being performed. The above description uses the phrase "over a relevant range" because, over long periods of time, most things can be changed (e.g., building and equipment can be sold or put to alternative uses) and thus are variable.
- *Variable costs* are costs that vary in intensity as time or level of activity in a unit of service changes. Costs often considered variable in a patient care setting include caregiver costs such as nursing or therapist costs; labor costs in areas such as dietary, lab, and radiology; and nonlabor costs such as drug and medical supply costs. Variable costs are usually divided into two types: direct and indirect.
- *Direct variable costs* are "hands-on" costs or costs that are closely related to performing a given unit of service. For example, nursing professional and therapist expenses are direct costs for patient care units of service, such as a patient day, whereas phlebotomist, technician, and lab supply expenses are direct costs for lab tests.
- *Indirect variable costs* are costs that are not "hands-on" in nature and are less closely related to a given unit of service. In the above examples, the phlebotomist, lab tech, and lab supplies are direct costs to producing a lab test, but are indirect costs related to the patient day unit of service. Other indirect costs for patient care include admitting, materials, supplies, drugs, and imaging. Indirect costs tend to vary less directly to changes in units such as patient days.

Cost accounting systems typically model costs according to these fixed versus variable and direct versus indirect relationships, with total cost being the sum of a set of fixed and variable (direct and indirect) costs. The relationship of changes in cost to changes in unit of service volumes for these types of cost is illustrated graphically in Figure 18–1.

Information concerning types of cost is frequently used in financial performance improvement discussions and thus is important to understand. These are important distinctions when considering the scope of, or accountability for, improvements in clinical performance.

Recall from the discussion in the previous section that in cost-related performance im-

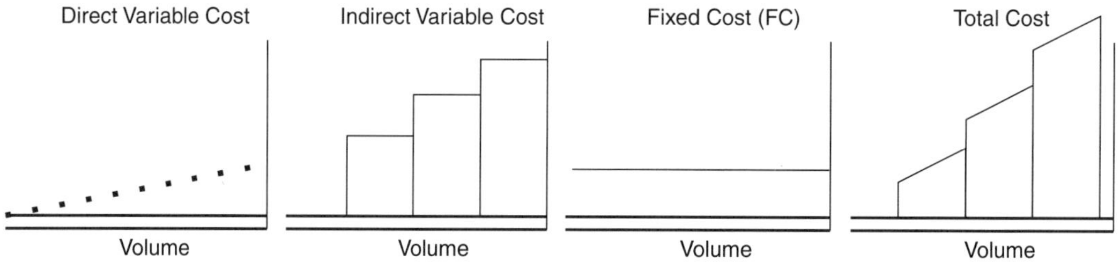

Figure 18–1 Relationship between Type of Cost and Unit of Service Volume

provement efforts, case managers are more able to impact cost through changes in utilization (changes in units of service, such as patient days, or tests per admission) than through productivity (changes in hours per unit of service or cost per unit of service). The implications of fixed/variable/direct/indirect/cost on performance improvement efforts are the following:

- To the degree that costs are considered direct variable costs (and to a lesser extent, indirect variable costs), then the greater the ability to impact or reduce costs through those volume changes. Conversely, to the extent that costs are considered fixed (and to a lesser extent indirect), then the less the potential to impact cost through changes in utilization.
- To the degree that costs are direct versus indirect, then the greater the ability of case management function to impact cost through changes in utilization. Or, conversely, to the degree that costs are indirect versus direct, then to the greater extent ancillary and support departments outside of patient care areas need to adjust their operating practices to realize short-term cost improvements through changes in utilization or unit of service volumes.

As stated earlier, the designation of a cost as fixed versus variable or direct versus indirect is based on judgment and will vary based on how aggressively the cost estimate developer considers cost to vary over changes in time and unit of service volume. Based not on empirical evidence, but on observations of cost estimates from a number of hospital cost accounting systems and discussions with cost accounting professionals, the following rules of thumb concerning types of costs are offered:

- Forty percent (30 to 50 percent) of an organization's costs are typically considered fixed in the near term.
- Of the remaining 60 percent variable costs, half can be considered direct versus indirect. This implies that 30 percent (25 to 35 percent) of hospital cost can be considered direct variable cost.
- Case management improvement efforts can generally impact variable cost and, to the extent they gain the active participation of key ancillary and support department directors, these efforts can impact total variable cost (where total variable cost equals direct variable plus indirect variable costs).
- What a typical hospital considered as direct variable, indirect variable, and fixed costs are summarized in Figure 18–2.

As a final note in this section for case managers, it is not necessarily important to know the details of how your cost accounting system esti-

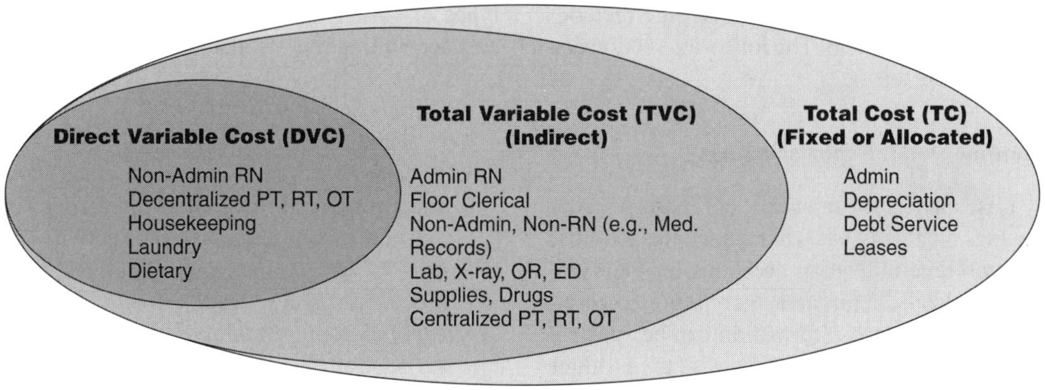

Figure 18–2 Typical Classification of Hospital Cost

mates costs; however, if you are involved in a case management-related cost improvement effort, it is important to gain an understanding of what you are to be accountable for in terms of the scope of the costs, what is included and excluded in cost estimates, and the magnitude of improvement. For example, many cost accounting systems report cost in patient care areas as "fully absorbed costs." This term implies that all costs from nonrevenue-producing areas, such as administration, housekeeping, plant operations, capital costs, and so on are allocated to revenue-producing areas, such as patient care units. In this situation, a manager should make sure he or she is not being considered responsible for impacting fully absorbed costs, because a significant portion of these costs are beyond the control of the clinical manager. This example illustrates the importance not only of understanding cost accounting concepts, but also understanding the reports produced by a cost accounting system, which is the focus of the next section.

A CASE MANAGER'S USE OF A HOSPITAL'S COST ACCOUNTING SYSTEM

A case manager's primary use of a cost accounting system will be in the use of its reports. These systems generate a series of routine and ad hoc reports containing information at varying frequencies and levels of detail. To effectively use a cost accounting system in making decisions, the case manager must understand its reports and, at least at a high level, the methods used to produce them. The following section discusses these topics.

Routine Detail Reports or Logs

Case managers can use detail reports or activity logs on a daily basis to manage the activities and resource utilization decisions for their current caseloads. In this area, more is not necessarily better. As such information can be substantial, it is often advantageous to produce *exception reports* to flag the occurrence of activities outside of the plan or norm that may require case manager intervention. Systems will have some degree of reporting flexibility, and reports should be developed to support or mirror the case manager's daily activities; for example, segmenting and sorting information in the order that work would be conducted by the case manager.

Routine Variance Summary Reports

Cost accounting systems also generate a series of summary reports to support the systemic or higher level decisions of a case management function. Most routine summary reports document (1) actual versus planned (or targeted) performance, (2) for a given period of time, and (3) summarized for a particular level of accountability in an organization.

Reporting Planned versus Actual Performance

Planned performance can represent a budget, an industry benchmark or "best practice," or an agreed-on set of targets (such as would be found in a critical pathway). Comparing an area's actual performance to that planned over a period of time will produce differences or variances. These differences are usually stated in total dollars for a given period. Cost accounting systems can measure, track, and report a number of planned versus actual variances to help the user not only in identifying that there is a difference and the magnitude of that difference, but also to understand the source of the difference. Typical types of variances a case manager may see in cost accounting reports include

- *Total cost variance*—the overall difference in planned versus actual cost.
- *Volume or utilization variance*—the variance attributable to the difference in planned versus actual levels of activity for units of service such as patient days, tests procedures, and so forth.
- *Efficiency or productivity variance*—the variance attributable to the difference in the planned versus actual cost per unit of ser-

vice, such as differences in nursing cost per patient day or radiology cost per procedure.

- *Mix variance*—the variance attributable to differences in the mix of activities in an area. For example, part of the variance in the planned cost of a service line is attributable to the difference in the planned versus actual mix of patients and DRGs within it.

Reporting Time Periods

Variance reports summarize information over a period of time, generally a day, week, or month. Most also report results on a period-to-date and year-to-date basis. This allows the manager to see how an area is performing both in the near term and in the long run. Also, if there is a major difference in period-to-date versus year-to-date performance, it gives the manager an indication that there may be a fundamental change in performance requiring intervention. Finally, some reports may show performance over a number of periods (e.g., months) to indicate trends in performance that merit the manager's attention.

Reporting by Levels of Accountability

The standard performance reports are designed toward a specific audience with unique responsibilities. A department director will receive information that has department-specific detail and rolls up to the department level. For the case manager, reports should have detail that rolls up to a level that corresponds to the manager's level of responsibility, such as service line, unit, or given patient population.

Ad Hoc Reports

Finally, cost accounting systems generally have ad hoc reporting capability. This type of reporting should be considered in addressing focused issues or questions being pursued by the case manager. In these cases, to the extent the case manager can be specific about the required information, level(s) of detail, subtotals, and desired formatting, the more useful the output will be in addressing its intended purpose.

Cost Estimating Methods and Implications for the End User

At the core of a cost accounting system are the methods it uses to estimate hospital cost at a detailed level. These estimates are not seen by the user, but are the underlying measures that, when accumulated, produce the cost estimates for a patient, a hospital department, or a service line that appear on the reports previously discussed. Different systems and organizations use different methods to estimate cost. The method used, though not essential for the case manager to understand at a detailed level, will have implications on the intended uses and limitations of the system. We will discuss three cost estimating methods, the strengths and weaknesses of each method, and the implications for case managers.

Use of Ratio of Cost to Charges (RCC) To Estimate Cost

The ratio of cost to charges (RCC) method of estimating cost is a high-level approach that estimates cost by the relationship of the total expenses to the total charges for an area. At the highest level, if a hospital's total annual expenses (costs) were $500 million and its total annual charges were $900 million, then its overall RCC would be $500/$900 or .56. This ratio could be used to estimate the cost of any case or any DRG by multiplying the total charges for a case or DRG by this ratio. Similarly, one could determine an RCC for any hospital department and use these ratios in a similar way to determine the lab or radiology costs for a given patient or DRG.

This method is attractive because it is simple and inexpensive to implement, can generally be supported with a hospital's existing system, and allows comparisons to a wealth of historical and comparative information from other hospitals. For example, hospital information publicly available for all hospitals through Medicare cost reports and Medicare billing files has all of the information needed to estimate any hospital's Medicare patient population costs at a DRG level using this method.

With its simplicity, however, comes a number of weaknesses. The method (1) does not differentiate between fixed and variable costs because it estimates total cost only, (2) is based only on dollars and thus cannot provide hours-related information that would support the analysis of staffing or productivity-related issues, and (3) has limits on its accuracy. Concerning its accuracy, the method assumes that costs closely resemble charges. Although this is generally true at the hospital level, it is not always true at the departmental level, particularly in cases where hospitals have adjusted charges to improve reimbursement. These limits should not affect most decisions or conclusions made from the information/reports they produce.

Use of Relative Value Units (RVUs) To Estimate Cost

A second method of estimating costs is through the use of relative value units (RVUs) or recognized industry standards that are available through outside sources, such as professional societies or hospital associations. This method is similar to that used in the RCC method, but the method is performed at a detailed procedure level and can be applied to estimate both hours and expenses. Where the RCC method estimates overall cost at the departmental or hospital level, RVUs can estimate both hours and dollars (cost), and can be conducted at a detailed procedure level (such as a chest X-ray, a CBC test, or a patient day). Using this method, both labor and nonlabor costs can be analyzed at a detailed level and accumulated to estimate cost at a patient case, service line, or departmental level.

The benefits of the RVU method are that, although more complicated than the RCC method, it is still fairly simple to implement using available industry standards and existing hospital systems, while having the added benefits of labor-related and more detailed procedure analyses. Its limitations include that (1) it becomes very difficult to use for cross-hospital comparative analyses using publicly available information because the information is built at a hospital's procedure level and (2) there are some limits to its accuracy because cost estimates are based on industry standards versus actual hospital experience. Again, these limits should not affect most decisions or conclusions made from the information/reports they produce.

Use of Detailed Hospital-Specific Cost Estimates

Some cost accounting systems, particularly those in large multihospital systems or academic medical centers, have costs based on hospital-specific estimates. This method can estimate costs at the procedure level, as with the RVU method, but will do so by making estimates (either by some measurement technique or by the technical estimates of a subject matter specialist) specific to the hospital and its unique facility, equipment, supplies, and operating practices. The strengths and weaknesses of this method are similar to those of the RVU method, with one added cost/benefit tradeoff: This method provides greater accuracy and allows more detailed levels of analysis than other methods, but is very time consuming to implement and maintain. The decision to use this method depends on the magnitude of the financial results expected to be gained through its use (which is why its use is generally limited to multihospital systems and academic medical centers).

What Do Case Managers Need To Know about Costing Methods?

Gratefully, the answer in a practical sense is "not very much." It would be helpful for a case manager to have a general awareness of cost and how it is determined in his or her organization's cost accounting system. Beyond awareness, a high-level understanding will be an asset when having discussions with members of finance or budget areas. Finally, if a case manager makes extensive use of reports from these systems to make decisions, such as changes in care plans or the development of treatment guidelines, it would be important to know the strengths and potential limitations of the information they are using. On this final point, all methods do a good job of making "directional" estimates of cost (estimates that support prioritizing improvement efforts), and in making relative decisions at a high level, such as comparing hospitals' DRGs or service lines. However, as these systems support more detailed decision making, as in the procedure level, or other decisions that require a highly accurate measure of financial impact, then the more sophisticated methods become more important.

WORDS OF ADVICE IN USING COST ACCOUNTING INFORMATION

This chapter concludes with some practical issues to consider, as well as pitfalls to avoid, when using cost accounting systems and data in general.

Set Goals and Learn from What Others Have Accomplished

The successful use of cost accounting information will involve establishing challenging but achievable goals (e.g., for cost, quality, and utilization) that, on an ongoing basis, can be measured and tracked against actual performance to gauge an organization's progress and improvement. In assessing its potential for improvement in this area, hospitals can look to what is being accomplished elsewhere in the industry. The wealth of publicly available cost and utilization information provides hospitals with an excellent opportunity to compare their current performance in these areas against those of their peers, competitors, and/or groups of recognized leading performers. This information will have limitations (e.g., it will be available for Medicare patient populations only for some hospitals), but will be an excellent source for identifying what levels of performance others have achieved and can help an organization "set the bar" for its own improvement efforts.

Prioritize: Focus on the Larger Things

Cost accounting systems can and do produce large amounts of information regarding an area's costs. This is good news and bad news for the clinical manager—the information can identify large numbers of possible improvement opportunities to investigate; however, the manager has limited time to pursue, validate, and act on these opportunities. The key for the manager is to prioritize, and when looking for a starting point, start with the big things. There is an industrial engineering rule of thumb referred to as the 80/20 rule, stating that 80 percent of any total is generally contributed by 20 percent of the items. The rule can be applied to a hospital with statements such as 80 percent of the admissions (or DRGs) are made by 20 percent of the physicians, or 80 percent of the radiology volume comes from 20 percent of the procedures, or 80 percent of the cost opportunities comes from 20 percent of the cost issues. In actual experience, the percentages vary somewhat (70–30, 80–20, etc.), but the relationship holds and the implication to the manager is clear: Spend your limited time on the small number of issues that will have the largest improvement potential. Use your cost accounting system to help in finding those issues. Use reports to find the highest cost patients, DRGs, service lines, physicians, supplies, drugs, and so forth. Determine which exhibit the greatest potential for improvement and focus your energies there.

Start with Summary Level Information and Drill Down for Detail as Needed

Cost accounting systems not only produce large amounts of information, but they also produce it at multiple levels of detail. This is more good news for the manager who is "prioritizing on the big things," and the advice is to start at the top and drill down as needed. This will keep you from being overwhelmed with too much information and make sure that, at each level, the focus is maintained on the most costly items or issues. For example, if you are working to improve cost performance in a particular service line, look first at the high-volume DRGs or physicians in the service line, then, within a DRG, look into the physicians or services that consume the most resources for cases in that DRG. For example, if pharmaceuticals are a large contributor, you should identify which drugs make the highest contribution, and so on. How far you will need to drill down will depend on the decisions being made. The manager should use information at as high a summary level as possible and stop when he or she has enough information to support the decision.

Reasonableness Test Your Information before Using It To Make an Important Decision

Clinical managers will likely use cost accounting information to address the issues they face, the questions they are asked, and the decisions they make. Once comfortable with the information produced by these systems, managers may have a tendency to request information and then quickly make conclusions and decisions based on the information they are provided. The advice here does not consume much time and is very basic, but will maintain credibility and avoid mistakes and headaches if followed: Reasonableness test your information. Cost accounting systems are powerful in terms of the analyses they can produce, based on the parameters, time frames, and assumptions provided by the analyst using the system. An analyst can misunderstand a report requirement, or make an assumption not intended by the requesting manager, that can produce results different from what managers thought they were requesting.

Make sure you understand the assumptions made in producing the information, what is included, and what is excluded. Test the results with some high-level tests. Include a "totals" line in reports where possible and test these totals against experience or against another familiar report with similar totals. If reports produce variances, calculate the variances as a percentage of the total to assess if they are reasonable. High-level tests of a report's reasonableness will give the manager some assurance concerning the accuracy of the report or point to some questionable findings in need of follow-up and validation. Either way, the tests will reduce the risk of mistakes and better prepare the manager for decisions to be made with the information.

Don't Get Too Caught Up in the Details

It might appear to be contradictory advice: Reasonableness test your work, but don't look too closely, especially at the details. However, these statements are consistent if they are restated as pay attention to the details when developing the system (especially the important details), check your work at a high level whenever using the system, and, finally, don't spend too much time on details that may be insignificant and that are diverting your time from the big, important things.

This advice is particularly relevant if one is working with cost accounting information at the system's base-level detail. Anyone working hard enough can find issues with some of the detailed measures or estimates of a cost accounting system. However, because the system consists of a large number of such estimates over long periods of time, these issues become immaterial or do not change the results and associated decisions that managers make based on that information (unless the issue is this one of the "big things"). The 80/20 rule mentioned previously applies here and is generally applied by organizations in developing their systems; the cost accounting system will be effective if it accurately characterizes the cost behavior of the small number of activities that account for the largest portion of cost and is reasonably close in characterizing the behavior of the remaining activities.

Be Careful in Using Averages To Estimate Economic Impact

Cost accounting systems often state costs in term of their average. These average costs are used in estimating the financial impact of performance improvement activities. In most cases, the use of averages will produce accurate and reliable results; however, there will be times when averages will misstate results. For example, when estimating the financial impact of reductions in LOS, an average cost per day factor is often used. On closer inspection, the true economic impact of the reduced days is often lower than estimated because they are achieved by eliminating the less costly days at the end of patient stays. Some activities during eliminated days are similarly eliminated, whereas others are merely shifted to earlier in the stay. The advice for case managers relative to this point, particularly if the manager is to be accountable for achieving the estimated economic impact, is to be aware of situations where averages do not accurately reflect the activities being estimated and use a more conservative cost estimate.

Consider Both the Revenue and the Cost Side of Economic Improvement

Cost accounting systems measure, track, and report an organization's costs. However, the economic and financial impact of the case management function in a hospital needs to consider both the cost and the revenue side of the picture.

Previous chapters have presented the various reimbursement arrangements that hospitals share with their payers and how changes in inpatient utilization and LOS impact the reimbursement for each. In estimating the economic impact of inpatient utilization-related improvements, reducing costs could (depending on the payer) produce a corresponding reduction in revenues. These lost revenues should be netted against any cost reduction savings to estimate the true economic impact to the organization. Inpatient utilization reductions for payers with fixed or capitated reimbursement arrangements, such as Medicare or most managed care plans, will not have a corresponding revenue impact loss. On the other hand, inpatient utilization reductions for payers with discounted fee-for-service, charge-based, or per diem reimbursement arrangements will have a corresponding revenue loss, which should be netted against utilization-related cost savings to estimate the actual economic impact. This will require assistance from someone in the finance department who can help the manager work through and, at a high level, model the reimbursement methods and associated contract payment rates.

In other situations, such as those where a hospital may be operating near its capacity in some of its units or service lines, inpatient utilization or reductions in LOS will free up capacity to admit elective patients that would otherwise need to be scheduled at a later date. In these cases, there will be an additional favorable revenue impact from these additional admission volumes that should be included in any estimates of economic impact.

Understand the Difference between "Implemented" and Realized Impact on Savings

This is an important distinction for clinical managers who are responsible for achieving "bottom-line" savings through their improvement efforts, particularly those working to achieve those results through reductions in clinical resource utilization and LOS. Let's assume you are a nurse manager working to achieve savings through reductions in LOS. You may have reduced the LOS in your area of responsibility by one day per stay. According to the cost accounting system, the impact of that "implemented" reduction is $400 per day for the 2,000 patients admitted in your area, or an impact of

$$\text{2,000 admissions} \times \text{1 day saved/admit} \times \text{\$400/day} = \text{\$800,000}$$

This estimated $800,000 implemented impact is also a realized "bottom-line" savings if these reduced days were accompanied with a similar reduction in direct patient expenses, such as nursing hours, ancillary support hours, supplies, and drugs. The point here is to illustrate the difference between an estimate of implemented savings and actual bottom-line savings. The take-away for the case manager or director of a utilization management effort is that achieving bottom-line savings in utilization and LOS reduction efforts will generally require an accompanying capacity management program (i.e., a program to manage per unit expenses to changes in volumes of patient days, tests, procedures, etc.).

Maintain a Balanced Scorecard for Improvement

Cost accounting systems provide hospitals with the tools needed to effectively assess and manage the cost objectives of their organizations. The systems are most effective when they are used in the context of an organization's overall performance improvement effort that includes a balance of clinical effectiveness, quality, and financial objectives. The development of a "balanced scorecard" to measure and track an organization's progress on all fronts will help the organization to maintain its focus on all dimensions of performance improvement.

SUGGESTED READINGS

C.T. Horngren et al., *Cost Accounting: A Managerial Emphasis* (Englewood Cliffs, NJ: Prentice Hall, 1999).

J.G. Nackel et al., *Cost Management for Hospitals* (Rockville, MD: Aspen Publishers, Inc., 1987).

Chapter 19

Decision Support for Case Managers

Magdalen M. Hunssinger and Carole Neff

TAKE THIS TO WORK

1. Decision support systems aggregate clinical, financial, and administrative data in a repository.
2. Case managers should participate in care system design sessions and upgrade activities to maximize their knowledge of data origins.
   - Clinical data come from medical records abstracting and coding, as well as order processing and patient accounting.
3. Decision support should allow the case manager to determine pathway adherence or variance without a need for paper chart reviews.

Decision support in its simplest form involves fact-based patient data being available in a format that is easily understood and quantifiable and that can be interpreted in such a way that the next logical action or sequence of events with regard to clinical care is known, understood, and usually considered accepted practice. Core clinical systems such as patient management, order management, clinical documentation, pharmacy, radiology, and lab provide the foundation on which clinical data are extracted, retrieved, and spun into a picture that enables the clinician to determine the steps in care planning and, if those steps are not readily known, alert the clinician to a potential catastrophic case and/or exception to a predefined standard of care.

SOURCE DATA

How are core systems key to decision support? Systems that capture data at the time of the event are considered core or source systems. The process of where, when, and how the data are captured and entered, the amount of subjective leeway allowed during data entry, and the underlying culture of the institution and its staff all influence data residing in their core systems. The above external elements affecting data capture are especially true for patient management, order management, and clinical documentation, and have less impact on pharmacy, radiology, and lab systems that deal with management of an order originating from a patient care area.

In order to understand the validity and types of data available to provide a reliable data foundation for decision support systems, the clinician must become intimately involved with how the source systems were designed, how staff are being taught to use them, and how they are actually used in the clinical setting. The majority of hospital staff are taught to use core systems in the classroom, and instruction is often in close alignment with the facility's vision and best-known clinical practices. However, outside of the classroom, theory often gives way to reality, and staffing deficiencies, high patient acuity, and other contributing factors endemic to the facility may compromise data entry.

An example of how data may be misrepresented during data entry is found in the following true case: A critical care unit clerk is entering multiple orders for a patient into the order management system. The clerk has already faxed the physician orders to the receiving departments of lab, radiology, and respiratory care. The faxed physician orders don't contain specific ordering detail information required by the order management system. During order entry, the clerk is required to enter a series of qualifiers that will be sent with each order to the receiving department. One field requires the clerk to enter the reason for the test. The reason for the test field is currently "hard-linked" to a predefined list of specific diagnosis codes that in theory make sense for that test to be ordered. The clerk has been instructed during classroom training to find the latest working diagnosis and enter that into the "reason for test." It is noted that physicians at this facility do not write the reason for test diagnosis with each order set and physicians are not phoned to amend the order after the fact, even though the field is required. After reviewing the chart, the clerk determines that the listing of diagnoses for this test code does not include a code that matches the patient's current admit or working diagnosis. The clerk chooses a code from the list, giving it a "best guess" because the field is required and further data entry will be halted until a value is entered. The patient in this example is truly in the diagnostic phase of care, and the presenting condition and diagnosis do not fit any of the pre-defined reasons for this test criteria hard coded in the core system. At this juncture, the clerk's best guess diagnosis choice is linked to that order entry session and those records are now stored on the system. There are many other questions about this facility's current practice pattern that arise from the above example. However, our focus will be limited to how data may be inaccurately entered into a source system and not truly reflective of actual events of a case. It is noted that the above is a good example of this sequence of events.

Each hospital is unique in respect to core system design, the reasoning behind each element required, why the element is needed, and which department requires the data element and requested its capture. Also unique is the type and amount of core data readily available from year to year. When developing and implementing a solid decision support model, you must conduct a thorough assessment of the core systems and understand the type of data available, the current system platforms, the core system data architecture, and how data integration occurs between disparate systems at the facilities. Each of these factors is unique at each hospital. Without taking into account how current systems are used, who uses them, how data are qualified at time of data entry, and how data are eventually captured and stored, the case manager's perspective may be out of alignment with what is achievable at that particular facility with regard to any planned decision support system implementation and/or interpretation of data retrieved from a core system and spun into decision support reports.

Case management staff should actively participate in core system design sessions, upgrade activities, and enhancement works at their facilities. Gaining a broader perspective on the types of data available and the history on why data are included in the core data set will assist in providing meaningful reports from which to base decisions and track variance. The core data need to mean what they say and be valid. Data integrity means consistent data entry from core systems. This is essential. Core data need to help people make decisions and not cause confusion over meaning or origin.

DATA MINING

What are the business drivers at your facility? Data mining requires the decision support team to have a clear understanding of current business drivers. In addition, it helps if a business analyst with a solid systems background is included. Designing a support decision model requires the team to focus on a vision that incorporates key business drivers into solid reports for outcome analysis. Decision support systems require a vision that results in practical and achievable measurements.

The business analyst can easily inundate the audience with too much data and too many reports. Capturing reports that track all variances may overwhelm clinicians with a lot of data and create hours of needless analysis and meetings to determine what is meaningful and what isn't. Narrowing the initial focus can help the team build on measurable successes as they gain expertise with their system and understand source data at their institution.

One quick approach to data mining is to focus in on ordering patterns for specific diseases and manage to an expected outcome. For example, certain medications used in the first few hours following myocardial infarction are considered effective in preventing further and more extensive heart damage. However, missing the window of time for administration decreases effectiveness. In addition, the medication is fairly expensive. It may make sense to report if the drug is prescribed within the appropriate time frame and within appropriate guidelines for managing myocardial infarction. Tracking patient outcomes using specific pharmacy medication ordering trends as a baseline can be a good starting point. Decision support technology can be used effectively to measure outcomes combined with a focused disease management strategy by determining business drivers that are measurable and those that can be managed effectively using the current system.

TYPES OF DECISION SUPPORT SYSTEMS

Decision support systems available in today's market fall primarily into two categories. The first category includes systems that aggregate clinical, financial, and administrative data from core systems and provide tools to support analysis and reporting on these data. The second category includes systems that are focused on managing select functions such as authorization management. In addition, there are some Web-based systems that would fall into this second category. The remainder of this section will focus on the first category of decision support systems, describing how these systems work and the basic functionality available within them.

Decision support systems aggregate clinical, financial, and administrative data in a repository. The financial data come from the payroll/human resource systems as well as general accounting and patient systems. The data from the payroll/human resource systems include job codes and job grades within departments. The account codes, along with revenue and expense by account, are gathered from the general ledger. In addition, data used to determine cost per unit of service are gathered. These data allow the identification of service units along with the budgeted volume, actual volume, unit charge, and unit cost. By combining the unit of service data and the job level and account level data, the cost per unit of service can be defined by category of expense. An example of this is as follows:

Unit of Service	Cost/Unit	Budgeted Volume	Actual Volume	Variance
Chest X-ray	2.00	100	110	10%

Cost by category of expense:
- variable direct cost 1.28
- fixed direct cost .55
- indirect cost .17

The clinical data come primarily from medical records coding and abstracting, but may also come from the order processing system and patient accounting. These data answer two basic questions: Who was the patient, and why was he or she receiving care. These data would include data elements such as patient age, gender, zip code, primary payer, primary and secondary diagnoses, primary and secondary procedures, and physicians involved in care as attending and admitting physicians. Finally, data from the order processing or patient accounting systems would indicate care activities and timing of these activities with regard to day of stay. For example, we would know that a 63-year-old male with probable myocardial infarction was admitted by

Dr. Jones. On day one of a five-day stay, one chest X-ray, two sets of blood gases, and two sets of cardiac enzymes were performed. When this patient level data is combined with the financial data, the patient, the care activities, the resources consumed, and the cost of these resources can be identified.

Some decision support systems also gather data about payer mix and contract arrangements. These data allow for net revenue to be estimated. Because each patient encounter will have payer information and the admit and discharge dates, it is possible to link this encounter with the contract terms in effect at that time and therefore estimate the net revenue associated with that episode of care.

Decision Support System Functions

The above describes the data requirements for building the repository associated with decision support systems. Next, it is important to understand the functional requirements associated with decision support. These systems generally provide decision support tools and support for the following: cost accounting, resource utilization management (UM), clinical process management, reimbursement modeling, and contract management.

The most basic form of decision support tool involves providing case managers easy access to data—access to detailed information about patients, the care they received, the resources utilized, the course of care, and the costs associated with this care, as well as the estimated reimbursement associated with the episode of care. In addition, the actual care delivered can be compared to the "expected" care with the variations identified. Understanding these variations in care can help case managers identify opportunities for improvement or current best practices. Enhanced access coupled with reporting capabilities including the ability to filter, subset, and graph data enable informed decision making by delivering the right information at the right time and place.

Cost accounting functionality supports decision making by allowing case managers to identify costs of treatment patterns. By supporting various costing methodologies, standards can be developed that accurately reflect the actual cost of providing care and the elements that make up these costs, including direct and indirect materials and labor. This allows case managers and care providers to understand the financial impact of treatment choices.

Resource UM requires the ability to capture, measure, and analyze resource utilization, costs, and outcomes, as well as the relationships between them. By studying resource utilization for populations of patients, case managers can predict utilization and identify at-risk populations requiring case management. Likewise, an analysis of historical patterns of resource utilization promotes enhanced planning for resource allocation and future programs/service based on demand.

Clinical process management involves the development of clinical pathways or protocols and a comparison of actual treatment patterns with these guidelines, as well as the identification of variations in the process and outcomes of care. Decision support systems must allow case managers to report on outcomes and to analyze the factors in care delivery that affect outcomes. By identifying and reporting on areas of excessive variation from standard practice, case managers and care providers can define strategies to move toward more uniform quality care delivery.

Reimbursement modeling allows case managers to estimate reimbursement for various payment arrangements. By tracking and analyzing reimbursement by individual contract or payer and comparing expected reimbursement with cost for these same populations, case managers can understand the impact of contract arrangements. Providing reports on the care required to treat various conditions, the costs associated with that care, and the estimated reimbursement can be invaluable for individuals involved in contract design and negotiations. Likewise, the ability to model changes to the care activities, cost of care, or reimbursement methodology and resulting change to aggregate reimbursement can be useful contract design.

Another common function of decision support systems is contract management. Contract management includes the ability to track and analyze expected versus actual reimbursement by individual contract or payer. The ability to monitor reimbursement contracts to ensure that the contracted terms with various third-party payers are being appropriately applied can be invaluable in an environment of tighter margins. Although this is a function that would probably not be performed by the case manager, the case manager may be called on to assist reimbursement analysts to interpret data associated with care received or care required by particular patient populations.

Clinical Pathways

Decision support systems can provide the data needed to develop clinical pathways. Clinical pathways are a planning mechanism geared toward developing treatment plans based on knowledge and experience. Developing and using clinical pathways or guidelines can help improve clinical outcomes, standardize patient care, and trim costs by assisting clinicians in delivering optimal treatments and tests in a timely manner.

Developing clinical pathways requires easy access to accurate information about the care activities, resource utilization associated with these care activities, and resulting clinical outcomes for a homogeneous population of patients. Decision support systems provide access to these data and may provide tools that support analysis and reporting on these data by case managers. These systems provide tools that allow users to "slice and dice" the data in ways that allow them to identify relationships that may not otherwise be evident.

Some decision support systems provide for "what if" analysis, allowing case managers to predict treatment activities that will contribute to the achievement of desired results. Decision support systems are not, however, intended to take the place of judgment by the clinician. Instead, by presenting meaningful data at the right time and place, decision- making can be optimized. By using "what if" models, case management teams can design clinical pathways that reflect best practice leading to desired outcomes instead of simply documenting the way things have always been done.

Retrospective Analysis

Retrospective analysis is an important component of decision support. Analysis of historical data to identify variation in care delivery and outcomes can serve two important purposes: It provides insight into processes and practices such that improvement opportunities can be identified, and it can be used to provide feedback to clinicians to reinforce desired behavior. However, retrospective review lacks the "vision" to design the desired future state.

Retrospective analysis typically involves reviewing data collected for a specific time period, for a particular population of patients as determined by the case management team. Analysis of these data helps case managers and care providers understand clinical practice, including the care activities, costs associated with these care activities, and reimbursement implications. This information can be combined with clinical research data and used to design clinical pathways or guidelines that embody best practice and will lead to desired outcomes.

The ideal approach is to plan care activities that will lead to desired outcomes and to measure and monitor the results. If desired results are achieved, reporting these results and the practices that lead to them can be useful in promoting or reinforcing the desired behaviors. If, on the other hand, the desired results are not achieved, it is important to identify opportunities and strategies for improvement. This retrospective analysis should be performed on a periodic basis because care guidelines should be revised to reflect newly acquired knowledge based on experience and research.

Although many organizations are using decision support systems to research current practice patterns during initial guideline development, few have automated these guidelines to the point that they can compare expected care and outcomes with actual care and outcomes. Some decision support systems allow case managers to build care guidelines into systems as standards, automating the comparison of actual care to expected or standard care and the identification of variances. If this functionality can be integrated with point-of-care systems to alert care providers to variations in care, it may be possible to more effectively influence decision making. Most organizations are just not there yet.

TODAY'S TECHNOLOGY

Current-state hospital technology architecture is very complex and highly unique at any given facility. Even though a hospital may have the same system as another nearby hospital or have a popular architecture, each facility will usually be configured and customized according to its particular needs, given the skill set of its information system (IS) staff and any outside help procured to complete the configuration. Hospitals typically have a patchwork of systems in place that are both automated and manual. Rarely is a facility able to work through a single vendor solution for systems, and it is the norm to have complex integration as part of the basic technology scenario. Case managers often aren't strategically aligned with IS staff. Case management staff are often unfamiliar with the complexities of their system and require help from IS staff. In many instances, there is a "tunnel vision" effect at UM strategy and design sessions convened to drive out solutions that will effect change and reduce costs for the organization. The challenge for case managers is to effectively manage expectations for decision support solutions and change given a less than optimal technology environment, coupled with limited time, resources, and budget. The more automated solution usually equates to a higher dollar expenditure in order to achieve it. However, a highly automated solution has the potential to have the biggest benefit to the organization overall.

Technology by itself doesn't produce solutions: People drive decisions and produce results. It is imperative to narrow the decision support technology focus down to what is doable today in your organization. Focus efforts on aspects of care that are manageable. Clinical pathways can be prioritized to determine which ones to manage. Significant barriers to decision support technology include the lack of a firm foundation with regard to core systems. Many systems exclude large chunks of the patient's episode of care. Other barriers include coming at the design from an operational perspective with a blurred corporate vision centered on business goals. Decision support requires a visionary perspective concerning outcomes. Design requires a vision and a plan—achievable in phases. Decision support implementation requires more than an operational focus. Once the decision support model is in place and reports are produced, the team should ask if the results are effecting change. If not, should the team continue to look at this particular area?

In conclusion, careful planning is required for any project that encompasses decision support. Alignment of the decision support team with the information technology services team will strengthen outcomes and provide a solid foundation on which to draw out key source data for analysis. Understanding what is realistically possible and balancing this against the overall decision support project goals and vision will ensure success for the organization.

SUGGESTED READINGS

C. Broverman, "Standards for Clinical Decision Support Systems," *Journal of Healthcare Information Management 13,* no. 2 (1999): 23-82.

P. Fisher et al., "Decision Support Tools in Health Care." (Papers commissioned by the National Forum on Health, Ottawa, Canada, 1998.)

G. Gillespie, "Online Clinical Guidelines Help Trim Costs," *Health Data Management* 8, no. 1 (2000): 39–45.

J. Metzger, "Cross-Continuum Care Management Information Management Challenges," *Strategies for Integrated Health Care: Emerging Practices in Information Management and Cross-Continuum Care,* eds. E. Drazen and J. Metzger (San Francisco: Jossey-Bass, Publishers, 1999).

L. Perreault and J. Metzger, "A Pragmatic Framework for Understanding Clinical Decision Support," *Journal of Healthcare Information Managment 13,* no. 2 (1999): 5–22.

Part VI

Models from Medical Centers Redesigning Case Management

CHAPTER 20

Rapid Design

David W. Plocher, Kathleen L. Meredith, and Hilary M. Lawn

TAKE THIS TO WORK

1. Rapid Design permits more effective planning than conventional series of committee meetings.
2. Rapid Design is *not* brainstorming. As the extensive prework describes, there is creative coaching involved, preserving participants' complete ownership of the new architecture.
3. Patient populations historically considered "highly complex" can be successfully managed using standardized pathways, guidelines, and algorithms that can then be customized to the individual patient.
4. Collaborative design sessions that involve key physicians and caregivers can produce effective tools and practices for managing patient care.
5. Data analysis is useful for identifying key areas for improving care and for determining optimal practices during the design session. Follow-up data can then be used by case managers, physicians, and hospital management to measure the effectiveness of design outputs and determine where iterative changes are needed.
6. Implementation of new tools and practices must occur immediately to ensure that momentum continues.

Over the past decade, the health care industry has experienced unprecedented consolidation. The competition for patients and the ensuing revenues is fierce. The number of acutely ill patients with shorter hospital stays is escalating. The window of opportunity for profit realization is becoming increasingly shortened. Proactive behavior is being threatened by reactivity; uncertainty is the norm. For industry leaders, this brings a new set of challenges as they grapple with the urgent realities of revamping strategic plans, integrating operations and processes, and managing within a compressed time frame. As a result, multiyear planning, design, and implementation has given way to four- or five-week timelines for decision making. These are the new realities of the health care industry today, and the pace is only going to get more harried.

EVOLUTION OF RAPID DESIGN

Hospitals and health systems have, until now, used a "traditional" approach to decision making by creating small, multidisciplinary teams of people who meet for two to three hours per week over a six- to nine-month period of time. The pace is slow and relaxed, and the outputs typically result in incremental changes to microprocesses within the organization. Invited attendees often miss key meetings, and momentum is difficult to sustain. The design work is often completed without a clear plan for implementation; in fact, those individuals participating in the design phase are not usually accountable or involved in seeing the implementation of their ideas come to fruition.

An alternative approach is to use an accelerated design process, referred to as Rapid Design. This methodology is an intense and focused facilitated process that empowers groups to reach decisions and develop action plans, which enable implementation. Accelerated design is accomplished through group sessions structured to achieve high-performance results in a reduced time period with active participation of key stakeholders. Based on their involvement, the Rapid Design participants become committed to the session outcomes. This methodology provides value and speed to solutions by using information about the health system, along with industry leading models and best practices (Table 20–1).

This chapter describes the advantages of using the Rapid Design methodology, specifically for case management model development. The various components are outlined, as well as the critical success factors involved in the process.

THE ACCELERATED SOLUTIONS METHODOLOGY

Rapid Design uses large-group facilitation to accelerate the delivery of value to business solutions. This innovative approach is uniquely suited to any complex business change requiring the involvement of a large number of stakeholders.

The foundation of Rapid Design includes design sessions that reduce the decision-making cycle from months to days, while maximizing stakeholder involvement and commitment. This involves getting the right people in the right place at one time to expedite their response time and decision making. Careful use of leading practice models, knowledge objects, subject matter specialists, and highly structured time management techniques enables participants to make quality decisions quickly. Individuals trained in unique large-group facilitation techniques conduct the sessions.

The schematic for the Rapid Design model is depicted in Figure 20–1.

Methods and Features of Rapid Design

- *Whole systems approach*—Involving all stakeholder groups in the design process

Table 20–1 Rapid Design versus Traditional Decision Making

Key Factors	*Traditional*	*Accelerated*
Decision making	• Confined to one site • Nominal user involvement	• Multiple sites • Users responsible for design
Predetermined content	• Decision making starts from scratch	• "Best practice" examples accelerate decision making
Momentum	• Meeting spans many weeks • Limited to 2–3 hours • Users do not complete assignments • No clear link to implementation	• Design occurs in dedicated, focused sessions • Time-boxing ensures completion
Representation	• Frequently do not have the right people at the table • Delay getting input from others	• All key stakeholders participate • No need to delay process

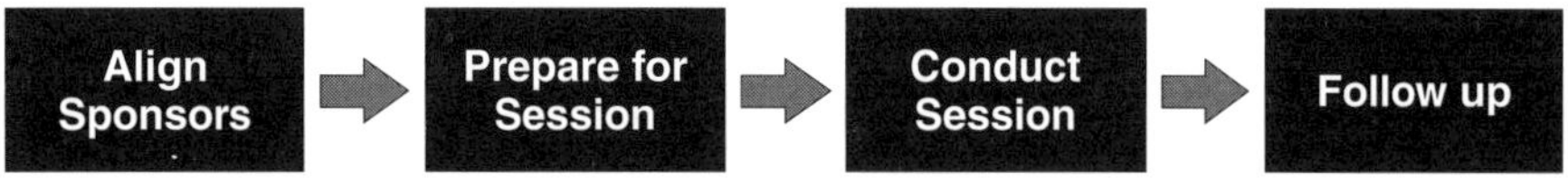

Figure 20–1 The Rapid Design Process Model

develops commitment to change and ensures that the right information is available during the design process. Stakeholders representing the "entire process" are physically together in one location, working collaboratively on the design.

- *Simultaneous tasks*—Simultaneous activity speeds the solution definition process. Teams work in parallel on separate aspects of the design. No two teams work on the same thing.
- *Straw case solution model*—The teams begin with a straw case. This avoids the "blank sheet of paper" and "reinventing the wheel" and speeds the tailoring process. Teams have the choice of rejecting the straw case, but seldom do.
- *Scalability*—The technique can be adapted for use on a wide range of projects, from system installations to full-blown multi-entity initiatives.
- *Time-boxed milestones*—Teams are provided clear expectations, or milestones. These milestones, which serve as checkpoints, are established at specified intervals throughout the process. Teams work freely over blocks of two to three hours to accomplish their milestones.
- *Tool kits*—A collection of leading practice tools and templates is available to facilitate the teams in reaching the necessary design decisions.

Enablers of Rapid Decision Making

There are many reasons why the Rapid Design technique works. Exhibit 20–1 lists a few key enablers that empower a large diverse population of individuals to achieve decision-making goals in an extremely compressed time frame. Compromising these enablers will put the Rapid Design session at risk of falling short of desired goals.

Benefits of Rapid Design

The Rapid Design acceleration technique can bring tangible and intangible benefits.

- increased speed to value
- accelerated decision making
- closure on decisions
- consensus and buy-in of key stakeholders
- collaboration across business units
- accountability and ownership of decisions

INDICATIONS FOR USE IN CARE MANAGEMENT

The development of a comprehensive, integrated care management program incorporating the array of components described in the previous chapters requires a large investment. Return on this investment can best be realized by using the Rapid Design methodology (Figure 20–2).

Design of the care management model will include both a high-level design to achieve clinical integration across multiple sites and also key care management infrastructure development, including the organizational structure and reporting relationships. The infrastructure design will be tailored to the specific market characteristics, organization maturity, and current business case objectives. The components of the desired future state goals and potential solutions will drive the actual Rapid Design agenda development.

A dashboard of integrated care management components across the continuum includes the items shown in Exhibit 20–2).

CASE MANAGEMENT INFRASTRUCTURE CASE STUDY

The Rapid Design process creates an environment that is conducive to developing improve-

Exhibit 20–1 Enablers for Decision Making

- Sponsorship
- Dedicated time and place to conduct design activities
- "Best practice" recommendation
- Especially developed decision-making tools
- Extensive time-boxing
- Results-oriented facilitation
- Effective decision-making rules
- Design broken into discrete sets of design activities
- Full participation of stakeholders
- Concurrent design activities
- Focus on tangible work products
- Defined accountability for implementation

ments over a short period of time through the use of group processes, structured exercises, experienced facilitators, and motivated participants. Success at a Rapid Design session requires that all of the people and resources instrumental to the process undergoing evaluation convene at one time, in one location, with strong support from their leaders and peers. It was in this type of environment that one group of health care system participants embarked on the process of designing care management in their hospitals.

The project sponsor organized the care management initiative, and a steering committee comprised of representatives from the health system was formed to direct and support the initiative. The steering committee began the design process by focusing on the care management model and the organizational structure. Next, the steering committee developed a model of continuum-based care management and organized a two-day Rapid Design session. The purpose of the Rapid Design session was to enable stakeholders from the health system to design the care management infrastructure for the organization.

A high-level agenda for the two-day session included the activities shown in Exhibit 20–3 with related time-boxing.

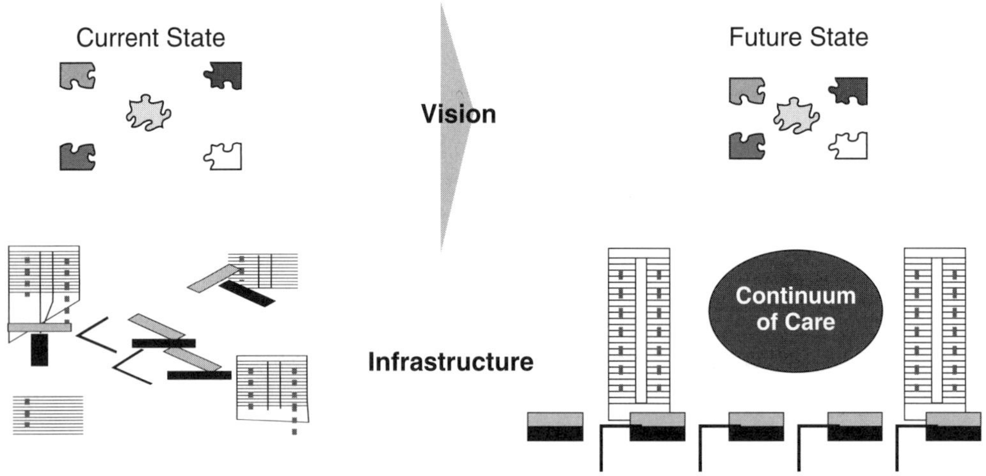

- Multiple processes and systems lacking integration
- Fragmentation between concurrent review and discharge planning
- Fragmentation of utilization and case management
- Inconsistent risk identification with poor integration into care coordination
- Lack of process in monitoring resource utilization

- Integrated processes and structure
- Focus on integration across the continuum
- Coordinated patient and cost management
- Seamless system of risk identification for care coordination
- Strong measuring/monitoring of pathways

Figure 20–2 Rapid Design: The Case for Change

Exhibit 20–2 Integrated Care Management Components

Inpatient	*Nonacute*	*Outpatient*	*Managed Care*	*Risk Assessment/ Wellness*	*Community-Based*
Goal: Effectively and efficiently manages inpatient lengths of stay and resource utilization	*Goal:* Effectively and efficiently transitions the patient to a cost-effective level of postacute care	*Goal:* Manages the long-term and chronic health care and social needs of at-risk and capitated patient populations	*Goal:* Meets managed care and payer requirements	*Goal:* Understands and manages the health care priorities and needs of patients	*Goal:* Manages the long-term and chronic health care and social needs of at-risk and capitated patient populations

Exhibit 20–3 Agenda for Two-Day Rapid Design Session

	Day One
8:00–8:30 am	Registration and Continental Breakfast
8:30–8:35 am	Welcome
8:35–9:15 am	Session Orientation • Leadership Kickoff • Overview of Care Management Initiative • Session Goals –Purpose –Overall Agenda –Ground Rules, Guiding Principles, Boundaries
9:15–10:00 am	Team-Building Exercise
10:00–10:45 am	Current State Assessment Activity and Report
10:45–11:15 am	Care Management Model Presentation
11:15 am–12:15 pm	Breakout Groups (Policies, Procedures, Tools)
12:15–1:00 pm	Working Lunch
1:00–4:00 pm	Breakout Group to Design the Components of the Case Management Model
4:00–5:00 pm	Breakout Groups Report to the Large Group Reaction to and Validation of Output of Breakout Groups to the Large Group (Including Physicians)
5:00 pm	Closing Comments, Wrap-up, Evaluations
	Day Two
8:00–8:30 am	Continental Breakfast
8:30–8:40 am	Day 1 Recap
8:40–11:00 am	Day 1 Breakout Groups, *cont.*
11:00 am–12:00 pm	Breakout Groups Report to Large Group (Including Physicians)
12:00–2:00 pm	Physician Session Breakout
12:00–12:30 pm	Lunch
12:30–4:00 pm	Breakout Groups (Action Plans)
4:00–5:00 pm	Breakout Groups Report to Large Group Reaction to and Validation of Output of Breakout Groups to the Large Group (Including Physicians)
5:00 pm	Closing Comments, Wrap-up, Evaluations

During the Rapid Design session, critical success factors for the design of the initiative were shared with participants. The success factors of the design were as follows:

- a functional organizational structure to support the clinical care coordination processes
- a clearly defined case management infrastructure that addresses roles, relationships, and accountability for essential care management functions
- integrated case management, discharge planning, utilization management, and quality management functions to ensure that key clinical and resource utilization variances are consistently monitored, reported, and analyzed for the ongoing review and improvement of patient care pathways
- physician sponsorship to address the sustainability of changes

Session Participants

Because the participants are the most vital component of a Rapid Design session, careful determination of who was invited and expected to attend was made. The individuals asked to participate represented the key stakeholders of the entity—a microcosm of the organization. This included individuals from several departments and from all levels of the organization. The selected participants possessed specific characteristics, such as the knowledge and experience to perform at a high level, the respect of their colleagues, the ability to be both creative and critical thinkers, strong interpersonal skills, and the desire and commitment to improve the organization. Perhaps the best example of individuals possessing the desire and commitment to improve the organization, specifically the care management process, are the project sponsors. Therefore, their participation in the session was critical in that it increased the support, commitment, and buy-in of the other session participants.

For the health system, the following individuals attended the design session: steering committee members, case managers, social workers, nursing administrators, physicians, case management director, unit operations manager, staff nurses (from medical–surgical, intensive care unit, emergency department), nurse manager, and pharmacist. In addition, the following departments were represented as well: admitting, bed control, respiratory therapy, rehabilitative therapy, cardiology, lab, stroke team, transplant services, call center, utilization review, outpatient services, clinics, home health, medical records, information systems, managed care, health plan, finance, reimbursement services, patient accounting, financial counseling, and insurance verification.

Because the health system is made up of several facilities that were involved in developing the recommendations during the design session, it was imperative that individuals from each facility be invited to participate. Additionally, it was necessary for the project sponsors and the other session planners to determine how many individuals from each discipline or department were needed in order to achieve the session goals. Inviting at least two individuals from the same discipline or department ensured those areas representation and input in the event that one of those individuals was unable to attend.

Once the participant list was confirmed, preparation of the participants for the session took place. Preparation activities included written communication well in advance of the session, containing logistical information, the purpose and goals of the session, expectations of participants, the list of participants, relevant research and prereadings, or other assignments that needed to be completed prior to the session.

Session Rules, Guiding Principles, Assumptions of Model

Specific boundaries or design rules were agreed on by the steering committee and shared with the participants at the beginning of the session. Exhibit 20–4 depicts excerpts of the boundaries of the session.

Because participants from several disciplines and departments were working together in one

Exhibit 20–4 Design Rules

What's In	What's Out
• Process flows	• Organizational structure
• Policies and procedures	• Staffing levels
• Care management tools	• Compensation

location for extended periods of time, it was necessary to establish ground rules to ensure the most successful results. The agenda allowed for a brief discussion of the ground rules. To focus this discussion and keep it concise, session leaders proposed a list of ground rules and allowed the participants to react to the list. Participants suggested revisions, additions, and deletions and ultimately reached consensus on what rules they would abide by throughout the session. Below is the list of ground rules the health system used during their care management design session:

- Design decisions will be based on what is best for the system as a whole, not on what is best for individual stakeholders.
- We commit to the process and to the design decisions that are made during the session.
- Design decisions will be based on the 80/20 rule (i.e., sufficient for 80 percent of the situation vs. a perfect solution).
- Leave titles at the door: Fully leverage all of the expertise in the room.
- Teams will complete their work products on time and be prepared for presentations.
- We will openly accept facilitator guidance and input when teams are having difficulty reaching a decision.
- Deliverables will be comprehensive and detailed.
- Respect the agenda: Arrive on time for each session, after meals, and breaks.
- Turn off all pagers and cellular phones during the session.
- Manage your own energy.

Guiding principles, assumptions, components, roles, and functions that supported the case management model are provided in Exhibits 20–5 and 20–6.

Work Groups

Several times throughout the session, the agenda called for the participants to be divided into small work groups of 15–20 individuals who were charged with a task to be completed within a specified time frame. These breakout sessions allowed critical work to be done simultaneously by session participants. Each group focused on specific decision points, thereby ensuring that all of the key processes were covered during the session. These multidisciplinary teams each had accountability for the development of processes and related tools. Work prod-

Exhibit 20–5 Guiding Principles

- Care coordination will be patient and family focused.
- Physician involvement and multidisciplinary communication, coordination, and collaboration along the continuum will be established as key cornerstones of the model.
- The integrated model will be positioned to be responsive to the changing payer and health care environment.
- The care management model will preserve the uniqueness of the health system.
- Industry leading practices will be used to design essential critical care coordination function, including a common set of definitions, processes, policies, and procedures.
- Customized methods, tools, and indicators will be used to track patient clinical measures, service measures, and efficiency in resource utilization.
- Current information technology systems will be maximized and additional technology enablers will be identified to support efficiency and communication throughout the continuum of care.

Exhibit 20–6 Care Management Model Assumptions

In preparation for the Rapid Design session, a framework and set of assumptions were developed. Initial assumptions of the model include the following:

- Care management resources will be deployed by patient population.
- On-site coverage will be provided 7 days a week, including the Preservice Center and emergency department.
- The focus will be on multidisciplinary collaboration.
- Results or status of activities will be measured and information will be used to enhance processes.
- Care management will ensure effective transitions between all levels of care (preacute, acute, and postacute) and include key linkages to payers and hospitals.
- The model will improve the processes and communication among payers, physicians, and the health system with regard to concurrent review and discharge planning.
- Consistent, timely, and optimal physician support will be constructed within the model to ensure buy-in and timely resolution of clinical care coordination issues.
- The model will ensure knowledge transfer to the health system to ensure successful implementation in other facilities.

ucts included process flow diagrams, screening templates, payer grids, relevant care management policies and procedures, job descriptions for individuals participating in the care management process, a communication plan, and an education plan.

To produce quality deliverables in the specified time frame, facilitators and recorders supported each group. The facilitators had a clear understanding of the content being discussed, as well as the tasks the groups were charged with completing. The facilitator's main role was to keep the group focused on the task at hand and foster an environment in which the pertinent issues could surface and reach resolution before time expired. The facilitator also assisted the small groups in preparing a summary of their work to present to the large group.

The recorder was responsible for capturing the ideas and outputs of the group once group members reached consensus on a particular issue. Like the facilitator, it was helpful for the recorder to be knowledgeable about the content and understand the deliverable(s) the groups were expected to produce. However, the recorder's main role was to document the information in an organized format using electronic templates for the process flows, policy and procedures, matrix, spreadsheets, and so on. The work products were then presented to the small group for validation and later shared with the large group for input and clarifications. The actual documentation from the entire session was collated and captured in a journal that represents an exact account of all of the decisions and recommendations to be taken forward into implementation.

On the second day of the Rapid Design session, the participants were reconfigured into new teams to develop the high-level implementation plan for the new case management model.

Education Plan Summary

After a large-group discussion around the purpose and goals associated with creating an education program for the new case management model, an education plan was developed for the health system staff in three specific areas of care—inpatient, preacute, and nonacute/community-based services.

Among each of the groups, it was generally agreed that the overall goal would be for all staff, including physicians, to be educated about the new case management model, specifically the goals of the model. In conjunction with a target date for implementation, the education group felt that the education plan should be rolled out over a three-month time period. The three subgroups devised educational components in the form of video learning, classroom teaching, and computer-based training modules.

A discussion took place regarding the need for physicians to "buy in" to the health system's overall vision and goals for the new case management model. It was generally felt that without buy-in, there would be very little change in how the health system currently operates. Participants felt that physicians have been educated about issues, such as denial management, in the past, and there has been little or no change in behaviors as a result of this education. There was strong agreement that for the new case management model to be effective, there would have to be some formal education for physicians.

Communicating the new case management model to all stakeholders within the system is key to the successful implementation and ongoing support of the program. The communication work group identified and prioritized all stakeholder groups and then brainstormed ideas related to the message, the method, and the timeline for systemwide communication. Additional plan design will be required by the implementation subteam; however, it is imperative to initiate and roll out the initial phases of the communication plan immediately.

A team was convened to address human resource issues pertaining to the case management redesign. Two issues were addressed: minimum qualifications for the key positions for case management and the construction of a typical case management team in terms of ratio of staff to patients.

Each work group from day one identified and documented the technology requirements that will be necessary for successful implementation of the new care management model.

SUGGESTED READING

P.E. Plsek, *Creativity, Innovation, and Quality* (Milwaukee, WI: ASQ Quality Press, 1997).

CHAPTER 21

Improving the Care of Complex Populations: A Case Study in Clinical Redesign of Patients with Acute Myocardial Infarction

Nancy L. Brennan

TAKE THIS TO WORK

1. Collaborative improvement in acute myocardial infarction management requires large-scale participation of cardiac services stakeholders.
2. Design emphasizes optimal medication orders, intensive care unit use, transfer criteria, and data monitoring.

Most health systems have invested energy in creating clinical pathways with variable success. Such approaches, even when successful, are primarily applicable to the care of the uncomplicated patient. Improving the care of a complex population and successfully implementing the design to achieve results is more difficult. The purpose of this chapter is to describe a highly customizable approach to redesigning the care of complex populations using accelerated large-group facilitation (Rapid Design). This approach achieves improved performance while maintaining or improving quality and service delivery. A case study will be used to illustrate the approach: clinical redesign within a multihospital health system.

INITIAL BUY-IN

A large-scale redesign of the care management infrastructure was completed so that it would be operative when implementation was ready to begin for the clinical redesign initiatives. Many interactions with the physicians had already occurred when the clinical redesign initiatives were begun.

The primary motivating factor for both the system and the physicians was financial. For the first time in this system's history, physician incomes had begun to fall. For the individual hospitals, a decline in margin had been noted as well. Without a dramatic change in practice, a net revenue loss was anticipated within three years. The recent financial plight came as a result of the Balanced Budget Act, with commercial payers moving increasingly to basing their rates on Medicare allowables. The clinical redesign initiatives were constructed to produce financial advantages for both the hospital and physicians.

IDENTIFICATION OF AREAS NEEDING IMPROVEMENT

Following the initial cultural work to create necessary agreement on approach, a series of one-on-one meetings with key stakeholders in the cardiology service line occurred. Beginning with the chairman of cardiology, an in-depth discussion with an Ernst & Young consultant focused on the probable areas of improvement.

The deliverables that would need to be created in order to harvest the improvement and set the stage for implementation were also preliminarily defined. This highly customized approach allows for the unearthing of sensitive issues, which are cultural blocks to the effective delivery of care, as well as more direct straightforward issues, which are more logistic in nature.

Following the initial interview with the key physician(s), one-on-one or small group meetings were held with other key stakeholders. In this instance, the nursing director, nursing manager, nurse practitioner, respiratory therapist, and staff nurses were all interviewed in depth. With each succeeding interview, the list of probable areas for improvement and key deliverables evolved. Prior to the actual design session, the refined lists (probable areas for improvement and key deliverables) were again reviewed with the key sponsor to finalize them and incorporate the input from the remainder of the team.

Following is an excerpt of anticipated opportunities for improvement at this multihospital system:

- Develop a systemwide therapeutic approach to the management of patients with acute myocardial infarction (AMI, DRG 121), which accomplishes the following:
  - Align care to be consistent with best practice.
  - Streamline patient management and movement throughout the system.
  - Reduce variation in physician practice patterns.
  - Eliminate medically unnecessary days.
  - Provide a "one standard" of care reputation within the community.
  - Provide program differentiation for competitive advantage.
  - Reduce variation in hospital utilization and costs.
- Develop clinical algorithms to expedite treatment decisions and expand treatment options.
- Develop systemwide clinical guidelines to facilitate reperfusion therapies.
- Establish a consistent approach to patient and family education.

In addition to defining the probable areas of improvement, the key deliverables of the session were also defined through the iterative interviewing process, but they are beyond the scope of this chapter.

DATA COLLECTION AND ANALYSIS

The above-defined areas for improvement and anticipated deliverables were used to drive the data collection and analysis. Data were drawn from several sources in preparation for this Rapid Design session in order to allow team members to understand their own current practices from a national perspective. The group began their discussions by looking at national benchmarks and then proceeded to review data from "like" hospitals. Once the group reviewed external benchmarks, they then looked at internal variability within their own practices. Although most "findings" and recommendations were a product of discussion among participants, comparative data were used to both stimulate thinking and validate findings of current practices.

Although some of the hospitals practiced within benchmark ranges, the data showed that variability existed throughout the system, with opportunities for improvement. The hospitals' length of stay (LOS) drawn from hospital financial databases ranged from 4.4 to 8.4 days for AMI (Figure 21–1).

Cost per case ranged from $5,306 to $10,476 (Figure 21–2). Team members were able to review their own data reflecting current practices during the Rapid Design session. The data proved to be useful in stimulating discussions among the team members.

Chart abstraction was done on 20 percent of the annual patient volume for DRG 121 during calendar year 1998.

DESIGN GROUP AGENDA

Prior to the actual design session, several preparations occurred in addition to the interviews and data analysis. An exhaustive literature search was completed to illustrate leading practices in both cost reduction and heightened quality/service delivery. The actual agenda for the

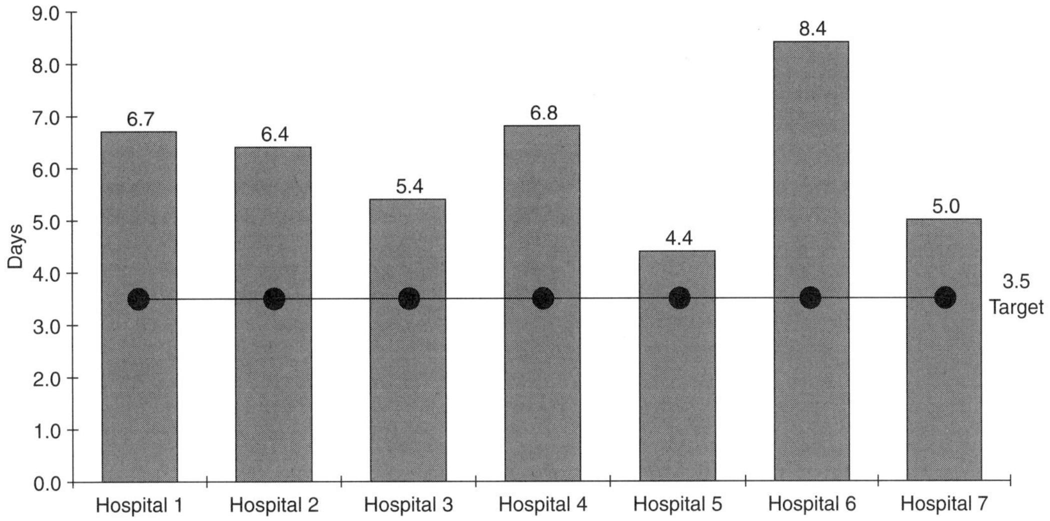

Figure 21–1 Comparison of Average Length of Stay for Acute Myocardial Infarction

session was designed with the key sponsors and customized to the system's specific situation and culture.

The session was scheduled to span two days.

- Day one: 8 AM to 6 PM
- Day two: 8 AM to 6 PM

Cardiology, cardiovascular, family practice, internal medicine, and emergency physicians attended from each of the hospitals within the system and shared their collective expertise and experience while contributing to the design.

ACTUAL DESIGN SESSION

During the actual design session, the data were initially reviewed in detail by the design team. The group was surprised at the variation in physician practice across the system, especially LOS, cost per case, throughput times, and the number of tests performed on each patient. The literature was reviewed for key ideas to be used in design, and those potential ideas were summarized and prioritized. Then the design phase began, with the group focusing on the creation of the specific deliverables that would result in achieving their target. The overall design team included approximately 25 persons, was multidisciplinary in nature, and represented physicians, nursing, care management, respiratory therapy, social services, home health, pharmacy, and laboratory services.

In order to achieve the deliverables, considerable negotiation was necessary to finalize the design. These sessions typically involve not only intellectual work, but also discussion regarding varying interests.

Deliverables, as they evolved over the session, were targeted to affect high leverage points for quality of care and cost savings. Clinical algorithms detailed the flow of patients from onset of symptoms to definitive treatment and ultimately discharge. Clinical flows, care guidelines, protocols, and orders sets were designed to enable "one standard" of care that promotes best practice, service, and cost awareness. A systemwide definition of clinical endpoints together with variance tracking will reinforce "one standard" across the system. The standardization of treatment technique in conjunction with pharmacologic and diagnostic testing guidelines is anticipated to reduce discretionary variability in resource use. In general, the bulk of cost savings results from a reduction in throughput times and in avoidable days.

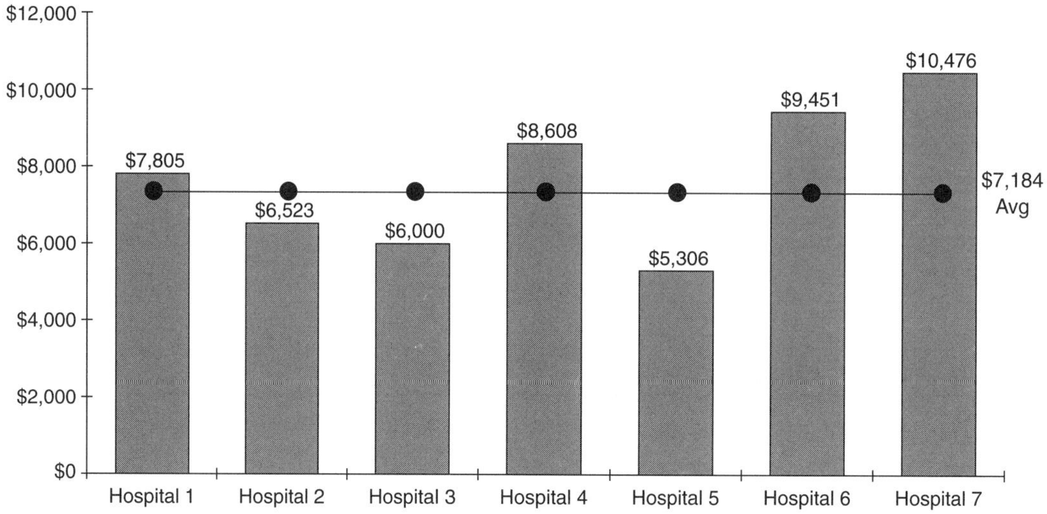

Figure 21–2 Cost per Case Comparison for Acute Myocardial Infarction

Some cost savings could eventually accrue from a reduction in supply costs, certain pharmaceuticals, and the use of laboratory tests and imaging.

PROBABLE COST SAVINGS

Based on benchmarking analysis and what the team believed could be achieved with the new "designs," it was determined that approximately 1,773 patient/bed days could be reduced. This LOS reduction took into consideration AMI, angina, and chest pain. The decrease in LOS, after considering revenue impact, translated into an opportunity of approximately $289,000.

IMPLEMENTATION

An exciting momentum is generated during these sessions. In order to avoid loss of that momentum, preliminary implementation team membership is established prior to leaving the session. After the Rapid Design session is completed, implementation begins. Implementation support typically includes putting together a service-based implementation team that is co-led by the chairman of cardiology and a nurse manager. The team defines and initiates the implementation work plan, timeline, roles and responsibilities, and education plan, and finalizes the deliverables produced during the Rapid Design session (e.g., policies and procedures, etc.). Ideally, the first implementation team meeting is held within two to four weeks of the session.

In conclusion, this approach allows for redesign of the care of complex populations through a customized definition of the key areas of improvement and deliverables based on both the specifics of the organization and the population of patients. It requires rigorous analysis of data and the provision of leading interventions in care design. It results in exciting synergy within organizations and highly customized designs, because, unlike conventional planning, a greater number of multidisciplinary stakeholders is in the session, time compression allows completion of the same process ordinarily requiring several months, and *independent professionals who have done this in multiple sites around the country are able to accelerate decisions with unique skill in large-group facilitation.*

Chapter 22

Improving the Care of Complex Populations: A Case Study in Clinical Redesign on Extremely Immature Neonates

David W. Plocher and Lana S. Peters

TAKE THIS TO WORK

1. Lessons learned with immature neonate study include a lack of precision around diagnosis-related group-based benchmarking.
2. Clinical redesign and patient management should be targeted at high leverage points for cost savings, including intubation time, neonatal intensive care unit length of stay, and postneonatal intensive care unit length of stay.

Most health systems have invested energy in creating clinical pathways with variable success. Such approaches, even when successful, are primarily applicable to the care of the uncomplicated patient. Improving the care of a complex population and successfully implementing the design to achieve results is more difficult. The purpose of this chapter is to describe a highly customizable approach to redesigning the care of complex populations using accelerated large-group facilitation (Rapid Design). This approach achieves improved performance while maintaining or improving quality and service delivery. A case study will be used to illustrate the approach: clinical redesign within a large academic health system for extremely immature neonates.

INITIAL BUY-IN

A large-scale redesign of the care management infrastructure was completed so that it would be operative when implementation was ready to begin for the clinical redesign initiatives. Much interaction with the physicians had already occurred when the clinical redesign initiatives were begun.

The primary motivating factor for both the system and the physicians was financial. For the hospital, a net revenue loss was anticipated within three years. Historically, the hospital had been relatively untouched by managed care. The recent financial plight came as a result of the Balanced Budget Act, with commercial payers moving increasingly to basing their rates on Medicare allowables. The clinical redesign initiatives were constructed to produce financial advantages for both the hospital and physicians.

Acknowledgments: We wish to express our gratitude to A. Patricia Johnson, Vice President, Operations/Chief Nurse Executive; Caroline Gentleman, Director, Inpatient Case Management; and Mary Ann Anderson, Director of Nursing, North Carolina Baptist Hospital of Wake Forest University Baptist Medical Center.

IDENTIFICATION OF AREAS NEEDING IMPROVEMENT

Following the initial cultural work to create necessary agreement on approach, a series of one-on-one meetings with key stakeholders in neonatal care delivery occurred. Beginning with the chairman of neonatology, an in-depth discussion with an Ernst & Young consultant focused on the probable areas of improvement. The deliverables that would need to be created in order to harvest the improvement and set the stage for implementation were also preliminarily defined. This highly customized approach allows for the unearthing of sensitive issues that are cultural blocks to the effective delivery of care as well as more direct straightforward issues that are more logistic in nature.

Following the initial interview with the key physician(s), one-on-one or small group meetings were held with other key stakeholders. In this instance, the neonatal nurse coordinator, nursing director, nursing manager, nurse practitioner, and respiratory therapist were all interviewed in depth. With each succeeding interview, the list of probable areas for improvement and key deliverables evolved. Prior to the actual design session, the refined lists (probable areas for improvement and key deliverables) were again reviewed with the key sponsor to finalize them and incorporate the input from the remainder of the team.

Exhibit 22–1 provides an excerpt of anticipated opportunities for improvement at this medical center.

In addition to defining the probable areas of improvement, key deliverables of the session were also defined through the iterative interviewing process.

Exhibit 22–1 Probable Areas for Improvement

- Management and movement of neonates through the system
- Discharge planning/discharge criteria
- Ventilator weaning and oxygen support
- Utilization of ABGs and other lab tests
- Utilization of routine chest X-rays and other tests
- Fluid management
- Family teaching

DATA COLLECTION AND ANALYSIS

The above-defined areas for improvement and anticipated deliverables were used to drive the data collection and analysis. Data were drawn from several sources in preparation for this Rapid Design session in order to allow team members to understand their own current practices from a national perspective. The group began their discussions by looking at national benchmarks and then proceeded to review data from "like" hospitals. Once the group reviewed external benchmarks, they then looked at internal variability within their own practices. Although most "findings" and recommendations were a product of discussion among participants, comparative data were used to both stimulate thinking and validate findings of current practices.

Because it was important for the team to review data that benchmarked "similar" institutions, University Hospital Consortium data were reviewed. This was drawn from a comparative database for cost and length of stay (LOS) that is made up of 63 of the nation's leading academic medical centers (AMCs). These data excluded outliers and represented 1997 experience. Although this hospital practiced within benchmark ranges for other AMCs, the data showed that opportunities for improvement still existed. University benchmarks ranged from 23 to 53 days average LOS for diagnosis-related group (DRG) 386. This hospital's LOS, according to the same source, was 38 days. Benchmarks for cost per case ranged from $20,000 to $55,000. This hospital's average cost per case was $38,000. The data proved to be useful in stimulating discussions among the team members. Subsequently, the team agreed that the DRG classification system was a crude measurement scheme for this population. More accurate patient segmentation (e.g., by grams) was initiated using the Vermont Oxford database (this analysis was ongoing at the time of publication).

Team members were able to review their own data reflecting current practices during the Rapid Design session. Chart abstraction was done on 20 percent of the annual patient volume for DRG 386 during calendar year 1998. Data points that peaked the team's interest regarding their own practices included number of blood gases performed, units of packed cells administered, days on ventilator, and days in the neonatal intensive care unit (NICU).

DESIGN GROUP AGENDA

Prior to the actual design session, several preparations were made in addition to the interviews and data analysis. An exhaustive literature search was completed to illustrate leading practices in both cost reduction and heightened quality/service delivery. The actual agenda for the session was designed with the key sponsors and customized to the medical center's specific situation and culture.

The session was scheduled to span three days.

- Day one: 3 PM to 7 PM
- Day two: 10 AM to 7 PM
- Day three: 10 AM to 7 PM

The chairman of neonatology arranged for key physicians to be present for selected hours in the session and then for a review and validation session one week after the initial design session.

ACTUAL DESIGN SESSION

During the actual design session, the data were initially reviewed in detail by the design team. The group was surprised by it, especially the number of tests that were being performed on each neonate. The literature was reviewed for key ideas to be used in design and those potential ideas were summarized. Then the design phase began, with the group focusing on the creation of the specific deliverables that would result in achieving their target. The overall design team included approximately 20 persons, representing such areas as nursing, case management, respiratory care, social services, home health, pharmacy, and lab.

In order to achieve the deliverables, considerable negotiation was necessary to finalize the design. These sessions typically involve not only intellectual work, but also considerable discussion regarding varying interests.

The design session ultimately resulted in the completion of multiple specific, practical outputs ready for implementation, which are beyond the scope of this chapter.

These deliverables, as they evolved over the session, were targeted to affect high leverage points for cost savings and appropriate treatment for patients. Respiratory support protocols to allow for more effective weaning and NICU discharge criteria will allow for earlier discharge from the ICU. Standing order sets in conjunction with pharmacological and diagnostic testing guidelines are anticipated to reduce discretionary variability in resource use. In general, the bulk of cost savings will result from a reduction in intubation time, NICU LOS, and post-NICU LOS.

Some cost savings could eventually accrue from a reduction in supply costs, certain pharmaceuticals (especially parenteral), and use of laboratory tests and imaging.

PROBABLE COST SAVINGS

Based on benchmarking analysis and what the team believed could be achieved with the new "designs," it was determined that approximately 1,400 patient/bed days could be reduced, or approximately 10 days per case. This LOS reduction took into consideration both transfers from the NICU to a lower level of care and overall LOS reduction. This decrease in LOS, after considering revenue impact, translated into an opportunity of approximately $300,000.

One year after the Rapid Design session, LOS performance measurements were ascertained. As Figure 22–1 illustrates, LOS was reduced by approximately 43%, surpassing the original goal for FY 2000.

IMPLEMENTATION

An exciting momentum is generated during these sessions. In order to avoid loss of that mo-

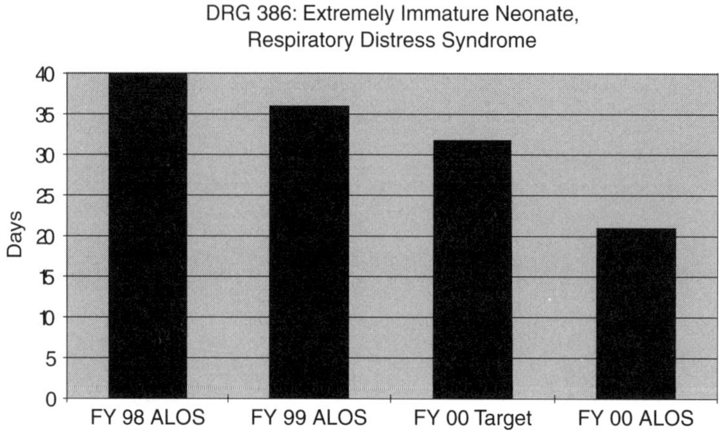

Figure 22–1 Length of Stay Performance Measurements

mentum, preliminary implementation team membership is established prior to leaving the session. After the Rapid Design session is completed, implementation begins. Implementation support typically includes putting together a service-based implementation team that is co-led by the chairman of neonatology and the nurse manager. Two one-day sessions were conducted initially to produce the implementation work plan, timeline, roles and responsibilities, and education plan, and begin finalization of the deliverables produced during the Rapid Design session (e.g., policies and procedures, etc.).

Ideally, the first implementation team meeting is held within two to four weeks of the session, with finalization of the first draft of the journal from the session by two weeks postsession for review. Implementation is optimally begun within a month postsession. Because of competing organizational initiatives, implementation was started three months post-Rapid Design session. By this time, team participants were anxious to begin implementing their "designs."

In conclusion, this approach allows for redesign of the care of complex populations through a customized definition of the key areas of improvement and deliverables based on both the details of the organization and the population of patients. It requires rigorous detailed analysis of relevant data and the provision of leading interventions in care design. It results in exciting synergy within organizations and highly customized designs, because, unlike conventional planning, a greater number of multidisciplinary stakeholders is in the session, time compression allows completion of the same process ordinarily requiring several months, and *independent professionals who have done this in multiple sites around the country are able to accelerate decisions with unique skill in large-group facilitation.*

SUGGESTED READINGS

D. Adamkin, "Issues in the Nutritional Support of the Ventilated Baby," *Clinics in Perinatology 25,* no. 1 (March 1998): 79–96.

Committee on Fetus and Newborn, "Hospital Discharge of the High-Risk Neonate—Proposed Guidelines," *American Academy of Pediatrics 102,* no. 2, pt. 1 (August 1998): 411–417.

L.M. Doyle and P. Davis, "Assisted Ventilation and Survival of Extremely Low Birthweight Infants," *Journal of Pediatrics and Child Health 32,* no. 2 (1996): 138–142.

"Management of Pediatric Patients Requiring Long-Term Ventilation," *Chest 113,* suppl. 5 (May 1998): 322S–343S.

P. Kongstvedt, "Using Data in Medical Management" in *Best Practices in Medical Management*, eds. P. Kongstvedt and D. Plocher (Gaithersburg, MD: Aspen Publishers, Inc., 1998), 440–451.

P.H. Perlstein et al., "Physician Variations and the Ancillary Costs of Neonatal Intensive Care," *Health Services Research 32,* no. 3 (August 1997): 299–311.

CHAPTER 23

Improving the Care of Complex Populations: A Case Study in Clinical Redesign on a Trauma Service

Wendy L. Wilson

TAKE THIS TO WORK

1. Trauma care redesign requires collaboration with multiple surgical specialties.
2. Key opportunities for improvement are found in intensive care unit use, drug use, supplies, discharge planning, and data monitoring.

Most health systems have invested great energy in creating clinical pathways with variable success. Such approaches, even when highly successful, are only applicable to the care of simple populations. Improving the care of a complex population and successfully implementing the design to achieve results are much more difficult. The purpose of this chapter is to describe a highly customizable approach to redesigning the care of complex populations using accelerated large-group facilitation (Rapid Design). This approach achieves improved financial performance while maintaining or bettering quality and service delivery. A case study will be used to illustrate the approach: clinical redesign at a major trauma center within a large academic health system.

Acknowledgments: We wish to express our gratitude to A. Patricia Johnson, Vice President, Operations/Chief Nurse Executive; Caroline Gentleman, Director, Inpatient Case Management; and Mary Ann Anderson, Director of Nursing, North Carolina Baptist Hospital of Wake Forest University Baptist Medical Center.

INITIAL BUY-IN

Initially, buy-in must be created among the key stakeholders. A large-scale redesign of the care management infrastructure was completed so that it would be operative when implementation was ready to begin for the clinical redesign initiatives. Much interaction with the physicians had already occurred when the clinical redesign initiatives were begun.

The primary motivating factor for both the system and the physicians was financial. For the hospital, a net revenue loss was anticipated within three years. Historically, the hospital had been relatively untouched by managed care. Its recent financial impact came as a result of the Balanced Budget Act, with commercial payers moving increasingly to basing their rates on Medicare allowables. These changes had impacted both physician and hospital financials, an impact that was expected to increase over time. This provided a strong platform for change. The clinical redesign initiatives were constructed to produce financial advantages for both the hospital and physicians.

IDENTIFICATION OF AREAS NEEDING IMPROVEMENT

Following the initial cultural work to create necessary preliminary buy-in to the approach, a series of one-on-one meetings with key stakeholders in trauma care delivery occurred. Beginning with the chairman of surgery (leading trauma surgeon), an in-depth discussion with an Ernst & Young physician consultant focused on the probable areas of improvement. The deliverables that would need to be created in order to harvest the improvement and set the stage for implementation were also preliminarily defined. For each system and patient population, it is expected that these areas of improvement and key deliverables will vary to some degree.

Following the initial interview with the key physician(s), one-on-one or small group meetings were held with other key stakeholders. In this instance, the trauma nurse coordinator, nursing director, case manager, and physical therapist were all interviewed in depth. With each succeeding interview, the list of probable areas for improvement and key deliverables was further refined. Prior to the design session, the refined lists (probable areas for improvement and key deliverables) were again reviewed with the key sponsor to finalize them and incorporate the input from the remainder of the team.

For this medical center, the areas listed in Exhibit 23–1 were defined as probable areas of improvement.

Exhibit 23–1 Probable Areas for Improvement

- Time and initial process through emergency department
- Length of stay/Bounce Back Rate/Intensive care unit length of stay/Use or lack thereof of intermediate care status
- Discharge planning
- Time for C-spine clearance and initiation of mobilization of patient
- Documentation of minimal cognitive deficits and postdischarge needs
- Utilization of key drugs (antiembolic protocol, Zantac, antibiotics)

In addition to defining the probable areas of improvement, the key deliverables of the session were also defined through the iterative interviewing process. Those deliverables were defined before the session.

DATA COLLECTION AND ANALYSIS

The above-defined areas for improvement and anticipated deliverables were used to drive the data collection and analysis. A sample was taken from the trauma registry, including all patients who met trauma triage criteria for the previous year for the months of January, April, July, and October. This sample totaled 500 admissions. Additional detailed data analysis was done by completing chart abstraction. In addition to the analysis of the trauma registry sample and the chart abstraction, extensive benchmarking data were analyzed and displayed.*

All of the above data revealed a high quality of care and good efficiency in terms of cost per day. However, in every set of data examined, the length of stay (LOS) was long versus benchmarks, and the intensive care unit (ICU) LOS was also prolonged. Their opportunity clearly rested in reducing general LOS and ICU LOS.

The data set was also used to calculate the actual revenue versus costs from the previous year. From these data, on the trauma service for the year, the losses (hospital side) were large, totaling more than $7 million. When referenced to benchmark data, if this group could reduce LOS to a best practice level, it was likely that those losses could be largely eradicated, with anticipated savings on the order of several million dollars annually.

The trauma registry data were sorted by several small populations (e.g., upper extremity/shoulder/chest fractures, hip/pelvic/lower extremity fractures, brain injury, spine injury, multiple trauma). The payer mix was calculated for all of these groups, as well as for the overall sample. Their payer mix was favorable with re-

---

*UHC data provided by the medical center and regional trauma data courtesy of Bishop Consulting.

gard to LOS reduction. In greater than 80 percent of cases overall, a financial advantage would occur with a reduction in LOS, with high proportions of self-pay, Medicare, and managed Medicaid (diagnosis-related group [DRG]-like payment mechanism). Therefore, even when the revenue impact was calculated from losses in per diem payments, it was anticipated that the savings would be considerable. In conjunction with their work with another consulting firm (Bishop Consulting), they were also renegotiating the payer contracts from a per diem basis to a DRG-like or case-rate payment (or other arrangement that favored LOS reduction).

DESIGN GROUP AGENDA

Before the actual design session, several preparations were made in addition to the interviews and data analysis. An exhaustive literature search was completed to illustrate best practices in both cost reduction and heightened quality/service delivery. The actual agenda for the session was designed with the key sponsors and customized to the medical center's specific situation and culture.

The session was scheduled to span three days.

- Day one: 3 PM to 7 PM
- Day two: 10 AM to 7 PM
- Day three: 10 AM to 7 PM

ACTUAL DESIGN SESSION

During the actual design session, the data were initially reviewed in detail by the design team. The group was surprised by it, especially the magnitude of current financial losses. The literature was reviewed for key ideas to be used in design and those potential ideas were summarized. Then the design phase began, with the group focusing on the creation of the specific deliverables that would result in achieving the target. The overall design team was large, totaling more than 50 persons for the trauma clinical redesign event.

In order to achieve the deliverables, considerable negotiation was necessary to finalize the design. These sessions typically involve not only intellectual work, but also considerable discussion regarding varying interests.

Deliverables, as they evolved over the session, were targeted to affect high leverage points for cost savings. In general, the bulk of cost savings result from four key areas.

1. reduction in LOS
2. venue of care (reduction in ICU LOS)
3. drugs
4. supplies

Some cost savings eventually accrue from a reduction in the use of laboratory and radiology tests, but until sufficient reduction occurs to impact full-time equivalents (FTEs), the cost savings are minimal. So although these (lab and radiology tests) are addressed above, the primary targets are the noted higher leverage areas.

In particular, the spine clearance process, the team communication process, and the setting of functional/medical and LOS targets on admission to the floor are anticipated to have a large impact on overall LOS. Short-term restructuring to create intermediate care beds with additional respiratory support, increased respiratory care support to allow for more effective weaning, and ICU discharge criteria will allow for earlier discharge from the ICU. Standing order sets in conjunction with pharmacological guidelines for key drugs will impact utilization. Additionally, the sedation protocol is intended to reduce oversedation to allow for earlier weaning and discharge from the ICU. Some key quality issues were also addressed (such as screening for minimal cognitive deficits previous to discharge).

In this institution, the attending trauma surgery staffing was limited. To achieve the best practice targets, it is likely that they will need to double their attending staffing from two dedicated trauma surgeons to four. With the likely savings that will result, this becomes financially feasible.

PROBABLE COST SAVINGS

On benchmarking versus average practice, approximately 5,000 patient/bed days can be re-

Table 23–1 Anticipated Financial Benefit with Reduced LOS

Improvement Level	*Necessary Changes*	*Anticipated LOS Reduction*	*Range of Anticipated Savings*
Average	Short-term delivery reconfiguration; immediate process changes	5,000 patient bed days	$2.5 million to $3.75 million
Best practice	Addition of two trauma surgeons	10,000 patient bed days	$5 million to $7.5 million

duced. This equates to a decrease in the average LOS of three days. On benchmarking versus best practice in the trauma resource network (done by Bishop Consulting), approximately 10,000 patient/bed days can be reduced. This decrease in LOS translates to the approximate financial targets listed in Table 23–1.

IMPLEMENTATION

Exciting momentum is generated during these sessions. This particular clinical redesign session was especially dynamic. In order to avoid loss of that momentum, implementation team membership is established before leaving the session. The first implementation team meeting is held within two to four weeks of the session, with finalization of the first draft of the journal from the session by two weeks. Implementation is optimally begun within a month postsession.

In conclusion, this approach allows for redesign of the care of complex populations through a customized definition of the key areas of improvement and deliverables based on both the specifics of the organization and the population of patients. It requires rigorous analysis of data and the provision of leading interventions in care design. It results in exciting synergy within organizations and highly customized designs, because, unlike conventional planning, a greater number of multidisciplinary stakeholders is in the session, time compression allows completion of the same process ordinarily requiring several months, and *independent professionals who have done this in multiple sites around the country are able to accelerate decisions with unique skill in large-group facilitation.*

Glossary

Abuse—incidents or practices of physicians or other providers or suppliers of services that are contrary to sound medical practices; that directly or indirectly result in some improper gain or unnecessary costs to the program; or program payment for services that fail to meet recognized standards of care or are medically unnecessary.

Access—the availability of services through the admissions process, emergency center presentation, outpatient services including day surgery, and all other services offered by a specific facility.

Administrative denial (Technical)—denials issued by the payer on the basis of noncompliance with technical or administrative contract requirements unrelated to patient care.

Admitting diagnosis—an initial impression/diagnosis made by the physician.

Ambulatory patient classification (APC)—the unit of payment (similar to the diagnosis-related group inpatient payment) used in the outpatient prospective payment system that groups outpatient services that are alike from a clinical and resource utilization perspective.

American Health Information Management Association (AHIMA)—the national professional organization that credentials registered health information administrators (RHIAs), registered health information technicians (RHITs), and certified coding specialists (CCSs); one of the four cooperating parties.

American Hospital Association (AHA)—the organization that houses and staffs the Central Office on *ICD-9-CM* and publishes *Coding Clinic for ICD-9-CM*; one of the four cooperating parties.

Appeal—a verbal or written request by the provider for the payer to reconsider an earlier denial decision and issue payment for the claim.

Avoidable days in service—a patient day at a level of care that is higher than the treatment needs require. Reasons include inability to deliver treatment or provide testing when required, lack of information to carry out treatment, lack of coordination or planning for discharge, and patient/family or attending physician disagreement with the plan to discharge or transfer.

Care management—the processes used by the case manager to facilitate care and manage resources throughout the patient's course of illness, with equal emphasis on the management of care outside of the acute care setting.

Case management—the processes used by the case manager to facilitate care and manage resources during the acute episode of care.

Case mix index (CMI)—the calculation reflecting the cost of treating all Medicare inpatient cases in a particular facility relative to the national average cost of treating all Medicare inpatient cases in the United States.

Clinical denial—denials issued by the payer on the basis of the absence of documented medical necessity or failure to meet severity of illness and intensity of service criteria that would justify the services provided, either for the entire admission or for individual days.

Coding Clinic for ICD-9-CM—the publication of the American Hospital Association's

Central Office on *ICD-9-CM* that provides coding information and official *ICD-9-CM* coding guidelines as unanimously approved by the four cooperating parties (the American Hospital Association, the National Center for Health Statistics, the Health Care Financing Administration, and the American Health Information Management Association).

Coinsurance—the percentage or dollar amount of the provider fee the member pays for a service rendered. Most commonly arises in prospective payment systems with the health plan paying 80 percent and the member paying 20 percent.

Comorbidity—a condition that coexists with the principal diagnosis at the time of admission that can, with the specific principal diagnosis, affect the treatment received, the length of stay, or the cost of care, and, consequently, the Medicare payment.

Complication—a condition arising after the time of admission that can, with specific principal diagnosis, affect the treatment received, the length of stay, or the cost of care, and, consequently, the Medicare payment.

Compromise—one party in an interaction acquiescing his or her interests and expectations to those of another party.

Cooperating parties—a partnership, consisting of representatives from the American Hospital Association, the National Center for Health Statistics, the Health Care Financing Administration, and the American Health Information Management Association, that is recognized as the official authority on *ICD-9-CM* coding in the United States.

Concurrent review—applies the same tools and process as the initial review, and is completed to identify the need for continuing the inpatient stay, or continuing care in the current level of care. Concurrent review allows for an evaluation of the use of clinical resources and is an essential component of care facilitation.

Consensus—implies a dialogue in which both parties are open to evaluating and adjusting their expectations during the course of the exchange. Rather than being forfeited, expectations are voluntarily moved toward a center point where a mutually acceptable outcome can be achieved.

Copayment—the established fee the managed care member pays for a service received. Most commonly arises in health maintenance organizations, with the member paying a small percentage of the fee up front.

Cost to charge ratio—a high-level approach that estimates cost by the relationship of the total expenses to the total charges for an area.

Coverage/benefits—those health care services that are paid for, in full or in part, by the payer.

Deductible—the dollar portion the patient pays for services rendered. This amount is capped. Once the member has paid the cap amount, the deductible has been met and the member pays a lesser amount for each service rendered. The deductible amount is generally inversely proportional to the amount of the established monthly premium. That is, as the monthly premium is reduced, the deductible generally increases.

Denial—a decision by a third-party payer to reject full or partial payment that then results in a discrepancy between expected and received reimbursement. This can include the payer decision to reassign the diagnosis-related group under which the claim was submitted.

Department of Health and Human Services (DHHS)—the government agency responsible for administrating all federally funded health programs.

Direct variable costs—"hands-on" costs, proportional to caregiver labor, for a given day of service. For example, nursing (nonadministrative) professional, therapist, dietary, and housekeeping expenses are direct variable costs.

Discharge planning—the processes used by the case manager and the multidisciplinary team to assess a patient's needs prior to discharge and make the necessary arrangements to transition the patient from the acute care setting to the most clinically appropriate setting capable of meeting the patient's needs.

DRG (diagnosis-related group)—the grouping of patients by clinical similarity and consumption of hospital resources, under the Medicare inpatient prospective payment system.

DRG grouper—a software program used by Medicare and other third-party payers to assign each hospital inpatient discharge to a DRG on the basis of information (principal and secondary diagnoses, procedures, age, gender, and discharge status) abstracted from the patient's medical record.

Elective—services that have no time urgency and could be optional. Some examples include tonsillectomy, breast reduction surgery, and bunion surgery.

Emergent—those services that must be carried out immediately, where life or limb is at risk. Examples include compound fracture, major trauma, and status asthmaticus.

EMTALA (Emergency Medical Treatment and Active Labor Act)—the statute that governs when and how a patient may be refused treatment or transferred from one hospital to another when he or she is in unstable medical condition or how he or she may be transferred if a higher level of care is needed that is not provided locally and if the benefits of the transfer outweigh the risks of the transfer.

External factor denial—the least common denial incurred by providers. It is based on factors outside of the organization's control or that are difficult to control. An example would include maximum benefit levels that have been incurred.

Fiscal year (FY)—the operating budget year (begins October 1 for the federal government).

Fixed costs—costs that remains constant over a relevant range of activity and relative time frame. Some examples include building or equipment depreciation, certain costs associated with maintaining the physical plant, and some management or administrative costs.

Fraud—the intentional deception or misrepresentation that an individual knows or believes to be false or untrue, and makes, knowing that the deception could result in some unauthorized benefit to him- or herself or some other persons.

Health Care Financing Administration (HCFA)—the branch of the Department of Health and Human Services responsible for administrating the Medicare program and maintaining the procedure portion of the *ICD-9-CM;* one of the four cooperating parties; cochair of the *ICD-9-CM* Coordination and Maintenance Committee.

Health maintenance organization (HMO)—the insurance for which the provider holds the greatest degree of risk and in which the member has the least degree of choice.

Home health care—covers a broad range of services and provides continuous or intermittent home care to persons recovering from illness or who are chronically or terminally ill.

Hospice—a Medicare-certified program that provides palliative care to terminally ill Medicare beneficiaries with a life expectancy of six months or less. Services include nursing care, medical social services, physician, counselor, home care aide, homemaker service, medical equipment and supplies, therapies, and bereavement counseling for families. Care can be provided in a variety of settings, including inpatient and at home.

Hospital blended rate—a regulated rate calculated for a hospital to reflect inflation, technical adjustments, budgetary constraints, geographic location, local wage variations, and other factors that affect the hospital's operating budget; when multiplied by a DRG's relative weight, the result is the Medicare payment for a case in that DRG for that particular hospital.

***ICD-9-CM* Coordination and Maintenance Committee**—the committee established in 1985 to provide a public forum for discussing possible updates and revisions of the *ICD-9-CM.* It is cochaired by the Health Care Financing Administration and the National Center for Health Statistics. Petitions for creation or revision of *ICD-9-CM* codes are presented to the committee for the purpose of being able to track diagnoses or procedures by specific codes and accumulate more meaningful data.

Indemnity—that insurance for which the provider has no risk. The payer holds the risk and the member has the greatest degree of choice.

Indirect variable costs—costs that are not "hands on" in nature, but are indirectly related to a given unit of service. Examples of indirect costs would include supplies, devices, materials, drugs, imaging, and lab. Indirect variable costs are less influenced by changes in units, such as patient days, than direct variable costs.

Initial review—review performed at the point of patient entry into the inpatient care setting. The review process applies the clinical necessity criteria for services and determines the level of care and the anticipated discharge needs of the patient.

In network—the providers that have accepted the payer's predetermined financial arrangement for services. They are the providers from which the members select to receive their health care services. Generally, in-network providers are listed in a health plan's directory that is provided to the members and providers as reference.

Intensity of service—the evaluation of the patient's condition to determine if the level of care and services are such that they could be provided in a less intensive setting.

Intermediate/extended care facility—provides care for older adults who are too ill or disabled to live independently but who are not ill enough to require hospitalization. These facilities provide basic medical services short of the need for 24-hour skilled nursing care.

Long-term acute care hospital (LTACH)—Medicare prospective payment system-exempt hospitals that provide intensive medical and rehabilitation services to patients who continue to require inpatient care. The patients in these facilities often have multisystem failure that requires intensive monitoring and gradual rehabilitative intervention. One distinguishing factor of an LTACH is that it must maintain an overall average length of stay of greater than 25 days.

MDC (major diagnostic categories)—the 25 mutually exclusive categories to which DRGs are assigned, most of which are based on a particular body system.

Medical necessity—the application of clinical criteria to determine that the patient/member requires the services that he or she is seeking, and that the services are being provided in the most appropriate level of care.

Medicare code editor (MCE)—a grouper screening editor who detects and flags coding errors that appear on billing claims, including invalid diagnosis and procedure codes, invalid fourth or fifth code digits, E codes as principal diagnoses, age and gender conflicts, manifestations used as principal diagnoses, nonspecific principal diagnoses, questionable admissions, unacceptable principal diagnoses, nonspecific operating room procedures, noncovered procedures, open biopsy verification, Medicare as secondary payer alert, bilateral procedures, and invalid discharge status.

Medicare special planned readmission (MSPR)—the rule that combines two admissions into one for purposes of billing if a patient is readmitted to the hospital on an elective basis for a procedure or treatment directly related to the prior admission. The MSPR is applied unless the patient's medical condition prohibits therapy or treatment during the initial patient stay, the patient is undergoing staged treatment (e.g., chemotherapy), the patient desires a second opinion or time to consider options, or an interim patient admission occurs between the first admission and the subsequent planned readmission.

Member—a person who receives health insurance benefits from a health plan.

National Center for Health Statistics (NCHS)—one of the four cooperating parties and the cochair for the *ICD-9-CM* Coordination and Maintenance Committee. It has responsibility for maintaining the diagnosis portion of the *ICD-9-CM.*

Notice of noncoverage—a formal mechanism of informing patients that they do not meet Medicare requirements for admission and that they will be held financially liable for the cost of the inpatient care.

Observation status—a hospital outpatient designation intended to specify a level of care associated with evaluation and decision making about a diagnosis that is more accelerated than inpatient care. Observation status is used to determine the need for possible inpatient admission or to resolve clinical circumstances such that discharge to a less intensive setting is appropriate.

Out of network—providers who have not accepted the payer's predetermined financial arrangement and are not available for member selection. If a member selects an out-of-network provider, the consequences may include the member assuming financial responsibility for services, or the out-of-network provider receiving no payment for services rendered.

Payer—the health insurance company that pays for the services provided.

Payment Error Prevention Program (PEPP)—a three-year plan designed to reduce payment errors and protect the Medicare trust fund by monitoring prospective payment system hospital claims and educating providers about payment errors.

Peer review organization (PRO)—the medical review agency within each state that is contracted by HCFA to review coding, DRG assignment, medical necessity, and quality of care for Medicare patients.

Penalty statement—an acknowledgment signed and dated by physicians who treat DRG-payment-based patients—usually when the physicians are granted hospital privileges—stating they have received the Notice to Physicians delineating the penalties for misrepresenting, falsifying, or concealing essential information required for payment of federal funds. The statement must be on file in the hospital before bills are submitted to Medicare or else the claims for payment may be denied.

Per diem—a negotiated rate of payment per day.

Per member per month (PMPM)—the monthly stipend the provider receives under contract with the payer in return for providing services to a set group of members.

Physician advisor—the role of a physician who serves as a clinical resource to the case managers and who facilitates the resolution of level-of-care and utilization issues when direct communication between the case manager and attending physician is ineffective or unsuccessful.

Point of service—the health insurance in which the member has a blended health plan, preferred provider organization and HMO. If the member obtains a referral for services and obtains those services from a participating provider, the financial burden is the lowest copay, as in the HMO. If the member self-refers to an out-of-network provider, a preferred provider organization-like level of benefits is available, although an actual preferred provider organization contract normally does not exist with the out-of-network provider. Therefore, this has also been referred to as the "indemnity wraparound."

Precertification—the requirement of a member to have permission from the payer to have a specific test or procedure. Generally associated with elective or urgent cases.

Preferred provider organization (PPO)—that insurance for which the provider holds some financial risk, generally in the form of predetermined, reduced fees.

Primary diagnosis—a term used to signify the condition that consumed the most hospital resources during an inpatient stay.

Principal diagnosis (PDX)—the condition established after study, to be chiefly responsible for occasioning the admission of the patient to the hospital for care.

Principal procedure—the procedure performed for definitive, therapeutic treatment rather than for diagnostic or exploratory purposes, or one necessary to treat a complication; the procedure most related to the principal diagnosis.

Prospective Payment Assessment Commission (ProPAC)—a panel of 15 members established by Congress to provide analysis of data from Medicare billing claims and recommendations for updating and modifying the prospective payment system.

Prospective Payment System (PPS)—the payment system for Medicare acute care inpatient services based on predetermined specific rates for each hospital discharge.

Provider—the person or organization that delivers the health care services (e.g., physician, hospital).

Referral—the authorization a member receives from the primary care provider to obtain services from a specialist for specific care. Generally, referrals have either or both time limits for the use and number of visits authorized. Some referrals are so restrictive that only listed tests or procedures can be carried out without financial penalty to the specialist or member.

Relative weight—the number assigned to a DRG to indicate the relative resource consumption associated with the DRG.

Resource center—a support center designed to allow case managers to leverage routine activities, payer referrals, communication, postacute service arrangements, benefit and eligibility verification, denial management, data entry, data analysis, and variance tracking to support and administrative staff.

Retrospective review—a review that is initiated after patient discharge and that is initiated for a variety of reasons, including payer request to validate services, quality reviews, audits to reconcile services rendered against the patient bill, and denial and appeal management.

Risk stratification—a method of classifying members who have been determined to need care resources, according to the expected intensity of case management needs and the anticipated time required to meet the treatment goals established by the case manager and the member.

Secondary diagnoses (SDX)—all medical conditions, other than the principal diagnosis, that are associated with the current hospital episode.

Severity of illness—the acuity of the patient's clinical condition and the evaluation of whether the clinical condition warrants the level of care or services provided.

Sixth Scope of Work—HCFA's expansion of its focus to achieve statewide improvement in seven areas of strategic importance to the Medicare population. The seven areas of focus can be found in Chapter 9.

Skilled nursing facility (SNF)—a facility that provides 24-hour/day nursing services to convalescing patients. Emphasis is on medical nursing care that is restorative in nature. They can be free-standing or hospital based.

Spend down—a provision that enables an individual to qualify for Medicaid assistance even if the person's income or assets exceed state-defined income eligibility requirements. Each state defines its own maximum income eligibility.

Subacute care—blends the technology of hospital care with the lower cost operations of a skilled nursing facility. Subacute typically provides a wider range of medical rehabilitative and therapeutic services than the traditional skilled nursing facility, including certain monitoring and parenteral therapy.

Subacute rehabilitation—focuses on short-term (average length of stay of 25–30 days) rehabilitation for patients with medical complexities and rehabilitation needs. Patients generally require 4.0–4.5 nursing care hours per day and therapies that extend up to 3 hours per day.

Subscriber—the person who purchases the health insurance and receives the health insurance benefits.

Therapeutic procedure—a procedure performed for definitive purposes rather than diagnostic or exploratory purposes.

Total cost—a summary of the labor and nonlabor resources required to produce a hospital's final product or service.

Transfer rule—a rule set up by Medicare to prevent hospitals and other health care organizations that also own Home Health agencies and other postacute care services from "double dipping." This would imply moving patients too quickly from the acute care setting to capture the DRG payment and then moving them into the provider's own alternative care settings where they can bill for additional services.

Uniform Bill-92 (UB-92)—a billing form, created in 1982 and revised in 1992, containing the patient's charges that is submitted to Medicare and other third-party payers for payment. It provides for the listing of up to 10 diagnoses and 6 procedure codes assigned to a particular case.

Uniform Hospital Discharge Data Set (UHDDS)—created by the National Committee on Vital and Health Statistics of the U.S. Public Health Service, the UHDDS contains 14 items recommended as basic data for hospital discharge statistics: the patient's personal identification, date of birth, sex, race, ethnicity, residence, hospital identification, admission and discharge dates, physician identification (attending and surgeon), diagnoses, procedures and dates performed, disposition (discharge status) of the patient, and the expected payer for most of the bill.

Urgent—services that must be carried out, but not immediately. Examples include closed reduction of a fracture or admission for simple pneumonia.

Utilization management (UM)—the process involving the application of tools and techniques to identify and anticipate patient needs and to support proactive coordination and management of clinical resources to meet those needs. UM spans the continuum of care and includes discussions around level of care and resource utilization.

Utilization review (UR)—the retrospective, reactive process that is used to justify a patient's hospital stay and level of care.

Variable costs—costs that vary in intensity as time or level of activity in a unit of service changes. Costs considered variable in the inpatient care setting include direct and indirect variables.

Verification of eligibility—the process that the provider uses to determine that the patient/member has coverage for the services that he or she is seeking to have rendered (i.e., the member is covered and the planned service is covered).

Write-off—the associated balance of a bill to be uncollectable; a general ledger entry is made to remove it from the organization's accounts receivable.

Sources

CHAPTER 9

Exhibit 9–1 Adapted from E.D. Hoffman, Jr., B.S. Klees, and C.A. Curtis, Brief Summaries of Medicare & Medicaid Title XVIII and Title XIX of The Social Security Act as of July 1, 2000/Medicaid: A Brief Summary/Basis of Eligibility and Maintenance Assistance Status, Office of the Actuary, Health Care Financing Administration, U.S. Department of Health and Human Services.

Exhibit 9–2 Adapted from Public Law 105–33, Balanced Budget Act of 1997, Subtitle J, State Children's Health Insurance Program.

Exhibit 9–3 Data from Coverage of Hospital Services/Duration of Covered Inpatient Services, Section 230.6, U.S. Department of Health and Human Services; Coverage of Services, Section 3112.8, Outpatient Observation Services, Medicare Intermediary Manual Part 3, U.S. Department of Health and Human Services; and 2001 Physician Fee Schedule, Program Memorandum, November 21, 2000, Health Care Financing Administration, U.S. Department of Health and Human Services.

Exhibit 9–4 Adapted from Medicare Inpatient Prospective Payment System, Report on the Effects of Implementing the Post-Acute Transfer Policy: Descriptive Analysis of PAC Policy Change, p. 2–14, Health Care Financing Administration.

Table 9–1 Adapted from Medicare & You 2000/Your Medicare Benefits, Medicare Part A (Hospital Insurance), Publication No. HCFA-10050, p. 5, revised January 2000, Health Care Financing Administration, U.S. Department of Health and Human Services.

Table 9–2 Adapted from Medicare & You 2000/Your Medicare Benefits, Medicare Part B (Medical Insurance), Publication No. HCFA-10050, pp. 6–8, revised January 2000, Health Care Financing Administration, U.S. Department of Health and Human Services.

Table 9–3 Adapted from Medicare & You 2000, Publication No. HCFA-10050, pp. 11–16, revised June 2000, Health Care Financing Administration, U.S. Department of Health and Human Services.

Table 9–4 Reprinted with permission from G. Hale, Outpatient Prospective Payment System/ Overview and Operational Considerations, Cap Gemini Ernst & Young Internal Presentation, p. 7, August 2000.

CHAPTER 11

Appendix 11–A Reprinted from The Official Coding Guidelines, American Hospital Association, American Health Information Management Association, National Center for Health Statistics, and Health Care Financing Administration.

CHAPTER 13

Exhibit 13–1 Courtesy of Cap Gemini Ernst & Young, Detroit, Michigan.

Exhibit 13–2 Courtesy of Dr. David Watkins, Fraiser Rehabilitation Hospital, Louisville, Kentucky.

Figure 13–1 Courtesy of Cap Gemini Ernst & Young, Detroit, Michigan.

Figure 13–2 Courtesy of Cap Gemini Ernst & Young, Detroit, Michigan.

CHAPTER 14

Figure 14–1 Reprinted from OSCAR Report 10, Office of National Health Statistics, Office of the Actuary, Health Care Financing Administration.

Figure 14–2 Reprinted from Office of the Actuary, Health Care Financing Administration.

Figure 14–3 Reprinted from Office of the Actuary, Health Care Financing Administration.

Figure 14–4 Reprinted from Office of the Actuary, Health Care Financing Administration.

Figure 14–5 Reprinted from 1997 Statistics, Health Care Financing Administration.

Figure 14–6 Reprinted from 1996 Statistics, Health Care Financing Administration.

Figure 14–7 Reprinted from Office of the Actuary, National Health Statistics Group, Health Care Financing Administration.

Figure 14–8 Reprinted from Office of the Actuary, National Health Statistics Group, Health Care Financing Administration.

Figure 14–9 Reprinted from Office of the Actuary, National Health Statistics Group, Health Care Financing Administration.

Table 14–1 Reprinted from 1997 Statistics, Health Care Financing Administration.

CHAPTER 15

Figure 15–1 Reprinted from U.S. Bureau of the Census, 1996.

Figure 15–2 Data from National Hospice Organization Fact Sheet, 1996.

Figure 15–3 Data from National Hospice Organization Fact Sheet, 1996.

Figure 15–4 Data from The Hospice Market, FIND/SVP, 1996.

Figure 15–5 Reprinted from Health Care Financing Administration Bureau of Policy Development, 1995.

Figure 15–6 Data from National Hospice Organization.

Table 15–1 Data from National Hospice Organization.

Table 15–2 Data from National Association for Home Care, 1997. Not for further reproduction.

CHAPTER 16

Exhibit 16–1 Courtesy of Cap Gemini Ernst & Young, Washington, DC.

Exhibit 16–2 Courtesy of Cap Gemini Ernst & Young, Washington, DC.

CHAPTER 17

Exhibit 17–1 Courtesy of Ernst & Young, Richmond, Virginia.

Exhibit 17–2 Courtesy of Ernst & Young, Richmond, Virginia.

Table 17–1 Courtesy of Ernst & Young, Richmond, Virginia.

GLOSSARY

Portions of the glossary have been reprinted from The Official Coding Guidelines, American Hospital Association, American Health Information Management Association, National Center for Health Statistics, and Health Care Financing Administration.

Index

C

I

J

Q